The Melody of Separa

Sylvia Zwettler-Otte

The Melody of Separation

A Psychoanalytic Study of Separation Anxiety

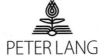

PETER LANG

Frankfurt am Main · Berlin · Bern · Bruxelles · New York · Oxford · Wien

Bibliographic Information published by the Deutsche Nationalbibliothek
The Deutsche Nationalbibliothek lists this publication in the Deutsche Nationalbibliografie; detailed bibliographic data is available in the internet at http://dnb.d-nb.de.

Cover Design:
© Olaf Gloeckler, Atelier Platen, Friedberg

Cover Illustration:
Alberto Giacometti, Homme qui marche II, 1960,
© VG Bild-Kunst, Bonn 2006;
Photograph: Ernst Scheidegger,
© Neue Zürcher Zeitung 2005.

For the German edition of Sylvia Zwettler-Otte
„Die Melodie des Abschieds"
© 2006 W. Kohlhammer GmbH, Stuttgart.

Printed with financial support of the Federal Ministry
of Science and Research in Vienna.

ISBN 978-3-631-58938-0
© Peter Lang GmbH
Internationaler Verlag der Wissenschaften
Frankfurt am Main 2011
All rights reserved.

www.peterlang.de

Some of my thanks and some of my reasons for the development of this book need to remain private. However, this certainly is the right place to thank my husband for his reliable presence, his intelligent, incorruptible and constructive criticism and for his patient acceptance of the priority given to this work over such a long period. My thanks to him also for his technical support in fixing difficulties with the obstinate computer.

When I have seen by Time's fell hand defaced
The rich proud cost of outworn buried age,
When sometime-lofty towers I see down razed,
And brass eternal slave to mortal rage.
When I have seen the hungry ocean gain
advantage on the kingdom of the shore,
and the firm soil win of the watery main,
Increasing store with loss, and loss with store.
When I have seen such interchange of state,
Or state itself confounded, to decay,
Ruin has taught me thus to ruminate
That Time will come and take my love away.
This thought is as a death which cannot choose
But weep to have, that which it fears to lose.

(William Shakespeare, Sonette 64)

This translation and publication has been made possible through funding from the City of Vienna Municipal Department of Cultural Affairs /Science and Research, (FWF Wissenschaftsfond)

Contents

The Melody of Separation

Introduction

It is with very great pleasure that I accepted Dr. Sylvia Zwettler-Otte's suggestion that I write a brief introduction to her book. In recent years, a number of publications have appeared on the topic of separation, but none to my knowledge has managed to write such an encompassing overview on the subject. Furthermore the author has a quite unique way of describing difficult and complex matters in a clear and flowing prose, bringing her vast clinical experience to the help of the readers by offering them a variety of telling examples to illustrate her points.

Parting is a universal and repeated event in human life, and I would be inclined to say that separation and separation anxiety are some of the earliest incentives towards psychic development. In the interaction and mutual responsiveness, which occurs from birth, between the infant and its mother, a specific and unique dialogue develops between them. We do assume that in the early stages of development, the baby's psychological boundaries with his mother are fluid and ill defined. However, in the space of a few months, the baby will become increasingly aware of what is need fulfilling, pleasure giving and familiar and what is not, and the mother-child dialogue will become increasingly more specific and more sharply attuned to subjective experiences. The 'mother', as an object, is becoming 'created' out of the subjective mother-child matrix, at the same time as parallel processes occur in which the baby builds up its own body-schema and self-representation.

In normal development, by about seven or eight months of age, every baby reaches a critical period in his psychological reaction to his mother, necessarily forced on him by the development of his self-boundaries. Other persons, particularly the mother, have thus far been to a significant extent a part of his own self, but the to-and-fro of his psychological development leads him to a greater degree of awareness of separateness. The ongoing dialogue with the mother suddenly acquires a new importance for him as a source of comfort, security, and well-being, as he feels the need to counteract his growing awareness of her as a person separate from himself.

It is at this time, that most babies display a fear of strangers, the famous 'eight months anxiety' so cogently described by Rene Spitz. This can be understood as the result of an unfamiliar, unsafe perceptual and emotional intrusion into the familiar expectable dialogue with the mother, a dialogue that normally enables the baby to bridge the gap of separateness and to restore the earlier feelings associated with the original close union, when mother and self were undistinguishable. At this point, the baby's own ego development and his increased perceptiveness and capacity for differentiation render him very vulnerable.

In 'Inhibitions, Symptoms and Anxiety' Freud describes how each of us experiences loss on a daily basis, an experience, which prepares us for that of separation and loss in general. Freud thought that the act of birth was the prototypical experience of separation and anxiety. But he insisted that there are other experiences, for example, when a child is left alone, or in the dark, or in the presence of strangers, instead of someone with whom he or she is familiar, like the mother. Freud writes: 'These three instances can be reduced to a single condition – namely, that of missing someone who is loved and longed for.' Freud goes on to draw a fundamental distinction between anxiety, pain and mourning as a consequence of separation.

The theme of separation and its concomitant anxiety and pain is so basic because throughout the life cycle, losses and partings are the order of the day. Every change brings with it a demand for the relinquishment of an aspect of a past state, which is now going to be altered. To be able to fully integrate changes, the ego has to be able to mourn the losses of the past and to adapt to the new in order to reach a satisfactory integration of the present. The state of our internal world, our relationships to our internal objects, will help or hinder us in this difficult task. In this book, 'The Melody of Separation', Dr. Zwettler-Otte tells us with precision and diversity about the many aspects of this basic human task.

Anne-Marie Sandler[1]

35 Circus Road
London NW8 9JG
Tel: +44 (0)207 2893655
Email: am@amsandler.co.uk

[1] Anne-Marie Sandler is training-analyst and supervising analyst in the British Psychoanalytic Society, whose president she was. She was also president of the European Psychoanalytic Federation, vice-president of the International Psychoanalytic Association and director of the Anna Freud Centre.

Preface

Separation can be taken as the starting point for considering our whole psychic life, since it necessarily calls to mind its opposite, *bonding* and *love* with its innumerable precursors and forms, all connected in diverse ways to *sexuality, tenderness, devotion, desire, passion, friendship, narcissism etc.*, which lead again - like love - to the painful counterpoint of *separation, loss, death, madness etc.* Separation also is a part of *development,* since it leads back – like love – to the origins of our lives as well as tapping into our ideas about their endings. Separation-anxieties pervade our life from birth to death in various nuances and intensities.

Separation-anxiety constitutes a psychic phenomenon that plays a role in the human struggle against transience – a transience that the production of children attempts to stem. It provides the impetus for the creation of works of art intended to outlive the artist: *exegi monumentum aere perennius – I have built a monument outlasting metal,* the Roman poet Horatius (Ode 3/30/1) wrote about his poems. Separation-anxiety also motivates the promulgation of religions that absorb such anxiety by promising reunion or eternal fusion.

Psychoanalysis offers a method for exploring and studying psychic processes to which there is hardly any another access. Psychoanalysis is a therapeutic technique for treating psychic disturbances and illnesses; it is a science with a complex theory of psychic functions, and it enables a critical understanding of cultural and sociological phenomena. Psychoanalysis can contribute much to the topic of binding and separating, to separation-anxiety and separation-pain, and to our responses to these trying experiences.

In psychoanalysis, past experience has the chance to develop in the present so that we can deal with its influence. This movement develops spontaneously in the transference of the patient and meets an echo in the counter-transference of the psychoanalyst. In this way, we grasp to some extent what emerges out of the large subterranean spaces of the unconscious.
Both separation as well as binding can be "healthy" or "ill", "good" or "bad". Both can provoke anxiety, thus signifying danger. While in separating fear appears to dominate, we are inclined to focus on the positive, comforting and pleasurable aspect, when we think of bonding.
It seems that we can approach the topic of separation only in a defensive way. The term "melody of separation" was used at International Psychoanalytic Conferences in workshops about „shuttle-analyses". These are analyses that for exceptional reasons cannot be conducted in the usual setting of four sessions weekly, but instead occupy a certain block of time. Such an exceptional reason might be, for instance, if somebody wishes to become a psychoanalyst, but there

is no psychoanalytic institute in his country and therefore he has to travel to do so. These analyses are characterized by lengthy interruptions due to the local distance between training-analyst and analysand. Since most people cannot live abroad several years in order to go through psychoanalytic training, it is possible to search for a training-analyst who will make a special individual arrangement for a blocked analysis. As psychoanalysts of different countries discussed their experiences of 'shuttle-analyses' at international conferences, it became evident, that even under such conditions it was possible to conduct a psychoanalytic process. Nonetheless, the issue of separation dominated these analyses, evoking what was termed a *'melody of separation'*. I was surprised by this romantic expression, because what I witnessed in a shuttle-analysis was the arousal of pure horror regarding every interruption. Over the following years colleagues adjusted their view: they had seriously underestimated the problem of separation and of the enormous extent of separation-anxieties and –pains. Speaking of a 'melody of separation' thus minimized the problem. The unavoidable breaks in shuttle-analyses call up not only early and often traumatic separations with a great intensity, they also seem to highlight all the shortcomings, defects and deprivation of the early environment, so that only unhappy blank spaces emerge exaggeratedly, and all benign aspects of the environment were apparently lost.

The romantic title "melody of separation", however, seems to meet very well my topic: it mirrored without conscious intention this tendency to deny the extent and horror of separation. A "melody" is a unit of following sounds, differing in pitch, interval, rhythm, time, colour, repetitions and variations. It can emerge and disappear; it can be folded, repeated and varied, encompassing a tender, soft voice of desire as well as a desperate scream of danger, as in the famous painting of Edvard Munch named 'Scream' (1895).

The book is dedicated to everyone who must grapple with separations: interested nonprofessionals, candidates of psychoanalytic training, and students of psychology, of medical, social and pedagogical sciences. The book will also be of interest for psychoanalysts and psycho-dynamically oriented therapists focusing on theory as well as practice for two reasons:

- The book considers the problem of separation-anxiety not only from a symbiotic aspect of the mother-child-relationship, but also the concept of triangulation. Most forms of separation-anxiety deal not only with the difficult solution of the mother-child-symbiosis, but also with the role of the father, the third figure, which matters from the very start. This figure is present in the desire of the mother and the realisation of the child; it becomes at the same time the cause of disturbing distractions of the mother's attention. This oedipal situation is the base of the triangulation and the attached conflicts that play an important role in separations.

- Psychoanalysts and psychotherapists today often are approached by patients who suffer from psychic illnesses characterized as 'Borderline states'. These people often suffer extensive separation-anxiety. Therefore, an expanded understanding of this psychic phenomenon might be helpful.

I draw examples from analyses, analytic psychotherapies and consulting sessions. The latter help us to recognize fluid transitions between healthy and pathological phenomena. The same is true of those analyses that are undertaken not only for curative reasons, but also for research and the development on personality. There is another contributing source too: personal experiences as an analyst. This does not mean that a psychoanalyst is always analysing outside the consulting room; this is only a fantasy of people who fear (and wish) to be caught and to attract the analyst's attention.

Case stories always raise the question of discretion. On principle, there are two ways to protect patients: either one changes details in a way that disguises the person; or one asks permission that his or her case be published with enough altered details to protect privacy. One of these two possibilities I have always chosen here.

Freud emphasized how important poets and writers contributed to our understanding of our psychic life. This debt is also acknowledged in modern psychoanalytic literature (for instance Kohon, 1999a; Green and Kohon, 2005). Green wrote that psychoanalytic models of the mind are rooted in "the inspiration of the literary giants of the past" (Green and Kohon, 2005, XIII), and he mentions, among others, Euripides, Shakespeare, Racine, Goethe, Stendhal, Baudelaire, Tschechow, Strindberg and Proust, calling them the "masters of psychoanalysts" (Green and Kohon, 2005, 10). Literature is an inexhaustible source of stimulation. The truths of poesies and literature still differ from those of the psychoanalytic science. Winnicott wrote: "Naturally, if what I say has truth in it, this will already have been dealt with by the world's poets, but the flashes of insight that come in poetry cannot absolve us from our painful task of getting step by step away from ignorance towards our goal" (in: Kohon, 1986, 173).

All translations - beside those mentioned in the Literature - were made by the author. Original quotations are marked as ", translated quotations as '.

Vienna, 2011

Sylvia Zwettler-Otte

1 Psychoanalytic bases

1.1 Bonding and separation as basic principles of life

Separation happens only where there was a unit beforehand. Thus separation and bond presuppose a duality. Separating and binding can be intended just from one side, from both (or more) sides, or from neither of them; it can be considered "good" or "bad", "normal" or "ill", and it can be painful or pleasurable. More often than not, separation carries a sense of pain and regret.

In focusing on separation as our central topic, we presuppose bonding as a matter of course. Also the child at the beginning forms a unity with the mother and at first hardly can grasp the separation that reaches a dramatic culmination during delivery. The baby will experience the mother, or just her breast, as part of his own body. And as soon as he experiences her absence, and the increasing tensions of drive (hunger and thirst), he protests against these unpleasant feelings by crying and weeping. We already recognize separation as a basic organizing principle of nature that we cannot influence; in dying, the final separation, we glimpse this organizing principle for the last time.

Adam Philips wrote a study of transience entitled "Darwin's Worms". There he compared Darwins's and Freud's theories[2]: "a life is synonymous with a body" described both of them. They describe our bodily lives "as astonishingly adaptive and resilient, but also excessively vulnerable, prone to many deaths, and shadowed by the reality of death" (Philips, 1999, 8). For Darwin and Freud, death was an organizing principle, and our efforts to escape – by religion or by trust to think of nature as being on our side – are misjudged, resulting from our wish fulfilling thinking. "Modern lives, unconsoled by religious belief, could be consumed by the experience of loss" (Philips, 1999, 14). The original meaning of the word 'religion' is "to bind."

---

[2] Although Freud chose his scientific career, inspired by Darwin's theory of evolution – as he said - he later connected psychoanalysis with Lamarck's theories. In October 1916 he explained to Karl Abraham: he wanted to demonstrate that what Lamarck called need, and according to him created and formed the organs, was the power of unconscious imagination regarding the own body: "Our intention is to base Lamarck's ideas completely on our own theories and to show that his concept of 'need', which creates and modifies organs, is nothing else than the power unconscious ideas have over the body of which we see the remains in hysteria—in short, the 'omnipotence of thoughts'. Fitness would then be really explained psycho-analytically; it would be the completion of psycho-analysis." But Freud never carried out this plan. (Jones, 1962, Vol. 3, 367).

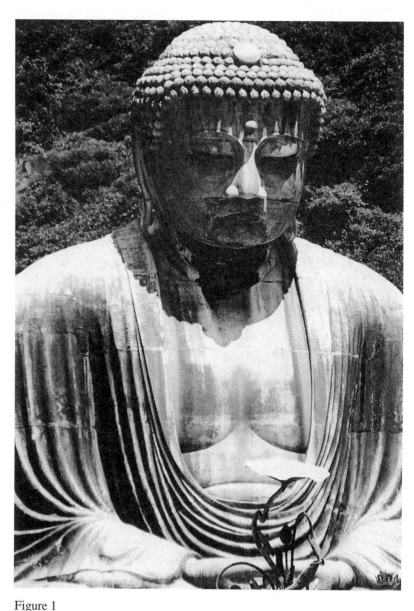

Figure 1
Buddha, Photo by Erla Maria Ammerer, Vienna
Religions, teaching about life after death or else offering a vision of regressive symbiotic fantasies about nirvana, help to absorb separation anxieties.

We can apply the perspective of natural science in a realistic way, if we keep apart the psychic experience connected with parting. In 1915, Freud stated in "Thoughts for the Times on War and Death" that our relationship to death is not an honest one. We maintain, that "death was the necessary outcome of life, that everyone owes nature a death and must expect to pay the debt – in short, that death was natural, undeniable and unavoidable. In reality, however, we were accustomed to behave as if it were otherwise. We showed an unmistakable tendency to put death on one side, to eliminate it from life." In reality, we are incapable of imagining our own death. If we try it, we nevertheless remain present as spectators: "At bottom no one believes in his own death, or, to put the same thing in another way, [...] everyone of us is convinced of his own immortality." (Freud, 1915, S.E. 14, 288)

This tendency is also revealed by cynical jokes – such as the words attributed to a husband: "If one of us two dies, I shall move to Paris." (Freud, 1915, 298) Thus, it is true that our attitude towards death is not honest. We behave as if we acknowledge death. We even make a last will in order to dispose of our goods, and we expand in this way our will. But again and again it is disclosed that actually we are incapable to extinguish ourselves in our thoughts – like in this joke.

Fear of death demands many renunciations: it prohibits many of us from embarking on great enterprises, like attempts at artificial flight, expeditions to distant countries or experiments with explosive substances. Many heroic and extraordinary achievements are only possible if the danger of death is denied. Freud quotes as an example for such an expulsion of death from all calculations the motto of the Hanseatic League: "Navigare necesse est, vivere non necesse." ('It is necessary to sail the seas, it is not necessary to live.'[3]) (Freud, 1915, S.E. 14, 291)

Those who are not ready to defy death can "seek in the world of fiction, in literature and in the theatre compensation for what has been lost in life. There we still find people who know to die – who, indeed, even manage to kill someone else" (Freud, 1915, S.E. 14, 291).

And in the realm of fiction we find the plurality of lives we need: we identify ourselves with the hero and we die with him. Yet we survive him and are ready to die again with another hero. *The secret of heroism is the denial of the danger that there is a final separation caused by death and the unshakable and unrealistically secure feeling that one can defy all dangers.* The rational argument for this attitude refers to abstract ideals that – according to our statements – are more valuable than life itself. However, our unconscious cannot

---

[3] This Latin translation of a Greek quotation by Plutarch was referring to a statement made by Pompeius, the Roman general who was said to have motivated with these words his sailors who were concerned about their lives because of a heavy storm. Thus, it might be successful to overcome the fear of death by intensifying the engagement to an ideal or to a charismatic personality. Of course, such inner fights between fears and wishes are to a large degree unconscious – independently how long they last.

believe in its own death and prefers to behave as if it were immortal: "What we call our 'unconscious' – the deepest strata of our minds, made up of instinctual impulses – knows nothing that is negative, and no negation; in it contradictories coincide." (Freud, 1915, S.E. 14, 296)

Our persistent memory of the dead became the basis for assuming that we continue in other forms of existence after we have apparently died. These subsequent existences were shadowy, often empty of content, as we can see from the old descriptions of the underworld. "It was only later that religions succeeded in representing this after-life as the more desirable, the truly valid one, and in reducing the life which is ended by death to a mere preparation. After this, it was no more than consistent to extend life backwards into the past, to form the notion of earlier existences, of the transmigration of souls and of reincarnation, all with the purpose of depriving death of its meaning as the termination of life." (Freud, 1915, S.E. 14, 295 f.)

Actually, nature harbours the final certainty of our individual death in its program and therefore deserves only our limited trust, a trust with limited liability, so to say. Nature sometimes treats its creatures carelessly and does not stir a childlike faith in a benevolent or divine authority. Nature often makes us – being part of nature – develop immense strengths and spurs creative possibilities, but this does not mean that nature is on our side. It is neither for nor against us, neither 'good' nor 'bad'. "Nature is astonishingly prolific, but it is a prodigal process going nowhere special, sponsored by destruction and suffering. What is wonderful and inspiring is the possibility of infinite variation and exquisite adaptation; what is daunting and terrible is the cost. Nature is abundant and unremittingly cruel from [...] a personal point of view." (Phillips, 1999, 40) Phillips underlines the paradoxical combination of undermining and conserving and shows that Freud and Darwin were interested in "how destruction conserves life; and in the kind of life destruction makes possible" (Phillips, 1999, 63).

Eventually one could accept the "kindness" of nature regarding the fact that we are equipped with the capacity to avoid some pain of separation by resorting to comforting imaginations and consoling feelings.

Devastation and maintenance, separation and binding, destruction and sexuality are functions of the antagonistic basic drives that Freud conceptualized as life- and death-drives. They are also named Eros (= love) and Thanatos (= death) according to their mythological origin. The aim of Eros is to establish ever greater unities and to preserve them – in short, to bind together. The aim of Thanatos, on the contrary, is to undo connections, to destroy things and to lead what is living into an inorganic state. So Thanatos is also called the *death instinct*. Freud explained: "In biological functions the two basic instincts operate against each other or combine with each other. Thus, the act of eating is a destruction of the object with the final aim of incorporating it, and the sexual act is an act of aggression with the purpose of the most intimate union. This concurrent and mutually opposing action of the two basic instincts gives rise to the whole variegation of the phenomena of life" (Freud, 1938, S.E. 23, 148). The analogy of the two basic instincts extends to opposing forces in the inorganic world – attraction and repulsion. Freud assumed that so long as this instinct operates internally, as a death instinct, it remains silent. But it comes to notice when diverted outwards as an instinct of destruction. Freud stressed that it is essential for the preservation of the individual that this diversion occurs. Some portion of self-destructiveness that remains internal finally "succeeds in killing the individual, not, perhaps, until his libido has been used up or fixated in a disadvantageous way. Thus it may in general be suspected that the *individual* dies of his internal conflicts but that the *species* dies of its unsuccessful struggle against the external world if the latter changes in a fashion which cannot be adequately dealt with by the adaptations which the species has acquired" (Freud, 1938, S.E. 23, 149).

In "The Ego and the Id" Freud had examined the distribution of the death drive in the individual. "The dangerous death instincts are dealt with in the individual in various ways: in part they are rendered harmless by being fused with erotic components, in part they are diverted towards the external world in the form of aggression, while to a large extent they undoubtedly continue their internal work unhindered. How is it then that in melancholia the super-ego can become a kind of gathering-place for the death instincts?"(Freud, 1923, S.E. 19, 53)

In 1937 Freud cited a historical forerunner in the 5th century BC, Empedocles. This Greek investigator, thinker, politician and physician, who later was compared with Dr. Faust, proposed a doctrine that approximated the psychoanalytic theory of the drives. Freud thought that Empedocles' cosmic fantasy was hampered only by the fact that it was stretched to an animation of the whole universe instead of restricting itself to the biological realm: "His mind seems to have united the sharpest contrasts. He was exact and sober in his physical and physiological researches, yet he did not shrink from the obscurities of mysticism, and built up cosmic speculations of astonishingly imaginative boldness". Freud suggested that Empedocles' theory about *philia* and *neikos* deserves our close attention. It "is one which approximates so closely to the psychoanalytic theory of the instincts that we should be tempted to maintain that the two are identical, if it were not for the difference that the Greek philosopher's theory is a cosmic phantasy while ours is content to claim biological validity". Empedocles taught that two principles governed events in the life of the universe and in the life of the mind, and that those principles were everlastingly at war with each other. He called them

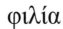

φιλία

(love) and

21

υεῖκος

(strife).

Of these two powers the one strives to agglomerate the primal particles of the four elements into a single unity, while the other seeks to undo all those fusions and to separate the primal particles of the elements from one another. Empedocles thought of the process of the universe as a continuous, never-ceasing alternation of periods. One or the other of these fundamental forces would gain the upper hand, so that at one time love and, at another, strife dominates the universe. Freud summarized: "The two fundamental principles of Empedocles –

φιλία

and

υεῖκος

– are, both in name and function, the same as our two primal instincts, *Eros* and *destructiveness*, the first of which endeavours to combine what exists into ever greater unities, while the second endeavours to dissolve those combinations and to destroy the structures to which they have given rise" (Freud, 1937b, S.E. 23, 244).

For the life-drive Freud coined the term *Libido,* but he found no analogue term for the death-drive. Later, sometimes *Destrudo* was used. While 'destruction' indicates a destructive act, the term 'aggression' (deriving from the Latin word *aggredi = approach)* offers a broader spectrum of meanings: one can approach somebody with hostile intention, but also in order to possess him or her, as in the sexual act that requires some aggression that normally is not regarded as destructive. Freud already showed that the mixture of the drives is decisive: too little aggression can render a man impotent; too much aggression turns him into a sex criminal.

In a comprehensive revision of Freud's theory of the drives and his structural theory Schmidt-Hellerau (1995, 316 ff.) suggested the term *Lethe* as a pendant to *Libido. Lethe* originates in the mythological Greek river that separated the living from the dead. The dead had to drink from the Lethe to extinguish memories of their lives on earth, before they entered Hades, the underworld. Thus, the term refers to the unconscious and the energy of the drive. This meaning is found in everyday language, in which we speak about 'lethargy'.

When psychic energy is invested in an idea or in an object, it is called *cathexis* in the psychoanalytic theory of the drives. Some clinical phenomena we can best explain by this economical term, such as mourning after the separation from an object. The impoverishment of relationships during the mourning process is due to an involuntary overcathexis of the lost object, resulting in a lack of energy for the cathexis of other objects, since there is only a certain quantity of cathecting energy available.

It seems apt that we apply two terms to the life-drive (Libido)[4] since the death-drive (Destrudo and Lethe) appears to us in two different forms. On one hand it is an aggressive-destructive form, on the other, it is a soft, invisible and perhaps therefore even more life-threatening form. Modern psychoanalytic theory can explain the seeming contradiction between Destrudo and Lethe. Andrè Green suggested a new conception of the death-drive, based on Freud's hypothesis of the death-drive. He argued for the importance of that form of destruction which consists in the decathexis of the libido from an object (Green, 2005a, 222).

Thus, we can intend destruction of an object by bundling cathecting energy into destructive actions as well as by turning away from an object, meaning a total decathexis. The latter way is somehow anticipating the successful destruction of an object as a factum: it no longer exists. Our language hints at this phenomenon, when we say about somebody: "For me he is already dead." It means that we consider him extinguished by ignoring him. We know very well that a child can experience the loss of love and attention as more destructive than a physical punishment.

Let us summarize: the life-drive produces bonding, based on the psychic energy called Libido. It enables us to cathect objects – as we say in psychoanalytic science, or to love somebody or something, as we say poetically. The cathexis of an object results in a differentiated perception of an object according to its individuality and singularity. Green termed this the objectualizing function, as opposed to the disobjectualizing function of the death-drive. While the objectualizing function enforces bonding, the disobjectualizing function of the antagonistic death-drive separates, dissolves, and destroys bonding; it diminishes the object's speciality and singularity as perceived in states of love.

Separation therefore is a function of the death-drive dissolving the bond to an object. It can be an arbitrary act or an involuntary, unconscious process; the latter occurs usually during the individual's development. An example is a child whose favourite toy becomes unimportant little by little: the child forgets more and more often the teddy, which was until now loved and which had to accompany the child everywhere; and one day the teddy remains for ever left in a corner. The child has dismissed the toy due to his normal, healthy development; he does not need it anymore as a "transitional object", as D.W.

---

[4] Not all psychoanalysts have accepted the theory of the death-drive; some ignore it, some have arguments against it. So argued for instance Laplanche that the term 'destrudo' rightly was not in general accepted, because there was no special energy of the death-drive: instead its energy was the 'libido' (Laplanche, 1985, 184).

Winnicott called this bridge between an important person of a child and the child itself. Transitional objects have the function to bypass the pain of separation by presenting themselves as substitutes that are more easily and permanently available.

However, not all separations develop in this painless way. There are, of course, different forms of separations, similar to forms of death, from a soft gliding into death, while body and soul seem to be in concordance, slowly releasing the world of objects, to a desperate death-struggle dominated by fear of death and savage pain of separation. The melody of separation can consist of silently longing tones or of ear-deafening dissonances. Libido and aggression are blended in this melody like in love that can take on tenderly soft forms or wild, untamed desire.

1.2   Psychoanalysis – a bridge between nature and culture

Before turning to the psychic work that separation demands I first want to sketch the position of psychoanalysis in considering the problem, which we can study from different points of view: from a biological, a sociological, a legal, a psychological-developmental point of view as well as from a psychoanalytical one.

It is not by chance that we have used terms of natural science, like "organic" and "inorganic", "drive", "instinct" and so on, but there also are allusions to art – paintings and poetry. Andrè Green writes correctly that psychoanalysis, being a method, a cure and a theory, "draws nourishment from both natural and cultural sources. It forms a bridge between nature and culture" (Green, 2005b, 632). Green defined psychoanalysis as "neither a science nor a branch of hermeneutics. It is a practice based on clinical thinking that leads to theoretical hypotheses." Elsewhere, Green writes: "Psychoanalysis is a fundamental science for knowing the human mind; it does not rely on other more basic disciplines of which it would be a by-product or application (Green & Kohon, 2005, 22)". Some of these remarks seem contradictory, but that impression might reflect an effort to clarify that neither psychoanalysis nor its subject – our conscious and unconscious psychic life – can be comprehended exhaustively by simple defined principles, which can be repeated and checked.

The question whether psychoanalysis is a science was raised from its beginnings repeatedly. I have no doubt that psychoanalysis can be considered a science, if its special subject is put into full consideration. Those who do not share this opinion, wish to define the term science more narrowly. This would not harm the immeasurable value of the kind of knowledge that psychoanalysis made available. I don't think that this question is essential, and I am not going to investigate it here in detail. Certainly, psychoanalysis is not a positive science. It differs from other scientific models, as Gregorio Kohon (1999a, 156) pointed out:

- The object of psychoanalysis exists at the limit "between the individual and the social, between self and others, between the inside and the outside, [...] between body and mind";
- "it operates through a different logic, the logic of the unconscious, where reasons and causes, pain and pleasure, past and present are inevitably entangled and implicated".
- It uses a specific language which is different from any of the so-called scientific disciplines, and
- the object itself determines the theory.

In an acute and subversive sense psychoanalysis turned our knowledge upside down by demonstrating the subjectivity of all our theories. Nevertheless, from another point of view it might be exactly this ability of psychoanalysis to study its own instruments and to gain objectivity out of subjectivity that we might consider truly scientific. It is a capacity to study the factors of our perception – a possibility not so easily available for other sciences.

This capacity of psychoanalysis to reach a high degree of objectivity regarding subjectivity is in my view, what renders it scientific. Especially during the last decades, it is clear that the criteria of the exact sciences are not necessarily certain themselves (Kennedy, 2002). The natural sciences are not so certain as some imagine, nor is psychoanalysis so uncertain.

We cannot expect, that this question can be soon settled, not among the psychoanalysts themselves, and not among the fans or opponents of psychoanalysis. Those concerned with quantified research and diagnostic criteria are facing psychoanalysts, who pursue "the subtle and sometimes contradictory meanders of the psychoanalytic process" (Green, 2005b, 632). I prefer the latter, but I respect the efforts of colleagues, who try to build bridges to other sciences; not because we shall find confirmations for our results outside of psychoanalysis, but because it opens a way to psychoanalysis for interested scientists of other disciplines and compels clarifications from us.

It might be useful to enlarge our conception of science and to find a new definition. However, we should not forget that it were we, who determined these systems of classification according to earlier states of knowledge; they are not dictated by nature, and we should not reject new and rich knowledge we find in a new way, just because it does not fit old systems. If a painting turns out to become bigger than planned, so that it does not fit a frame, one might rather change the frame instead of cutting the picture to size.

For Freud, who occasionally spoke about the 'psychoanalytic science', there was no doubt that psychoanalysis is "a part of the mental science of psychology. It is also described as 'depth psychology'. Psychology, too, is a natural science. What else can it be?" (Freud, 1938, S.E. 23, 281)

1.3   Separation – mourning and depression

> '…it is a matter of general observation
> that people never willingly abandon a libidinal position,
> not even, indeed, when a substitute is already beckoning to them.'
> (Sigmund Freud: Mourning and Melancholia, 1917, 243)

We have already distinguished between a soft, hardly noticeable form of loosening and detachment that often happens in a healthy process of development, and a painful separation from an object. If we are forced to separate from somebody or something, this is a psychic burden and challenge, which we call 'the work of mourning'. This difficult process of mourning is connected with the pain of separation and the feeling of an existential threat that emerges during a separation.

In 1917 Freud made in his paper "Mourning and Melancholia" a clear distinction between the 'normal' process of mourning and the psychic state that we call today a 'depressive state'. "Mourning is regularly the reaction to the loss of a loved person, or to the loss of some abstraction which has taken the place of one, such as one's country, liberty, an ideal, and so on." (Freud, 1917, S.E. 14, 242)

Mourning as well as depressive states are characterized by a deep and painful irritation, a reduction of interest in the external world, a loss of the capacity for love and an inhibition of efficiency. However, different from depression we can overcome mourning after a certain period of time. In a depressive state, however, we notice also a decrease of self-estimation, an inclination to self-reproaches and an anticipation of punishment. The depressive person sketches an extremely negative image of himself; nevertheless, he does not seem to be ashamed about all the failures he is listing. We can solve this contradiction, if we scrutinize the contents of such self-accusations: regularly we detect that these accusations are in fact reproaches that this person would have liked to address to the lost love-object. He has fetched this object somehow into his ego or – as we would say in our psychoanalytic terminology – he substituted the object by identification. Freud illustrated this process by an impressive metaphor: "Thus the shadow of the object fell upon the ego, and the latter could henceforth be judged by a special agency, as though it were an object, the forsaken object." (Freud, 1917, S.E. 14, 248) Due to a regressive development, identification with the object took over again. Identification had also been the first step in choosing an object, and it usually contains a high degree of ambivalence. Identification retains the lost object in the ego thus avoiding the separation.

In mourning, however, reality testing recognizes and acknowledges that the beloved object does no longer exist and that it is necessary to withdraw the libido – as we call the psychic energy – from this object, although we struggle against it. "Each single one of the memories and situations of expectancy, which demonstrate the libido's attachment to the lost object, is met by the verdict of reality that the object no longer exists; and the ego, confronted as it were with the question whether it shall share this fate, is persuaded by the sum of the narcissistic satisfactions it derives from being alive to sever its attachment to the object that has been abolished." (Freud 1917, SE 14, 254) Thus, mourning impels the ego to give up the object by declaring the object to be dead and offering the ego the inducement of continuing to live.

This development we can consider to be 'normal': the respect of reality triumphs, and after each memory is faced, first overcathected and then decathected, the ego is free again.

1.4   Anxiety as unpleasant state of affect

We now have looked at the polarity of life and death and at separation as the opposite of binding. We are turning now to the anxiety that very often accompanies separations. Separation-anxiety arises in the healthy development of the child who becomes independent, and also when a grown-up person fears to lose a beloved object; but also psychic diseases may hide separation-anxiety behind different symptoms.

In a paper about anxiety-neurosis Freud started with the assumption that an arousal of excitement, especially sexual tension, can be transformed into anxiety. Later on, he discriminated an automatic anxiety from anxiety as a signal. Automatic anxiety occurs in a traumatic situation, if the arousal of excitement caused by external or internal factors renders one helpless so that one feels incapable of coping with this excitement. Anxiety as a signal is the reaction to the threat of a traumatic situation that might become dangerous. Separation of a love-object we experience as the greatest danger; its loss or the loss of its love can accumulate unfulfilled wishes and thus make us feel helpless. Signal-anxiety tries to prevent an outburst of strong and very unpleasant anxiety and aims at a reduction or an avoidance of the danger with the help of intelligence.

We all know also the pleasure of thrill, which Michael Balint described: if anxiety can be kept on a low level, mastering provokes a feeling of triumph. Usually we have for instance little doubt that we shall very likely survive a ride on a switchback; thus overcoming anxiety can be delightful and pleasurable.

1.4.1 Birth as a "model" of separation-anxiety

The first great state of anxiety in the individual's life is birth, a sometimes dramatic separation during the parturition. Inge Merkel (Merkel, 1994, 48 f.) describes in her novel "Eine ganz gewöhnliche Ehe" ('A totally normal marriage') a normal delivery from the perspective of a woman being in labour:

'Penelope, the wife of Odysseus, was sitting in the chair for delivery. She knew, of course, that everything was happening, as it should. Exactly like the cattle that were foaling. However, this usually worked quicker. Nevertheless, beside this reasonable insight she was caught in the event that preceeded in her body. She was alone with her flesh. 'Like this it will be in dying', occurred to her vaguely. 'Then one also will be alone with oneself, in spite of all busy activity around.'...Paralyzed by tensed horror she was listening into herself to the struggle of the strangling vessel that was she herself, and simultaneously to the emergency of the suffocating struggling being in her, that also was still herself, but no longer totally herself. Synchronously she felt the suffering of the suffocated being fighting for breath, and herself strangling. Suddenly it came to her mind like a shining flash of a memory, how it was, when she was thrown into the water as a newborn baby. How long did it last until she re-emerged! Distress caused by flood, emergency of suffocating. Raving pain gripped her again, and a dreadful strangeness in herself. She experienced herself with strangulated breath creeping through the subterranean spaces of her own flesh, where in stifling gloominess, in the stench of blood and shit and putrefaction nature takes place in lively activity between loosening, metamorphosis and resurrection.'

Intuitive knowledge and vague memory are combined with a feeling of strangeness and impotence during the spontaneous dissolution of the unity and this first experience of separation.

We have to stress that these are impressive *fantasies* about birth and death. We are not capable of producing *memories* regarding those first and last events of our life, but a flood of ideas and images. Thus, we can study fantasies about birth and death, not the psychic processes themselves which occur during birth or death; there is no certainty whether and how our so-called psyche can already or still work in such moments.

"The act of birth is the first experience of anxiety, and thus the source and prototype of the affect of anxiety", Freud added in 1909 at the end of the 6th chapter of his 'Interpretation of Dreams' in a footnote (Freud, 1900, S.E. 4, 399). This remark was elaborated by Otto Rank 1924 in his book: "The Trauma of Birth". Rank was for a long time a close collaborator Freud's, but Freud[5] did not fully agree with Rank's view that all attacks of anxiety later on are efforts to get rid of the original trauma of birth. Of course, Freud first stated: "There is much more continuity between intra-uterine life and earliest infancy than the impressive caesura of the act of birth would have us believe. However, he then emphasized that the mother was not yet an object in intrauterine life:"But we must not forget that during its intra-uterine life the mother was not an object for the foetus, and that at that time there were no objects at all."He reminded us of the fact that: "the reason why the infant in arms wants to perceive the presence of its mother is only because it already knows by experience that she satisfies all

---

[5] At the beginnings Freud gave positive hints to Rank's book, but in 1926 he finally changed his mind in a radical way. According to Bion Freud was influenced in this by Ernest Jones (Bion, 2005, 2).

its needs without delay. The situation, then, which it regards as a 'danger' and against which it wants to be safeguarded is that of non-satisfaction, of a *growing tension due to need*, against which it is helpless." (Freud, 1926, S.E, 20, 136 f.) It is only after repeated experiences of satisfaction that the mother is created as an object[6] that is needed and longed for. And Freud specifies: "Pain is thus the actual reaction to loss of object, while anxiety is the reaction to the danger which that loss entails and, by a further displacement, a reaction to the danger of the loss of the object itself."(Freud, 1926, S.E. 20, 170)

1.4.2 Separation-anxiety and separation-pain

Two clinical examples will demonstrate how separation-anxiety can hide behind an inhibition or a symptom and how efforts to avoid conflicts and the pain of separation may look like. I have chosen deliberately two cases, which show how much parents and children are entangled. Both came with the diagnosis "school-phobia".

Peter, a six year old boy, was a very lively and sociable child before he entered school. He had become already very independent. However, in school Peter suddenly had great difficulties and did not learn to write and to calculate, in spite of high intelligence. The mother was upset and arranged a consultation. It was easy to make contact with Peter; he told me, that he just had to sing a song in the class, and that he had chosen the song of little Hans, because he had this melody always in his mind. This remark made me alert to the lyrics. When he came to the line: 'but mother wept very much', he was blocked, and finally said: 'she wept more and more'. The projective tests revealed feelings of anxiety and guilt concerning the danger somebody may feel desperately alone, while somebody else enjoyed being with others. Peter was regressing in his development. The fact that school demanded more time caused a conflict and a problem of separation for mother and child. The father, who travelled a lot for professional reasons and therefore was often absent, could not be helpful. The mother became more depressed, while Peter first connected with some children and even fell a bit in love with his female teacher. However, this soon caused guilt feelings. He unconsciously was afraid to betray his mother, and he pulled the brake by failing in school. He did not fail in reading; reading his mother had taught him, so it was okay to master it. Until now, Peter had managed to be independent from his parents according to his age. Now the separation-anxiety was rising, and his mother could no longer manage to let him go – to some extent also because her husband was often absent. Her clinging to the boy intensified his own separation-anxieties, which were intermingled with growing guilt, as he tried to overcome his fears. "Mother wept more and more...," the children song had reminded him of his anxieties. Partly he projected his

---

[6] A similar metaphoric formulation we can find in Laplanche, who wrote that life crystallizes the first objects to which desire adheres, even before thinking clings to them (Laplanche, 1985, 187).

separation-anxieties onto his mother, partly her unconscious fears activated his own. It was a vicious circle, which rather pushed him back to symbiosis than forward to development. Since Peter had developed properly before, out of his own strength, it seemed advisable to offer help to the mother. If only he would have got support in his detachment, her despair and her provocation of his guilt feelings might have accumulated. In a long consultation, the mother decided to enter psychoanalytic psychotherapy, which helped her to cope with her conflicts. As soon as she recognized the analyst as an object that was capable of standing and acknowledging her wishes for dependence and who could connect her feelings with her own history, her relationship to Peter normalized. Before, he often had to substitute the father, who had not been enough available – a problem, which the parents could now discuss and mitigate. Peter finished his first year at school with excellent success, as he told me, when I saw him for a follow-up consultation; the text of the song of 'Little Hans', however, he hardly remembered now – it seems that a strong rampart of repression had to be established against the seductive regression, to which he had been near to succumb.

The second case was also a "school-phobia"*:*
Isabella, 7 years old, refused to go to school. The scholarly success she experienced, and the school-friends she had, lost any attraction for her. The parents realized that this change was connected with the birth of the little brother. Isabella hid her intense jealousy behind a pseudo-caring behaviour. She feared that while she would be in school, the baby would become mother's only darling. Thus, she hoped the problem would be solved if she did not leave the house anymore. She pretended to suffer from headache, then her belly hurt, and later she refused to go out without offering any reason. The fear to leave the house was based on her urgent need to control the situation at home. The vague content of her anxiety was unconscious and had been misunderstood as school-phobia. A phobia usually has the advantage that one can avoid the frightening object, which apparently caused the anxiety. However, there is a price to pay: one has to tolerate many restrictions. Nevertheless, Isabella had another advantage: she made her parents pay her a lot of attention by her refusal to attend school. Impressed by her difficulties they decided that Isabella should undergo a child-analysis. In this analysis, Isabella soon gave up her symptom, but this, of course, was not the cure. It was rather a result of her relief, that she had her analyst totally for herself during the sessions, being alone in the limelight. However, her envy and her jealousy had to return, and it took some time, until these heavy feelings were worked through.

While in the first case separation-anxiety was covered by an inhibition to learn, in the second case the school-phobia was the symptom in the foreground. The separation-anxiety was not caused by the fear of loss of the object itself, but by the fear to lose a special relationship to the mother and to have to renounce the privileged position of being a single child. Thus separation-anxiety is a means to avoid pain of separation and to stave off a state of helplessness, loneliness and a flood of unfulfilled wishes. Sometimes the narcissistic aspect of unsatisfied needs dominates; sometimes it is the dreaded loss of the beloved object. The relationship is reinforced by both, by the emotional binding between the subject and the object *and* by the satisfaction of needs. Sometimes separation-anxiety centres round the fear of solitude; often this fear is connected with the feelings of having failed in some way – guilt feelings due to forbidden wishes for love or else murderous fantasies, which often cause serious irritations without the person becoming fully aware of them.

2 The danger of loss and our knowledge of transience

2.1 Consequences of separation-anxiety: binding devalued or overvalued

'...what is painful may none the less be true.'
(S. Freud, 1916)

Our awareness about the inevitability of separations is full of conflicts and splits, and this influences not only our relationship to death as final separation, it interferes with our valuing everything we consider desirable and good. This awareness of transience affects everything. Devaluation is an effort to protect oneself from the threat of separation by turning away from an unreliable object, which therefore deserves to be despised. Overvaluation, on the other hand, tries to find solace regarding unreliability of the object in an intensified attention and endeavours to love it as much as possible.

In 1916 Freud examined our reactions to transience in his essay "On Transience". Using the example of a poet and a friend who were his company during walks in a beautiful landscape and who were unable to enjoy magnificent nature because of its transience, Freud assumes: "What spoilt their enjoyment of beauty must have been a revolt in their minds against mourning. The idea that all this beauty was transient was giving these two sensitive minds a foretaste of mourning over its decease; and, since the mind instinctively recoils from anything that is painful, they felt their enjoyment of beauty interfered with by thoughts of its transience." Such a devaluating view can extend over the whole world and lead to a painful disgust. It is driven by a demand for immortality, which "is a product of our wishes too unmistakable to lay claim to reality: what is painful may none the less be true". Freud opposes to this dramatic pessimism a contradictory attitude, one considering transience an increase of value: "Transience value is scarcity value in time. Limitation in the possibility of an enjoyment raises the value of the enjoyment". Regarding the beauty of nature each time it is destroyed by winter, it comes again next year. Of course, this is not true for the beauty of human bodies, but "evanescence only lends them a fresh charm". Pictures and statues we admire today will crumble to dust, but this does not devalue them. "Epoch may even arrive when all animate life upon the earth ceases; but since the value of all this beauty and perfection is determined only by its significance for our own emotional lives, it has no need to survive us and is therefore independent of absolute duration." (Freud, 1916, S.E. 14, 305) Nevertheless, many sensitive minds must fight against the foretaste of mourning, because we instinctively shrink from pain, and that is why the prospect of loss disturbs enjoyment of beauty. However, even the most painful mourning "comes to a spontaneous end. When it has renounced everything that has been lost, then it has consumed itself, and our libido is once more free (in so far as we are still young and active) to replace the lost objects by fresh ones equally or still more precious." (Freud, 1916, S.E. 14, 306)

Thus, our awareness that enjoyment must be followed by separation can lead to devaluation or overvaluation of a possible enjoyment. In the first case one tries to renounce cathecting the object in order not to suffer a painful detachment later on; this is an obstinate-ascetic attitude. In the second case, one tries by overcathexis to delay the separation as far as possible and to find compensation for threatened separation by gaining especially intensive pleasure[7]. In analyses, we sometimes have the opportunity to study both mechanisms.

---

[7] An interesting example for overvaluation of lost attachments we can occasionally recognize in a special liking for antiquities: old objects allow a resurrection of old relationships one had – or would have liked to have – to parents, grandparents or great-grandparents. In fantasy, separations can be undone, and the highly idealizing appreciation of old things can be connected with an effort to repair old bindings and to work through outdated guilt. A patient, for instance, had considered his grandfather "an old beast", but he preserved his favourite pipe like something very precious – he tried to turn a "bad" object subsequently into a "good" one. By imagining a kind grandfather, the patient created him in his mind. .

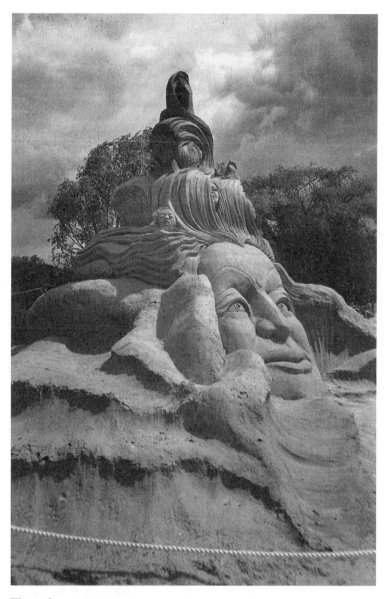

Figure 2
Sculpture made of sand, Neusiedl am See, Austria, Photo by Sylvia
Zwettler-Otte
Sand sculptures – in contrast to stone sculptures – seem to renounce the
demand to appear eternal.

2.1.1 Don Juan and the comfort of multiplicity

The following case demonstrates how repeated experiences of separation caused a devaluation of any close relationship in order to avoid further disappointments. Superficiality and multiplicity of relationships were a compromise settlement between the search for closeness and the struggle against it, and they were also a sort of comfort for the painful early separations that were "forgotten" and repressed.

A 30-year-old patient told rather proudly about his nickname "Don Juan". He thought that he had no difficulties in establishing relationships. He felt that he easily won all hearts, and he could not understand why he nevertheless often was depressed and saw no sense in his life. He compared himself with Midas, the mythological figure, who starved to death, because everything he touched turned into gold. 'Don Juan' regarded himself as lucky because of his popularity, but actually it was ultimately worthless. If his flirting skills would not function so well, he would withdraw totally. Soon he also in analysis established a superficial relationship to me, as he did with all his acquaintances. He did not mind, if he was late. He hardly noticed my holidays; it apparently made no difference to him, whether I was there or not. However, one day he went immediately after his session to a nearby shop, and when leaving he saw me passing in my car. The following weekend he felt uneasy without having an idea why. During the next sessions we analysed a nightmare he had: it revealed that secretly his relationship to me had changed. When he saw me driving away in my car, he had been flooded with fears of separation. He was anxious I might have an accident (a punishment for leaving him alone)! Or I might leave him for ever – like his first girl friend, whom he had loved idolatrously and who went abroad after they had a terrible quarrel about his jealousy. Or I might suddenly stop seeing him – like his nanny, whom he had loved more than his mother, who was so often ill. Nevertheless, the nanny left him. She married, cancelled her job and followed her husband to another city. All those disappointments neither he himself nor his parents took very seriously. The result was that he devaluated all relationships and so preferred to have as many as possible. The quantity seemed to him a guarantee that he never again would be alone, and he started to avoid any deep feelings. If he would never fall in love, he never again would be hurt by somebody leaving him and letting him desperately alone and helpless.

Like the poet in Freud's essay, 'Don Juan' was fighting against painful mourning, which would necessarily be the consequence, if he would devote himself to his positive feelings of love and desire. In analysis, he had to recognize that there are breaks and limits, and that he suffered from them. Somehow, he had hoped that he would be able to control his feelings even in analysis, which luckily did not work. Instead, working through his repressed traumatic separations changed a lot in his life; he had to learn to renounce absolute certainty. Finally, he became free enough to take up a new and satisfying love-relationship with a woman, who answered in return to his feelings. After quite a long time of reluctance, he had managed to devote himself to the psychoanalytic process and to tolerate the fear and the pain of separation that re-emerged in the transference.

2.1.2 The female restorer

Another example demonstrates how, in our mind, the fact of transience can be intermingled with guilt feelings due to our destructive fantasies. Sometimes this results in quite creative solutions, but often they are not good enough.

Saskia did not know why she had chosen her profession, but she loved it. It gave her the feeling that she could preserve precious pieces of art and preventing their decay, she somehow snatched them from transience. She had lived a bit dreamily, but content and reserved, devoted to her work. Only at weekends, she occasionally spent time with colleagues, with whom she was acquainted from her study of the history of arts. In her leisure time she had furnished her little flat so beautifully, that the few visitors considered it to be a jewel. However, when she – to her own surprise – fell in love with one of her customers, her quiet life became chaotic. Her feelings for this man, whose great knowledge in matters of art she admired, grew deeper and deeper. She enjoyed sharing aesthetic pleasures, but when he asked her to marry him, she panicked. When she became pregnant, the conflict seemed unsolvable to her. A colleague, who saw her desolate state, advised her to see me for a consultation. It was a heavy start, because Saskia hoped I would tell her exactly what to do to free her from conflict. She felt under pressure of time concerning whether she should have an abortion or not. Although I did not offer to her the relief she had expected and did not take over the responsibility for her decision, she remained in psychoanalytic psychotherapy. In my counter-transference it was difficult for me not to take the child's part spontaneously; but I managed to provide space for Saskia without influencing her. She allowed time to decide for her and was glad, when it finally was too late for an abortion. She began to share the anticipating joy of her partner. Nevertheless, her anxieties increased during her pregnancy and she was so terribly afraid of giving birth that she asked me to reserve a place for an analysis "in case I would survive delivery". In spite of this wish, it took four months after the birth to find an arrangement with her husband and a baby-sitter, so that she could start to come regularly to her analysis. Saskia had needed a Caesarean operation and therefore she felt that she had not really given birth herself. This she considered both disappointing and calming. She had been so afraid of giving birth because her mother nearly died during the birth of her sister, who was 7 years younger. Her mother was diagnosed with cancer during her pregnancy, and she died a few months after the delivery. The father assumed that the outbreak of the lethal illness had been caused by the hormonal change and felt guilty and depressed. He gave the baby to his sister, because he was unable to care for it. Saskia tried desperately to cheer him up. She became an excellent pupil so that he had no reason to be concerned about her. She cooperated with the housemaid in order to provide for her father a comfortable home. And unconsciously she and her father were connected by unbearable feelings of guilt. Saskia had hated the thought that she would have to share her room with a sibling. Secretly, she considered it the result of a "miscarried death-wish" that the mother, and not the baby, had died. A few sessions later she said in despair, that actually it had been even worse, because she had wished to get rid of both! She would have enjoyed being alone with her daddy! Actually, there were very few moments that she could enjoy: for instance, when she occasionally went with him to the museum. There it happened that she became aware of her wish to become a restorer. Her profession became a singular, great and successful attempt to undo the dam she felt she had built. However, to enjoy love she unconsciously had restricted herself, so that she was afraid, that this would be punished by penalty of death. This – in her view – had happened to her mother. All this material emerged in analysis and was based in the transference on unrealistic fears concerning my well-being. Every weekend, every holiday caused tremendous separation-anxieties. Saskia was sure that I soon would no longer be there for her. Only after she had revealed to herself and to me her death-wishes towards her mother and towards the baby, with whom she had been in rivalry so excessively in her fantasies, she could forgive herself. Now she could recognize, that she had transferred her unconscious conflicts, death-wishes and separation-anxieties to me. And she felt how much the early death of her mother had hurt her. She had to repeat the mourning that she had not been able to experience before, due to her guilt feelings, her confusion and her efforts to comfort the depressed father. -

In this second case, a creative choice of profession helped her to cope with unconscious feelings of guilt. The daily work had the meaning of reparation and restoration of objects that were endangered by loss and damage. Only when she fell in love a crisis did arise, provoking a wave of separation-wishes and anxieties as well as guilt feelings, upsetting her deeply.

2.2 Simultaneously knowing and not-knowing – a tricky compromise

> *'Death? An unavoidable and*
> *at the same time always missed rendezvous,*
> *since its presence means our absence.'*
> *(Anne Philipe: Nur einen Seufzer lang, 1969, 11)*

We may acknowledge at the outset that our relationship to death as final separation is deeply split. We know we shall die but it is a knowledge we cannot grasp emotionally. Our affect is split off from intellectual knowledge, it is not 'cathected' and therefore we often behave as if we do not know. The capacity to deny what we know differs greatly among individuals. Freud said that our relationship to death is not an honest one. In his essays about "Fetishism" (1927) and "Splitting of the Ego in the Process of Defence" (1938) he elaborated his thoughts on the sources of our insincerity. The compromise between our wish and the unpleasant recognition of reality results in contrary reactions. On the one hand the wish for immortality seems paramount; on the other hand reality must be taken into account too.

In the realm of infantile development we recognize such a split, as when discovering the difference between the sexes. The little boy, who already experienced his penis as a part of the body suited for pleasurable play, usually is confronted with stern warnings that he should – at least in public – renounce this entertainment. Otherwise he might risk punishment. Sometimes these admonishments amount to perceived threats that he might lose this highly prized body part – that is, threats of castration, which are taken seriously. In most cases such comments frighten little boys only too effectively because, when considering girls they have seen, there do exist human beings lacking this body part. They infer there is some truth in these threats and that it already has happened to girls. Fetishists maintain a belief in later life that women also have a phallus. They substitute – like little boys – for the missing organ a thing, a fetish, which symbolises triumph over castration anxiety. Of course the little girl also discovers pleasurable feelings between her legs early. She gets frightened and feels guilty that she might already have lost the penis she saw boys possessed, maybe due to forbidden play. Thus she acquires the illusion that she too has - or at least has had - a phallus.

A female patient had a yearning for a certain type of car which "looked the same at the front and at the back". In analysis an unconscious fantasy crystallized which originated in childhood: she imagined that men and women "looked the same at the front and at the back"; the nucleus of her fantasy was the denial of a difference of the sexes. After this discovery the patient's nearly obsessive shopping of high heel shoes vanished and the phallic meaning of her passion for high heels as a fetish became conscious. Freud had summarized already 1927in his paper about Fetishism: "Thus the foot or the shoe owes its preference as a fetish – or a part of it – to the circumstance that the inquisitive boy peered at the woman's genitals from below, from her legs up" (Freud 1927, 155). In little girl's curiosity how mother and father look like when undressed stems from the same motive.

So despite an intellectual awareness of genital differences the (often unconscious) fantasy can be maintained that all people are equipped similarly and that there is no 'castration.' This split in knowledge resembles our skittish stance regarding mortality too. We form a compromise between the force of an unpleasant perception and the power of our contradictory wish for eternal life. It is a compromise, which is only possible when tendencies of unconscious thinking are dominant – in the so-called 'primary process'.

Thus we enable a wish-conforming and a reality-conforming view to co-exist. But the price to be paid for this co-existence is what Freud (1937) in "Splitting of the Ego in Defence" viewed as an incurable rift in the ego. Such a psychic mechanism plays a key role in fetishism, in neuroses in general and most especially in psychoses which utterly turn away from reality. Due to a well developed synthetic function of the ego both attitudes can be integrated.

2.3   Our own death and the pleasure of extinction

An underlying awareness of threatened separations of beloved persons and things can make its way from separation-anxiety to separation-pain, and even then it is an anaesthetized pain. The pain is cushioned by a layer of cotton wool spun of denial regarding our own death. Even in fantasies about our own death and the mourning of it, the feelings of the *living* person infuse these imaginings, and so the prospect of dying remains emotionally incomprehensible. So concerns about the transience of the world often are rooted in the defence mechanism of projection: the others are vanishing, not ourselves; the "world" is fading, not us.

This outcome is not changed by reports of people who fell into a near-death coma and revived. Such experiences go back to the bible; witness Lazarus. A coma might have led those experiencing it far from their familiar lives, but it is followed by a return and a renewed contact with the living. These "Lazarus' people may believe they glimpsed the other side, but actually they were still on this side. These "peregrinations of the soul, just as it is getting ready to take leave of the body, are a feature of very ancient beliefs. But for those of us who cannot conceive of the soul as separate from the tomb called soma, they do no more than arouse our curiosity" (Green, 2002, 150).

Freud in "An Outline of Psychoanalysis" wrote that "it may in general be suspected that the *individual* dies of his internal conflicts but that the *species* dies of its unsuccessful struggle against the external world if the latter changes in a fashion which cannot be adequately dealt with by the adaptation which the species has acquired." (Freud, 1938, 150) He wrote this passage when he was preparing to flee from the Nazis in order to die in freedom in London. This signified a fight for an individual, personal death, from inside, and it was an escape from a death inflicted from outside. The internal world should hold sway over the external world. The unavoidable fact of dying is soothed by the satisfaction of dying in one's own way. In the fifth chapter of "Beyond the Pleasure principle" (1920) Freud assumed that every living creature dies out of inner reasons returning to an inorganic state.

The tension arising from the development from the inorganic to the organic substance seeks to extinguish itself. The first drive intends eventually to return to inanimate matter. Hence, the primal instinctual satisfaction is the extinction of the own existence. Here is a state of tension from which only death can release us. The organism wishes to die in its own fashion and on its own terms and so, paradoxically, it fights hard against dangers from outside which might help to attain its aims more quickly, by a kind of short-cut. The death-drive that Freud postulated late in his life proposes a compensatory award of pleasure for struggling successfully to undergo a special, personal, and self-fashioned death. As Freud summarized: "The pleasure principle seems actually to serve the death instincts." (Freud, 1920, 63) Adam Phillips calls us "artists of our own deaths" (Phillips 1999, 77 f.). The instincts, being sources of our suffering as well as of our satisfaction, promote the survival of the species and the death of the individual.

The twelfth fairy

There is a fascinating example of a child's spontaneous understanding that dying is an unavoidable, frightening and yet unconsciously intended process, This realization should not surprise us: Christopher Bollas stated: „[…] before the small child is capable of topographically significant representations, […] the child already 'knows' the basic essentials of human life, of his human life" (1987, 280).

The child who lived protected in an intact family, was confronted with the serious illness of the grandmother. The parents tried to prepare the child that the grandmother might die. But she recovered. Nevertheless, the child remained depressed. Beside this additionally two harmless "symptoms" appeared:
- *the wish to hear every evening the fairy-tale of Sleeping Beauty ("Dornröschen") and*
- *the habit to fall out of the bed every night.*

In long talks it turned out that the child was preoccupied with the following thoughts which were worked through again and again:

1. *All people have to die, even the grandparents, the parents and oneself.*
2. *One has to die, but one cannot die without one's agreement. At some point one has to want it. This paradox of a need to want what one rejects at the same time was the content of what the child was playing with, for instance, putting the dolls on a slide and explaining to them that they should move forward until the decisive moment comes when they will start to slide down more or less willingly. When the child fell out of the bed during the night, it was this moment, when falling was inevitable, that she evidently experienced with a mixture of pleasure and fear.*
3. *This depressing, but also fascinating new experience reminded the child of "The Sleeping Beauty": the thirteenth fairy, who had not been invited to the birthday-party of the princess and was full of jealousy, wanted the princess to die. But the twelfth fairy reduced this threat to a sleep of 100 years. This was a compromise between the death wish of the bad fairy and the reparation of the good fairy who wished to undo the death sentence. This – the child felt – was similar to the fact that one has to die, but not without one's agreement.*

It is remarkable, how early an awareness can unfold that is compatible with highly theoretical thoughts of a sophisticated person. Nevertheless, it is a knowledge that remains speculative since the science of death, so-called thanatology, never can be positivistic. We may wonder, whether we should admire the intuitive wisdom we sometimes find in children, or whether instead we should regret with ample humility that we do not progress very much as grown ups.

The intent to transform dying into a personal, individual death is an endeavour of the pleasure principle to catch up with the reality principle. It is a compromise between the reality of our transience and our desire for immortality; the unavoidable becomes covered by an adapted wish and shows up in the striving to die one's own death, if dying must happen anyway. Nevertheless, this attitude is similar to the behaviour of an inexperienced Sunday rider who behaves as if he had wanted to go where his steed is going, in order not to injure his reputation for horsemanship.[8]

The child who plays with those down-sliding dolls likewise reveals an acute sense of the plight that as soon as we are born we are put on a slide, and from a certain point we have to commit ourselves to the slipstream of gravity, even if we sometimes struggle desperately crawling back to delay extinction. Here one

---

[8] On the 7th of July 1898 Freud sent a first draft of what later became the 7th chapter of the 'Interpretation of Dreams' to his friend Wilhelm Fließ, and he remarked: „It completely follows the dictates of the unconscious, on the well-known principle of Itzig, the Sunday rider. 'Itzig, where are you going?' – 'Do I know? Ask the horse!' I did not know in any paragraph, where I would come." (Freud, 1986, 348)

also is forced to give in and to follow instincts rooted in the organism. To give up a futile effort, when there already is a decision in the fight between the life- and death-drive, is a relief, a reduction of tension that we also can call pleasure. That is why the metaphor of the slide that can also provide pleasure fits in; thus our last pleasure might be the pleasure of extinction.

2.4 Pleasure principle saved

We are dealing with the paradox that there is something in us, as in all organisms, pushing us back to an inanimate state and that we simultaneously know and ignore it. In our intellectual behaviour we fight for survival, but on a deeper, instinctual level we try to ensure our own individual 'customized' death. Dying cannot be a learned art; maybe that is why death might be considered the moment of our greatest individuality.

Freud had recognized two principles in psychic life:

1. *The pleasure-unpleasure-principle*, which usually is just called the pleasure principle, says psychic activity in general aims at attaining pleasure and avoiding unpleasure.
2. *The reality principle* modifies the pleasure principle by accepting detours during the search for pleasure in order not to fail, when reality challenges, and to avoid disappointments or other negative consequences.

Checking external reality and taking it into account protects the pleasure principle, even if some pleasure has to be delayed or perhaps surrendered due to dangers in the real external world.

But our task is not only to scan the external reality to check whether it is suitable for a secure satisfaction of needs. The internal world also has to accord with our psychic activity, an aspect emphasized by Anne-Marie and Joseph Sandler. They noted that "the ego makes every effort to maintain a minimal level of safety feeling" and that "this feeling of safety is more than a simple absence of discomfort or anxiety, but a very definite feeling quality within the ego." (Sandler & Sandler, 1998, 2 ff.) The Sandlers introduced the term "safety principle" which is connected with well-being and self-assurance. In the development of the child this positive aspect of the child's relationship to his superego becomes a splendid source of love and well-being. Usually a child prefers to renounce satisfaction, even sexual satisfaction such as masturbation, if this ensures the maintenance of the love of the parents.

In the grown-up individual alongside the search for pleasure the search for well-being remains. There is a strong pressure to find safety and, like the reality principle, the safety principle often leads to decisions to delay or to renounce the satisfaction of a wish, because it might prove too dangerous if fulfilled.

The safety principle plays a similar role to the pleasure principle as the reality principle does; but while the reality principle is scanning the external world to detect dangers, the safety principle is examining the internal world of internalized objects whose love must not be lost. Separation-anxiety and separation-pain must be prevented.

The conscious and unconscious psychic life form inner reality, so that one might incorporate the screening of inner reality into the reality principle. Nevertheless, it makes sense to reserve the term safety principle for this attention turned inside, while the reality principle concentrates on outside events. Freud was quite concerned with differentiating stimuli outside from those inside us when he introduced the reality principle. Both, the reality principle and the safety principle serve to promote the security of the individual. An ideal state of well-being is achieved, when the external and the internal world are in a homeostatic balance and when there are no signals of anxiety on either side. Such a state is a guarantee of harmonious biological and mental functioning.

Sandler's concept integrates ego-psychological and drive-theoretical aspects, since it is based on internalized object-relationships. These internal relationships to important objects are connected to drive-wishes and their elaboration. Freud saw anxiety as a signal regarding threatening dangers, which included external and internal dangers. He called the fear of loss of somebody's love the greatest internal danger, equal to the loss of a beloved person.

The safety principle contains the drive-aspect. Otherwise the concept might substitute instinctual satisfaction for stability, constancy and psychic equilibrium. Safety is a neutral platform from which one evaluates venturing wherever drive-wishes can be fulfilled. There are people who remain on this platform and renounce pleasure to avoid any risk. In such cases the only pleasure is perverse, a clinging to internal objects hostile to desires. Thus the safety principle offers an opportunity to balance internal relationships. But if this state of balance is not open to reconsideration the safety principle loses its function of regulation. A freezing within a relatively secure state might occur because the avoidance of unpleasure surpasses the search for pleasure. Our relationships are always in danger due to external and internal realities. Neither external catastrophes nor the sudden twist from love to hate or to silent dissolution can be banished for good. And often love and hate are totally intermingled in unsolvable struggles. Andrè Green said: "Freud's latest and greatest discovery concerned the inevitable fusion of love and hate and their possible defusion"[9] (Green & Kohon, 2005, 26; 16).

---

[9]Lacan introduced for this fusion of love and hate (no love without hatred) the term *hainamoration* (lovatred).

While the pleasure principle focuses on an object for instinctual satisfaction, the reality principle broadens our view of the surroundings and checks the environment regarding dangers possibly connected with the satisfaction. This process is reality testing. The safety principle pays attention to dangers coming from inside and checks, whether the loss of internalized objects, or a conflict with them, is truly a threat. If there are no serious threats noted, then pleasure can be pursued with alacrity.

The reality principle, like the safety principle, offers compromises according the notion: better less pleasure and more safety. The reality principle forces us to look at cold facts we must confront if we want to protect ourselves against danger. The safety principle, by contrast, concentrates on the positive side regarding comfortable security and maintenance of good relations to the objects. The homeostasis established by watching the external and the internal world vigilantly is useful from a biological point of view and is registered as a feeling of safety and well-being. This feeling is one you might call pleasant in a vague way, while "pleasure" hints at a higher degree of excitement and concrete contents. One might compare the pleasure principle to a zoom lens that draws satisfying objects nearer, while the reality principle and the safety principle can be compared to a scanner screening external and internal dangers. A sound psychic equilibrium is based on an integration of the reality- and the safety-principle and serves the protection of the pleasure principle, which avoids external or internal losses, if possible.

A young patient had understood in her analysis that she projected many inner dangers to her environment; in vain she tried to avoid them in a phobic way. She started to look at her internal conflicts and compared this new capacity with something she had learned in her riding sessions: one can – according Sally Swift's book about Centred Riding – look with "hard" eyes, exactly and with concentration on a fixed point; but one also can look in a comprehensive way with "soft" eyes, thus taking in the periphery, below and above, and achieving more awareness, less tension and an easier movement forward. Both perspectives are important, according to the need served. In this way – she felt – she no longer focused on an external danger, but she could now also listen to what was going on inside her and with free floating attention she perceived there a lot so that she recognized problems and often was able to solve them.

Of course, often even a very wary 'monitoring system' protecting pleasure as a basic principle of life becomes overstrained at times. Our defence mechanisms cause repressions and displacements that distort the information we get from the monitoring system.

A very disciplined and sportive man aged 50 made a trip with his wife on bicycle through an isolated area. It was extremely hot and he must have noticed the danger and the stress because he suggested to his wife that she get down from the bicycle, if the strain was too much. In the next minute, he collapsed and died shortly afterward. Apparently, he could not recognize his own strain; he had to shift it to his wife, whom he better could allow to be weak. His ambitious superego had not tolerated this self-perception.

3 Facets of separation

3.1. Summary of aspects already mentioned

We have covered many aspects of separations where it becomes evident how we try to escape separation-pain by shrinking from separations altogether:

- By binding as opposite pole and remedy for separation (for instance the teddy bear, a beloved transitional object, which helps the little child to endure separation from the mother),
- by denying death as a final separation (clinging to religious ideas or "eternal" ideals),
- by letting a lost object go in order not to lose one's own life (the work of mourning),
- or - if the process of mourning fails, as in the case in depression - by fetching the object into the ego, where it is held tight,
- by focusing on birth as prototype of separation, thus conjuring up symbiotic fantasies,
- by inhibiting performances and functions in order to avoid separation (case of Peter, who felt guilty, when he left his mother and could not stand her/his separation-anxiety),
- by a phobic avoidance of objects, which cause a separation from other objects (Isabella's "school-phobia"),
- by producing guilt feelings, which are connected with separation-anxieties and often are the other, hidden side of separation-wishes,
- by projecting one's own wishes to separate onto other persons, a mechanism that creates (unconscious) separation-anxiety,
- by regressing to a symbiotic relationship in order to avoid separations,
- by suffering narcissistic wounds due to the loss of a caring person,
- by devaluation or overvaluation of relationships regarding our split knowledge about transience and about the fact that separation-pain is the price to be paid, if one loves somebody, and
- by checking the external and internal reality in order to prevent the loss of beloved objects.

3.2 Examples of psychoanalytic literature considering separation-anxiety

Freud in "Three essays on Sexuality" (1905) understood that the core of fear in children stemmed from anxiety over loss of a beloved person. At that time Freud considered blocked sexual excitement as the main cause of neurotic anxiety.

This thesis he illustrated four years later in the case of little Hans, whose love of his mother turned into anxiety and a horse phobia; horses had become phobic objects representing the threatening phallus of the father.

In 1917 Freud mentioned in his introductory lectures that anxiety during birth was a prototype of separation anxiety. (But he did not support Otto Rank's extension of this idea nine years later.)

In 1920 Freud described in "Beyond the Pleasure Principle" his observations of his grandson, when 18 months old as he tried to overcome his separation-anxiety by a game using a wooden reel with a piece of string tied round it. He threw the reel and pulled it back again by the string so that he could control disappearance and return. With this simple game the child overcame separation-anxiety and could allow the mother to move around more freely.

In "The Ego and the Id" (1923) Freud continued his delving into separation-anxiety. He traced the fear of death back to earliest childhood, recognizing that for the ego life and being loved is identical; where love is in danger, life is in danger, too.

In "Inhibitions, Symptom and Anxiety" (1926) Freud once more dealt with the separation-anxiety of the child. The child cathects the mnemic image of the mother intensely, but being a hallucination it has no effect: "and now it seems as though the longing turns into anxiety. This anxiety has all the appearance of being an expression of the child's feeling at its wits' end, as though in its still very undeveloped state it did not know how better to cope with its cathexis longing. Here anxiety appears as a reaction to the felt loss of the object; and we are at once reminded of the fact that castration anxiety, too, is a fear of being separated from a highly valued object, and that the earliest anxiety of all – the 'primal anxiety' of birth – is brought about on the occasion of a separation from the mother" (Freud, 1926, S.E. 20, 137). The danger from which the child wants to be safeguarded is non-satisfaction, when tension grows due to unsatisfied need. The fear of this situation is displaced and turns into the fear of the loss of the object. Separation-anxiety becomes a warning signal about an impending situation of traumatic helplessness. Separation-pain is reaction to a real loss of an object, and defences try to reject instinctual needs in order not to get overwhelmed when the object is missed.

This summarizing we find also in Freud's late writings ("An Outline of Psycho-Analysis", a fragment published posthumously in 1940). Here Freud focuses on mourning and defence as linked with separation-anxiety, which now is seen as reaction to the threat of the loss of an object.

Psychoanalysts after Freud studied some aspects of separation-anxiety in more detail and discovered new facets. Without entailing a complete survey of those contributions[10] I want to highlight a few:

---

[10] An comprehensive survey can be read in Bowlby (1998, 423-448) and especially in Jean-Michel Quinodoz (2004).

Melanie Klein

connects separation-anxiety with unconscious fear of annihilation. She considers it a reaction to the death-drive. Its activity is experienced as persecution. The feeling of total dependence from the first love-object, as well as fear of having it erased by destructive impulses, contributed to development of separation-anxiety. For example, a little girl felt that when her mother kissed her 'Good-night', it was a separation forever because the child unconsciously wished and consciously feared that the mother should leave her alone with daddy forever. Another example is a little boy, who had similar but conscious wishes that his father go away and so expected to be punished for these thoughts by losing him forever. Thus Klein emphasized collusion of external and internal dangers, with the latter appearing as sadistic impulses and destructive fantasies causing depressive anxieties and guilt feelings that inhibit the drive.

Anna Freud

described in her papers, which she published with Dorothea Burlingham, how the form of separation rather than its fact is what provoked great anxiety. Often separation was experienced as punishment so that the child shows all the love they can to avoid separation. Anna Freud also discussed different ways that separation-anxiety is expressed during the phases of the child's development. Fear of annihilation might transform to separation-anxiety, castration anxiety, fear of loss of love and guilt feelings.

Max Schur

studied the learning aspect of separation-anxiety. The perception that an unpleasant feeling such as hunger can be stopped by an external object, introduces a shift so that it is not hunger itself that seems so traumatic, but the absence of the object that can stop it.

Ernst Kris

emphasized the difference between the loss of a love object and the loss of the love of the object. In the first case it is about the satisfaction of needs, in the latter about the personal relationship to an object that cannot be easily substituted.

Helene Deutsch

isolated the infantile separation-anxiety from sorrow and mourning as more mature forms of relationship. Thus she considered separation-anxiety during later phases of life in principle as regression to a state, where the ego is not strong enough for mourning.

Therese Benedek

dealt with separation and reunion of loving persons. She described anxiety as a general reaction to separation, which represents a trauma. The awareness or expectation of mourning causes an escalation of desire for the absent object or the object that is threatened by separation[11]. Beside anxiety as a signal, if the loss of an object is feared, there is also a fear of disintegration of the ego.

Margaret Mahler
attributed, like Benedek and Anna Freud, different forms of separation anxiety to different states of development and elaborated the phases of autism, of symbiosis and individuation. For all these phases the capacity of separation, of locomotion and the connected joy regarding the independence gained by it are decisive. During the symbiotic phase separation is experienced as annihilation.

René Spitz
concentrated on narcissistic trauma. He regarded separation-anxiety as a signal, that appears in order to prevent traumatic situations, which might threaten narcissism.

Anne-Marie Sandler, Joseph Sandler and Walter G. Joffe
also stressed the violation which the self suffers due to the loss of an object and the separation-pain. Thus the loss of an object that assures well-being causes a loss of a vital self-aspect. Joseph Sandler showed how infantile separation-anxiety in a traumatic situation lead to the need to provoke such a situation, if there was a perceived chance that one might struggle successfully against separation-anxiety. A female patient was so hard of hearing, that her analyst had to shout at her, as her grandmother had done, who in her lonely childhood had in this way made her feel that there was a sure presence. Joseph Sandler did not agree with Mahler that individuation with the need to overcome separation-anxiety is a phase of development; he rather saw it as a line of development running through the whole life.

H.S. Sullivan
pointed to the danger of inner separation, which the child feels if the mother disapproves of what the child is doing. The child's fear depends on the mother's behaviour and not only on physical needs. The need for contact is not less important. If it is neglected a painful feeling of loneliness arises. When the mother refuses or rejects tenderness, she provokes anxiety.

W.R. Fairbairn
picked up the hypothesis of Otto Rank that the birth-trauma is the prototype of all separation-anxiety, which Fairbairn considered the origin of all psychopathology.

---

[11] This mechanism a female analysand described with affection: she was shocked about her "falseness", that she approached her husband with tender gestures, as often as she felt really angry with him. She had a highly ambivalent relationship with him and often thought of a divorce. By showing signs of love she restored the balance between separation fantasies and closeness.

D.W. Winnicott
followed Melanie Klein in many aspects, but he also added that the earliest anxiety stems from being insecurely held and insufficiently cared for by the mother. He showed how children overcome their separation-anxiety by the use of transitional objects and that the capacity to be alone is primarily acquired in the presence of a protecting object.

John Bowlby
combined an empirical-behaviouristic approach with the introspection of psychoanalytic object-theory by developing *attachment-theory*. He studied separation-anxiety in the normal as well as in pathological development. He differentiated three forms of reactions: 1. the protest, which is connected with the effort to keep the object that threatens to go away; 2. the depressive reaction of despair and 3. the loss of interest in the lost object (= detachment).

We can already see in these examples in psychoanalytic literature that there is an oscillation between focusing on unconscious processes and looking at observable behaviour. There is either an emphasis on what happens within the person (intrapsychic) or between the persons involved (interpsychic), based on conscious and unconscious relationships. Although all these facets belong to the same phenomenon, it is plausible that not all of them can be seen from each point of view, which of course can lead to controversies.

3.3 Separation as achievement

When we consider psychic development of an individual, it is clear that the capacity of separation is a decisive criterion of maturity. Many psychoanalysts emphasized that separation is an achievement which depends on the development and creativity of the individual in finding solutions.

Anna Freud in 1965 elaborated psychic lines of development that include this capacity. There is development from infantile dependence to a grown-up love life, or the line of physical independence, which is seen in eating and washing oneself without help and in taking care for the own body with a growing feeling of responsibility.

Margaret Mahler studied carefully the transition from symbiosis to the individuation of the little child.

S. Freud, as mentioned above, described the creative solution of a child (cf. chapter 3.2), who managed his separation-anxiety by inventing a game: he made himself a wooden reel vanishing and reappearing by pulling it back with a string; thus he worked through the absence and the presence of his mother by controlling such a situation.

Also Winnicott stressed the creativity of the child, who is capable of accepting a transitional object as a substitute for the mother and of overcoming in this way separation-anxiety.

The growing capacity of the child to renounce the permanent real presence of the persons closest to him and to overcome his separation-anxiety is a very important step in development. It is the prerequisite for entering a kindergarten and later on a school; at least at this time the child should have attained enough independence regarding his social maturity.

But the capacity of separation remains a question of maturity, even if it is often concealed by all sorts of distracting noise. The boisterous behaviour of adolescents might mute this melody of separation, which they nonetheless hear because of their fast-fading childhood and their alienation of parents. And behind the loud quarrels of grown-ups there can be a desperate feeling of paralyzing impotence, for instance, if somebody can neither stand nor leave the partner. Finally the last stage of the life demands a special ability to give up what has been familiar for many years, and only those, who can manage this to some extent, succeed in adapting to the reality of their reduced physical strength by allowing changes, by overcoming losses and by accepting other forms of satisfaction.

Also in jokes about dying the aspect of separation as achievement is expressed: A lady asked her dying husband why he was so scared, even children can die. Here the joke's essence is the double meaning of the word 'can': it is used in the sense of achievement, but also in the sense of a possibility.

In "Thoughts on War and Death" (1915) Freud wrote: "Towards the actual person who has died we adopt a special attitude – something almost like admiration for someone who has accomplished a difficult task. We suspend criticism of him, overlook his possible misdeeds, declare that 'de mortuis nil nisi bonum', and think it justifiable to set out all that is most favourable to his memory in the funeral oration and upon the tombstone. Consideration for the dead, who, after all, no longer need it, is more important to us than the truth, and certainly, for most of us, than consideration for the living" (Freud, 1915, S.E. 14, 290).

But not only from the perspective of the bereaved does death often appear as an achievement. So, for example, Pontalis (according to Phillips, 1999, 78) spoke in connection with Freud's concept of the death-drives about "death-work", and M'Uzan (1976) wrote about the "work of dying". Similarly, when we read in the biographies of prominent persons about their agony, there is often the impression of a great effort during a process that needs be undergone. Frederic Chopin appears to have said in his last hours that people would not disturb dying individuals in their ordeal, if they knew its importance (Gavoty, 1977; Poutalès, 1964).

Here we might consider the problem of euthanasia, a Greek word for 'dying well', which seems an euphemistic term to hide the fact that often we ourselves hardly can bear to see somebody in dire illness or in agony. Great poets know this. Arthur Schnitzler regarded the word 'release' as tricky because "it turns the most terrible wish in dissembling compassion". If we say: 'he should be finally released', we mean that we want to be released, because we can no longer stand to witness helplessly how somebody dies. The forbidden wish that the agony should be over so that we are no longer forced to see it is projected to the dying individual who 'wants to be released'. More often than not we cannot know whether somebody near death has such a thought. Robert Walser spoke in the novel "Ohne einander" ('Without each other') about the "infection" with death. It is understandable that we flee from this danger as far as we can in order to save ourselves. It will remain an extremely difficult decision in each case whether we are allowed to take the 'own' death out of somebody's hands or not. We are not freed even if this person signed a declaration earlier, because at that time he could not know himself, what he might feel in his final hours. In many cases the 'decision' will settle itself – if possible with the agreement of the fatally ill – by providing as much pain release as necessary without directly ending his life.

We have dealt with mourning as a psychic achievement that is rewarded with the award of staying alive in a separate chapter.

If we speak of separation as achievement, there is the possibility that one fails in this achievement and that one may not develop this capacity sufficiently. In this case the other person is not really 'loved', but needed, because the incapacity to be alone does not allow choice. Winnicott studied the capacity to be alone (1984, 43 f.). He pointed out that this capacity can only be developed in the presence of somebody else. A facilitating environment supports the immature ego of the child and can be introjected, so that the ability can evolve to be really alone. If there are no persons who represent such a supporting and strengthening environment, the development towards independence becomes stuck, and sometimes the capacity to be alone and to separate is never attained.
Maybe one has the impression that such incapacity is not the exception but the rule. Innumerable guide books or articles try to help. Language itself hints at the difficulty of separation: one 'gets' a divorce, thus trying to delegate the labour of separating to a third person; nevertheless this does not spare a couple the own separation.

Not only to separate from other persons is difficult. Also things often cannot be dismissed even when their meaning and history is no longer clearly remembered. Sometimes this creates a chaos that mirrors on the outside the inner confusion. For such problems workshops are established. For instance 'Feng Shui against the every day junk,' which promises participants will develop the capacity to create free spaces by shedding old burdens. If such exercises succeed, this might be due to the attachment to the person who recommends or 'allows' such a strategy; this would mean that separation could be managed because of a new binding.

Some separations are inhibited by 'outstanding bills': unsatisfied desires and hopes, but also stubborn-aggressive insisting on unfulfilled wishes may retain objects in spite of experiences that had not been satisfying until now; 'gluey' libido continues to adhere to them. The positions of libido are not given up willingly, as Freud pointed out in "Mourning and Melancholia".

At the outset we wrote about separation and bond as the two basic principles of life. During normal development of an individual the capacity of bonding to an external object unfolds and, later, diminishes again. In the same way the capacity of separation increases until an optimal independence is achieved, and then during older age it decreases again.

If one separates from somebody – or in theoretical language: if the libido is decathected from an object – libido is taken back into the ego. In his 26th Introductory Lecture Freud illustrated the reversible transformation of ego-libido (this is libido concentrated on the ego) into object-libido by a metaphor from zoology: "Think of those simplest of living organisms [the amoebas] which consist of a little-differentiated globule of protoplasmic substance. They put out protrusions, known as pseudopodia, into which they cause the substance of their body to flow over. They are able to withdraw the protrusions once more and form themselves again into a globule. We compare the putting-out of these protrusions, then, to the emission of libido on to objects while the main mass of libido can remain in the ego; and we suppose that in normal circumstances ego-libido can be transformed unhindered into object-libido and that this can once more be taken back into the ego." (Freud 1917, 415 f.) As examples of extreme shifts of libido may serve states as the psychical behaviour of a person in love, when it seems that the whole libido is absorbed in the idealization of the beloved person; or states during an organic illness, when the whole libido is withdrawn from the external world back upon the ego. Such a state also the poet Wilhelm Busch knew, when he described the psychic state, if one suffers from toothache:

> 'Concentrated is his soul
> in his molar's narrow hole.'[12]

Modern psychoanalytic theory deals at length with the phenomenon that not only the ego and the objects get cathected with libidinal energy, but also the psychic process of cathecting itself. Green, setting out his conception of the

---

[12] Freud quoted these lines of Busch in regard to a sick man, who withdraws his libidinal cathexes back upon his own ego, and sends them out again, when he recovers. (Freud, 1914, 82)

death drive, describes how withdrawal of cathexis (disinvestment) attacks the objectalizing process,. He called this destruction due to a negative narcissism "disobjectalizing function" (Green, 2005a, 222). On the other hand, if a psychic function like the binding to an object is cathected, the psychic function is "elevated to the status of an object". If the dissolution of the bonds to objects serves a malign form of narcissism, the disinvestment destroys, what investment had built up. If negative narcissism destroys this way the objects, it is an attack against the own ego continuing destruction until the final escalation by suicide.

However, the notion that not only objects but also the process of cathecting itself can be cathected, is important. It allows greater flexibility and the change of objects. Then not only the beloved object but love itself is loved.[13] When libido is withdrawn from an object that is no longer available, the cathecting energy can continue turning to the objects in order to find a new love object. If this is successful, it is not necessary that the libidinal cathexis returns totally back to the own ego, as it happens in narcissism.

It is a balanced state, like the one that the safety-principle provides: the focus is more on the harmony with internalized representations of important persons than on instinctual satisfaction. Similarly, if loving and not only the beloved object is our focus, inner balance seems more important than conquering this special love object. It seems that in such a situation the decision has not yet been made whether libido will be invested in an object or whether the libidinal energy should be withdrawn. A total withdrawal includes the danger that the individual remains imprisoned in his narcissism and never again will turn to another object. In malign narcissism this withdrawal even goes on by decathecting and thus erodes the own ego. The balance between narcissism and love also can become frozen. Then the action of love is loved, and none of the objects, which can be easily substituted, has a value anymore of its own; the price to be paid is a lack of true satisfaction, as we have seen in the case of "Don Juan".

What is pathological, however, is not the balance but the fixation of the balance. It makes it impossible to turn the attention to objects, to choose and to have a lively exchange with them. Thus separation can be considered healthy if an unreachable or permanently unsatisfying object is given up and substituted by a new one. During such a process a passing withdrawal of libido will be followed by another phase, in which a love-object is cathected again.

---

[13] Also this discovery was already made in everyday life, when in chansons and songs love itself is praised. So sang for instance Jacqueline Boyer "Do me the favour to greet Love warmly from me; tell her I am permanently dreaming of her." But also in literature we find this thought: Hermann Bahr, for instance, presents in 'The Concert' (a highly successful theatre play) the lawyer Dr. Jura, who is very ready to give his young wife to an elder great pianist. He says (already peeping at the pianist's wife): 'Life with a woman is something so wonderful! I wonder whether it really matters, with which woman one lives.' (Bahr 1961, 56)

The capacity to separate plays a role in the choice of a profession. Sometimes it seems that one can see the degree of maturation in the distance a chosen profession has from early experiences which the child had. This concerns not only such cases where the profession of the parent(s) is taken without any consideration. Other activities the child gets to know in early years have often a shaping influence. Regression and fixation on previous periods of life can influence the choice of profession.[14] Thus, events which touched a child seriously in kindergarten, at school, at a physician or in a hospital, often influence a child deeply and unconsciously because of a heavy affect like anxiety or triumph. An analysand, for instance, told me that he had decided to become a medical doctor when he was four. At that time he was in hospital and was fond of a kind doctor who explained everything to him and called him the bravest patient he ever had. A strong emotional experience can prevent other professional possibilities from appearing; only the admired representatives of a special profession dominate the imagination.

Of course it would be wrong to judge a person's maturity only on the basis of choice of profession. Someone might try to escape early environment by choosing a job which is remote from what the parents did. But this choice also can be an unconscious disguise of continuing dependencies and might appear only on the surface to be a successful escape.

In close relationships the capacity to bear a certain amount of separateness is crucial for the stability of the bond. This is true for friendships as well as for marriages and indeed all forms of contact intended to last. But usually one does not know this, if one is in love - a state which is "a resurrection of a former state related to childhood", as André Green said (Green, Kohon, 2005, 20). Since no honeymoon is endless, later on different demands gain weight gradually. If they are repressed in one partner, it harms his/her personal development as well as their relationship, via hidden hate. Even if the dominant partner enjoys narcissistic triumphs, he or she will lose the lively exchange with the other one. If both try to suppress each other, a permanent power struggle arises; this eventually guaranties nothing but sadomasochistic pleasure. However, if enough common pleasure is maintained and if both are allowed also to devote themselves from time to time to separate interests, the relationship has a high degree of flexibility resulting in a high degree of stability, too.

In psychosexual development sexual identity requires a decision that means separation from one of two possibilities: defining oneself as a man or as a woman (cf. Kohon, 1999a, 18 ff.). If one feels the need to keep the option to identify with both sexes, the development of a clear male or female identity is inhibited. For an artist creativity can be so closely linked with ideas of female fertility, that he cannot develop an unambiguous male identity.

---

[14] Cf. Zwettler-Otte S., 1991

Transcending the level of relationships separation is also a prerequisite for the free development of intellectual abilities. For this the capacity to think must be evaluated higher than loyalty towards authorities, who may be idealized. Without an independent mind there is the danger of blindly following authorities and renouncing formation of opinions of one's own. On the other hand an immature stubborn opposition might manifest that it is only about contradicting others. Both options remain dependent. It is exactly the development of a high capacity for discernment that leads to high intellectual achievements; it is an ability, which contains the possibility of linking thoughts as well as of separating from given ideas. Such an independent mind is based on a stronger cathexis of mental functioning than a need to cling to an object.

3.4 Daily exercises in losing objects

Let us look at everyday life for a family experiencing all the usual mundane small separations and losses of objects. Here then is a kind of cross-section of a couple's life coping with a little child. To do so we return to Saskia, the female restorer, whom we got to know in chapter 2.1.2. Since her analysis a year and a half has passed.

From the comfortable depths of sleep the parents awoke early in the morning. This shift seems extremely difficult for Saskia, since vague memories of her early childhood had become accessible again. For instance, how cosy it was, when she curled up in her mother's arms while watching TV. Neither she nor her husband needed an alarm clock, since their little daughter announced her waking with remarkable precision every morning. Usually she does it with a whining voice, protesting that her mother was not lying next to her. She had separated, though only for a few hours and by just a few metres. Kurt and Saskia, of course, would prefer to enjoy more of the warm closeness before getting up, but they have to separate so that Saskia can nurse the baby and Kurt prepare breakfast. In the meantime, little Julia is satisfied because her mother is totally devoted to her, and pronounces loudly: "Gaga!" Thus she informs Saskia that she is ready to part with her excrement, a product she gives her mother as a present. Saskia accepts it with praising words. She is really glad that the good digestion of the child proves, how well the child is cared for and how it "functions" without any problems. Recently, when Saskia had been away for one day, Julia refused to give this "present" thus expressing her concern about the prolonged separation. During breakfast Julia tries hard to disturb her parents' conversation; she simply does not like it if they divert their attention from her – even that appears to be too much of a separation. However, she nearly had forgotten her protest, because the father gave her a little wooden duck. Her interest in this toy diverted her from her mission of defending her position as the centre of the family. For Kurt it is not easy to say goodbye to his wife and his daughter in order to attend to his professional tasks. For him to be happy within his own family is still something wonderfully new. Saskia takes Julia with her for shopping. In the supermarket Julia is attracted to the soft toy-dog of another child, with whom she starts to play. But in a little while she has to separate from that child and her little toy dog. She cannot do so without tears. Her mother quickly offers her another toy to console her regarding the loss. After lunch Saskia puts her daughter to bed, but although it is evident that Julia is tired, she hesitates to close her eyes. Only after Saskia sits down next to the baby cot with a book, the noises of the turned pages reassure the child that the mother is still there and that she can fall asleep securely. Saskia herself needs some time to shift from her role as mother to other tasks of the day. Later on in the afternoon the babysitter comes so that Saskia can go to her analysis. Julia is still too sleepy to protest vehemently against her mother's departure, and the babysitter skilfully engages her into a game so that there does not arise a great row due to the impending separation. After three hours, shortly before Saskia comes home again, Julia becomes worried. Soon she has to say goodbye to the likeable babysitter, with whom she just has got acquainted. This confused her a bit, but the joy of her mother's company again ended the conflict. When the father returns, the light irritation is repeated, because it disturbed the just renewed getting together with the mother. But Julia likes that her father greets her by throwing her carefully up in the air and catching her again with a laugh. She enjoyed this game of funny little separations, squealing with delight. Saskia notices, smiling, that now Kurt seems to be more interesting to Julia than herself. There had been evenings, when she became jealous and felt that it was unfair, if Julia turned away from her. It was she who had cared for Julia the whole day, sacrificing to the child - at least at the time being - her professional career - and when the father came home she was forgotten. When the child went to bed again after some grumbling, she hugged the teddy bear, which made it easier to say goodnight to the parents. Now a couple, who were friends, came for a short visit to show pictures of their holidays and advise Saskia and Kurt, because they had in mind a journey to the same place. The friends spoke so enthusiastically about their vacation, that Saskia forgot about her doubts regarding such holidays, which would mean to be a break from life in the familiar environment. She had little hope that her secret wishes for a chance to make up for the fact that she and Kurt had not had a real honeymoon. She dreamed of romantic dinners and dancing but she was afraid that all these things could not happen because of Julia. This thought created guilt feelings over a conflict between her love for her child and her love for her husband. Nevertheless, seeing the photos and brochures stirred her craving for a holiday. There was a fascinating discussion and the guests, although tired, stayed longer than planned, putting off departure with a few additional glasses of wine.

It had been a normal day, full of little separations. Some of them touched upon conflicts of loyalty, when the symbiosis of mother and child or the relations between the parents were upset by a third person. The child separates from the parents, the attractive toys from the other child; the babysitter and the returning father supplant the mother, and so on. It caused a conflict that is incompatible with devoting oneself at the same time totally to work or to the spouse or to the child. Even attending analysis created feelings of guilt. However, Saskia felt that without analysis she would remain entangled in her difficult history and so have less chance to be a good enough mother. The children of the visiting couple were older, a fact which encouraged Saskia and Kurt that they too will overcome the hurdles and balance their own needs with those of the child to whom they were attached, though sometimes with ambivalence. Their friends are models of good parents, but they also infringed on the closeness between Saskia and Kurt, who actually had not planned to live with somebody else so intimately. For them it was a considerable achievement to part with their life as singles by growing together into a family. The occasion was a plan for holidays. *Holidays are separations that are introduced on purpose; a mixture of pleasure and thrill plays a great part in imaginations regarding journeys: one parts willingly with the familiar environment hoping to come home again safely, which is mostly, but not always right.* Often one can detect the craving for just such a pleasant thrill, which means a triumph of the pleasure over the fear, when somebody discusses his holidays. This was the case with Saskia's and Kurt's friends, who, incidentally, had to overcome also a regressive moment of laziness when able finally to say goodbye.

I have emphasized the role of the third person also because this has theoretical implications. The third person is not only important for loosening the symbiotic relationship of a couple, thus facilitating further development. Especially if one studies separation-anxiety, there might be the inclination of overlooking the Oedipus-complex as nuclear complex of neuroses in favour of a two-person-psychology – thus denying the active potential of conflicts. Regarding triangulation and connected configurations of thirdness Green pointed out with some irony, that Freud described in detail pregenital structures and their full meaning in relation to the crowning of infantile sexuality with the Oedipus complex; but after his death the psychoanalytic community thought it had discovered something important in pregenital forms. Thus "the figure of the father was to fade increasingly until it became almost absent from the clinical picture. In the same way, castration anxiety saw its domain shrink in the face of anxieties linked to an exclusive mother-child relationship: anxieties of separation, intrusion, etc." (Green, 2005a, 187)
But this clinical example indicates that separation-anxiety cannot be fully understood clinically nor theoretically without taking into account the role of the third person. We have seen in the chapter on Saskia her terrible fear of death when she was about to give birth. Her relationship to her father was laden with heavy guilt after she lost her mother so early. These experiences influence how she feels as a mother and wife. Her infantile death wishes towards her mother, which in analysis slowly became conscious, seemed to her a catastrophic reality

she had caused by her magic thinking. Unhappily, her wish to be alone with her father was fulfilled, and this made her also highly attentive to any sign that her little daughter would turn to her father. But other moments also contributed: whether it was her husband, her stalled career or her analysis – a third person always was involved when incompatibilities and conflicts were arising, and those conflicts were always connected with separations and therefore with separation-anxieties and wishes for separation. So it is an unjustified simplification to reduce the problem to what goes on only between mother and child.

3.5 Chronology of separation-anxieties

Our lives are marked by innumerable separations, great ones and small ones, temporary ones and final ones, traumatic and easy ones. How a separation is experienced, is highly subjective and is not necessarily in accord with the judgement of others in the environment. A child put too early into the kindergarten might experience separation as trauma, if he feels in his inner reality that it is a punishment for bad wishes and fantasies. The parents, however, may misunderstand the child's desperate protest as a proof that it was indeed necessary to bring him there in order to foster his socialisation and integration in a community. Such a discrepancy between the feelings of the parents and of the child can be overcome, if the parents succeed in the difficult task of seeing what really is going on in the child. But it can also be a dramatic point in a disastrous development, even if the parents are very interested and aided by pedagogical guides because they want to do the right thing. If, for personal reasons, they are unable to understand the wishes, passions and fears that preoccupy the child, it can go very wrong. It is not possible to decide in advance, when a separation is "healthy" and when it is "endangering." Of course, it can be a good sign if a child separates without problems and just with a little hesitation. But in order to evaluate the uncertainty and complexity of all these processes one might take also into account the possibility that a child can behave well in this situation because he has already given up, adapted totally and no longer tries to resist. Then a "false self" – a term introduced by Winnicott – is established that hides true feelings, and the child is left alone with his trouble.

3.5.1 A "healthy" patient after traumatic loss

The previous chapter looked at the experiences of loss in the everyday life of a young family. Now I'll compare how a "healthy" person and how a "very disturbed" patient might respond to traumatic separations. I have chosen two cases of elderly people so that we can overlook longer periods of life.

Peter, 67 years old, and Iris, his wife, were returning home, along with an acquaintance, after they attended an open-air theatre. The road had sharp curves and they were suddenly hit by another car. The acquaintance was killed instantly. Iris succumbed in hospital to severe internal injuries. Peter had been hurled down the slope of a hill. Suffering a compound fracture of a leg he could not climb up to his wife. He recalled her hand dangling from the car wreck – a horrible image that persecuted him afterward during his sleepless nights and which he could not help but interpret as his wife beckoning him to follow her in death. Since these sleeping disturbances did not abate after several weeks, a general practitioner, whom Peter saw for the flu, prescribed sleeping pills. Peter declined and said that he simply felt incapable of dealing alone with his traumatic loss. Therapy was very likely Peter's actual quest, since he knew this doctor viewed psychotherapy positively, having seen leaflets in the waiting room offering addresses of psychotherapists. The doctor initially hesitated to suggest therapy because he was afraid his patient might worry about being classified as "abnormal". But when the patient himself made the request, the doctor was relieved, supported it and confirmed that this would be a better idea than medication, and he gave him my phone number.

The first sessions were filled with idealizations of Peter's and Iris' 35 year marriage. The common pleasures had always been given much more weight than the difficulties. Their greatest joy, however, had been their daughter. She was now 30 years old and happily married in France. She had visited them as often as possible. After the fatal accident she came immediately and tried to help her father although she herself was deeply shaken by the loss of her mother. After two months in psychotherapy Peter during a session suddenly started to weep bitterly. Although he felt that there was no reason to be ashamed nor to apologize, he explained at the end of the session – looking at me for the first time with full attention: "It seems that I needed you in order not to be alone in this moment, when I would be able to grasp the extent of this loss." During the following sessions his sense of guilt came up - that he stayed alive while his wife had died – and so did his gnawing suspicion that their acquaintance, who had been driving the car, might have prevented this accident. Memories of previous separations in his life emerged. None were as agonizing as this one, but some of these experiences demonstrated his remarkable strength and maturity. To acknowledge this fact was encouraging to both of us. The first painful separation he remembered was suddenly being moved to his grandparents because his mother gave birth to his sister earlier than expected. The father ran a small shop and had to find somebody to fill in for him before he could stay at home to look after him. The grandparents had not been very sensitive in dealing with Peter. His parents had tried to prepare him for the imminent birth but his feelings were very mixed, and now the new little rival's quick appearance combined with this unhappy separation from home. Nevertheless, the grandparents insisted in their naïve way that he show joy about his little sister and even make presents for her. Anyway, one day he and his grandfather were shooting arrows against a target; Peter enjoyed this game that allowed him to express his unconscious hate, and was the opposite of the demanded solicitous care he did not feel toward his sister. The grandparents praised his chivalry when, after a direct hit, he shouted: "I'll shoot anybody who might do harm to my little sister!" He was of course unaware that it was himself to whom this threat was directed. He transformed his feelings of inferiority, of being repelled, of anger and jealousy, into learning a sports skill. This new ability had phallic meaning and one can assume that Peter could use it to work through his oedipal struggles with his father, whom he considered guilty that the mother was in hospital with a newborn baby and that Peter was temporarily abandoned.

Soon after, Peter entered kindergarten. This separation from home was easier because he found a new realm where he quickly fit in. His start at school two years later occurred without problems. Only when his teacher, whom he liked very much and who facilitated his development, became pregnant after the first year, he had another bad time. He enjoyed nothing, quarrelled with everyone and although he had gotten accustomed to his little sister, he now considered her silly and useless. Looking back, Peter now thought: "I was mourning a double loss: the kind teacher, and subsequently also the mother of my early childhood. She had made me lose my position as an only child." He probably was right that part of his separation-pain regarding his teacher was a repetition of the loss due to his mother's delivery. At the end of this session he glanced at my waist, as if to check, whether I too would desert him due to pregnancy. I took this to be a sign of an intensified transference. He displayed stronger feelings toward me, feelings which might have recalled memories of his first teacher. Since his treatment was not an analysis but planned as a short psychoanalytically orientated intervention to help him to overcome his crisis after the accident, I did not immediately pick up this concern about me. We both expected that this short treatment would be adequate. We did discuss the fact that after the loss of his beloved teacher he responded with great learning achievements. He disliked the next teacher and he tried hard to prove that he could learn without her. He became the best pupil and easily won a place at grammar-school. Due to his success at school his relationship to his parents was without serious problems. Only when he stayed out with friends longer and longer, he began to quarrel with his father, who preferred him to act as protector of his sister, and was inclined to restrain their liberty. The mother often had the role of a mediator, and Peter's detachment from the parents evolved slowly. When his grandfather and, soon after, his grandmother died, his mourning was a general understanding of the course of human life and respect regarding his mother's painful feelings; he had not often been with his grandparents, only when his sister was born. He still thought of his arrow-exercises with his grandfather with a kind of triumph, as if this had helped him to acquire some virility and independence. Because of the grandparent's death he delayed plans to go for a year in a foreign country to study. He did not want to burden his parents just now with another departure and decided to do his *military service first. So it was possible to stay with his family, but also to withdraw a bit because he became so involved in the powerful dynamic of young men in the military. Afterward he went to France to improve his French. But shortly before he left he fell in love with a girl at the university, so that he suffered a lot from parting with her. Looking back, Peter had remarkable insight into what might have caused his falling in love: "Maybe it was exactly because my journey was already fixed, that for the first time I fell in love". His wish to separate from his family now had love as a counterbalance. But his girl could not remain faithful during his absence. She asked his sister to tell him this bad news as gently as possible. For Peter's sister this journey to France in order to bring him this dire message became a date with destiny. There she met a medical student, whom she married two years later. Peter was upset by the unfaithful girl friend, but soon he had to admit that their relationship could not be so deep after such a short time and that he himself wanted more experiences. Unfortunately he had to leave France earlier than planned, since his father died due to a heart-attack. He and his sister helped now their mother to rearrange her life, to find a leaseholder for the little shop, and to help her financially. Peter earned his living and his study of languages by doing diverse jobs. He did all these necessary things reluctantly and felt paralyzed, until he realized that this was his way of mourning his father. He felt guilty that he had not been closer to him, that he had not helped him in the shop and that he had not estimated highly enough all they had done together, the trips, the family-parties and the football-games. His mother saw his suffering and told him how glad his father had been about Peter's decision to go his own way and that he had appreciated this more than having a successor for the shop. Liberated from guilt Peter recovered. His sister had to go back to France, and so Peter became main carer for the mother. In some ways he enjoyed it, like being an only child again. He lived in a student community, but he regularly saw his mother, helped her in the house and garden and was there when a few years later she became ill and died. His greatest regret was that it was only in hospital that he could introduce to her his new girlfriend Iris and that she could not see this relationship develop into a solid bond. After her death Iris treated Peter with such a combination of support and tact that this trying time bonded them strongly. And now Iris, with whom he had lived decades and who was the mother of his daughter, was dead. They still had had so many plans: a longer stay with their daughter in France and so on. He did not allow himself to do these things now. Instead he visited the cemetery every other day. When he told me this he suddenly laughed: "Iris would shy me away from there if she could! She would prefer seeing me more among the living." "Then why don't you do it? Maybe it is her wish and yours as well", I answered. He looked at me shocked and remained silent, as if he was caught in a trap. The next week he brought a letter of his daughter, who invited him so persuasively that he planned to visit her and her husband in summer. It seemed he wanted to hear from me the permission which Iris no longer could give him. We planned the end of the therapy before his summer holidays.*

One year later I got a letter from him in France where he had found a little flat and even made arrangements with the help of his son-in-law that eventually he would go to a private home for aged people there. Thus he need not be concerned about burdening his daughter and her family yet remain near them. His greatest joy was that he would see a grandchild growing up. He was eager to care for this child. He ended the letter by reporting that he asked his best friend to look after his wife's grave until he would return – for a visit. In the dining-room of his new little flat he had now a huge beautiful photo of his wife.

This short psychoanalytic therapy lasted about six months and helped to induce a process of mourning and a shift to a new way of living where other, available bonds gained priority over the lost love object. Together with this achievement he would be able to maintain his introjected relationship to his late wife as a precious part of his psychic life.

This psychotherapy experience also had important technical results. The traumatic separation spontaneously stirred recall of former situations of separation, thus letting him tell his life story from a long-term perspective. Like a weaver's loom that heaves a special layer of threads to the surface, this tragic event evoked similar situations in his past, which showed an encouraging pattern of healing. Separation until now had been overcome with academic achievements and intensified bonding to available objects. This observation became key for my studies concerning the possibilities of psychoanalytic short-term psychotherapy, which first David Malan decades ago developed at the Tavistock-Clinic in London.

3.5.2 An "ill" patient

The following case was a psychoanalysis four times a week. The patient is now 59 years old. Five years ago his sister urged him to see me because she feared that he was suicidal after his wife's slow and painful death from cancer. Due to our issue I'll emphasize also in this case the situations of separation.

The sister called to arrange an appointment with me for her brother. I politely declined, explaining that her brother ought to ring me himself if he wished to see me. He called a few days later. The first interview mainly was about clarifying the fact that I had no interest if he himself had no wish for psychotherapeutic help. Harry – as I name the patient here – seemed to have expected anything but not that I would refuse the order of his sister. Confused and a bit annoyed, he said at the end of the first session that I was right not to try to persuade him to enter therapy. He said he had lost everything and had done the wrong things all his life. I answered that this was not how I saw his situation but that I knew that it would be fruitless to persuade him. He was silent a moment and then stood up. At the door he turned and asked whether he might call me later. This he did in a week. In his second session he told about his unhappy childhood, his failing at school and in his profession, and about frequent physical diseases. Now his asthma recurred, as in his childhood. When I suggested that he might enter analysis after the summer break, he asked: "Is this worthwhile at my age?" I said little. He said that in his family nearly everybody lived more than 87 years or more, thus he had about three decades to live. He knew that even a successful analysis could not give him back his wife or years of his life, but it might change his view and his suffering, thus giving him the chance to live differently the time he still had. This session he did not run away as he had done before.

Harry had a difficult task upon birth: he had to console his grieving mother over her first son, who had died after a few weeks. This was the aim of Harry's procreation. His elder sister (by 3 years) apparently was not enough comfort for loss of the boy. Harry's mother cared for him in an anxious and overprotective way, watched him night and day and was alert to his slightest indisposition, imagining she might lose him too. She discouraged contact with his father, and so he had few memories of him. The father withdrew more and more to a nearby inn and died, before Harry went to school. Harry remembered how excited his mother and his grandmother were at the father's funeral. Both women wept loudly and wore black, which frightened him. Actually there was another loss that was a real shock for him. He had a rabbit, which lived in the grandmother's stable. He loved it, fed it and watched it with devotion. One day his grandmother asked him whether he had noticed, that today at lunch he had eaten a part of his little rabbit. This scene was traumatic, but also typical of the grandmother's sadism. Harry vomited and soon had eating disturbances, which caused incessant quarrels between his mother and his grandmother. The overprotective mother was upset that he refused to eat. He just ate enough that he need not be nourished artificially - a threat he was afraid of. When he entered school, the eating difficulties improved, or more accurately, it shifted to the digestion of what he should learn. Harry remained shut in on himself. He had to repeat the 4th class, but did not mind separating from his classmates, since he hardly had contact with them. Once a new teacher said to his mother thoughtfully "What Harry is capable of and what not, we do not really know". From this moment Harry loved him because he had allowed that Harry perhaps might know quite a lot more than he showed in classroom performance. When he lost this teacher, who was transferred to another school, Harry fell again into deep lethargy which took months to overcome. One day a dog attached himself to Harry. He was happy but this did not last long either. His sister was allergic to animal-hairs, and he was forced to bring the dog to a pet-home. From that day on he ceased learning and just waited until he was no longer forced to go to school. He hated his sister, whom he believed to be rather jealous than allergic. He hated his mother, who demanded this renunciation, and he hated his grandmother, who had murdered his rabbit. He would have liked to become a veterinarian, but everybody assured him that there was no chance because of his bad school-reports. Then a relative, who pitied his poor mother, agreed to take Harry as apprentice in his joinery. Harry was not skilful at the trade, but as a seller he was worse since he avoided contact with customers. His main task became to draw drafts for made-to-measure furniture. He did this work carefully, but it was not appreciated by his master. Anyway, he could finally earn a living. It was, as if his life had now stagnated in this little room of the joinery. At the weekends he stayed home, looking at TV. His mother had given up hope that he might become "something reasonable". After her death his sister took over care for him. She was shocked, when he one day told her out of the blue, that he was engaged, and that he would move in his fiancée's house. After five years they married, because she felt pregnant – which turned out to be wrong. It remained a very quiet relationship, infertile in many ways but lasting. He would not say his marriage was happy or unhappy. His guilt feelings from past failures were too great. The suffering expression on his wife's face reinforced this conclusion. She was a muted reproduction of the brassy dominance he knew in his mother, his grandmother and his sister. Two years ago the wife was found to have cancer. The treatment was unsuccessful, and she died, Harry was left alone in his confused and bitter mood, only occasionally in contact with his sister.

In analysis it was touching to see how Harry – in spite of long periods of hopelessness and in spite of his age – became lively. It was new for him to find a special attention in a space where he wasn't pressed and manipulated. However, this was exactly what irritated him so that he tried to push me into the role of overprotective mother or sister. During the first two years he reacted to our separations during weekends and holidays with attacks of asthma. It was as if he unconsciously had to enact a scene of being crushed whenever contact was interrupted. He fantasised overwhelming closeness, when there was actually some distance between us. He experienced this symptom as very dangerous. It symbolised the greatest, but injurious, proximity. A longing for closeness, and his rage over its absence, had been mixed up. At this time he was not able to introject our relationship. His early experiences of bonds had ignored his needs and suffocated him in a symbiotic and sadistic way. In his mind mother, grandmother and sister seemed fused in one overprotective figure, overpowering, vital, but at the same time a danger to his life. There was no triangulation; the third figure was missing. Harry had no male model and nobody had helped him to cope with his feelings. The short contact with the sensible teacher was too brief to compensate for the lack of a father. His love for animals was based on identification with feeble creatures maliciously killed by strong women. In his nightmares his grandmother appeared gigantic and dressed in black. He saw himself as an immolated rabbit, a coward who was good for nothing. In the fourth year of his analysis Harry started drawing not only drafts for furniture for his profession, but just for himself. Once a female customer bought one of his drawings, he felt proud as if he had earned money for the first time. He devoted more time to his hobby and participated in a course for painting with water-colours in Greece. There he met a woman, with *whom he shared much of his leisure time. What connects them most is a young dog they fetched from a pet-home.*

This analysis showed clearly that even intrusive and burdensome relationships cannot be given up easily, but that similar variations of them are searched, if no other kind of relationship can be imagined. Although analysis often is experienced as overwhelming due to the high frequency of sessions, it can be the only chance to part with unhappy old bonds.

4 Separation and old age

'Death and sun
nobody can consider with a constant eye.'
(Greek sentence[15])

We return now to the point where we began: neither age nor the process of aging can be detached from the atmosphere of death, the final separation from our life. We were confronted with our split relationship regarding death: we know about it, we calculate it, but at the same time we repress and deny it. Age is the time, when death unavoidably nears and our fear of death becomes a more realistic anxiety.

Our everyday language exposes our defences. We say that people, who have passed the middle of their expected life span are "in their best years," We fix the "mid-life crisis" after the 50th year, which would suggest that there is an army of people aged 100, or we mark it earlier in order to make the middle of life time a prolonged season. We call the grave a 'place for rest', sometimes admitting that it is the very last one. We usually notice that others are aging and dying, but not ourselves too. The dead, we hear, are 'going to a better world'. Sometimes the joke is on us. If we avoid speaking of 'old' ladies by calling them 'elder' ladies, this feint actually is not a decrease but an increase.

We are afraid of age not only because of the unavoidable culmination in the final separation of death, but also because of all the losses along the way: the loss of youth, loss of energy, the loss of the capacity for love and for being loved.

How one can be enticed to enter the labyrinth of defences we find, for example, in Thomas Mann's "Death in Venice". The main character Aschenbach watches with a shudder how another traveller garishly dresses in a yellow fashionable suit with red tie and Panama hat, behaving rather strikingly like a doddering adolescent topped by a periwig and coated with make-up. A short time later he himself is seduced by the adulations of a coiffeur, who promises to make up his face to that of a glowing young man and who assures him that now he need not hesitate to fall in love.

Our inclination to go headlong into the trap of such illusions is a boost for the cosmetic industry and cosmetic surgery, going far beyond common sense. We often find a similar adamant denial in fashion. Sometimes it seems that the mirror has not yet been invented, let alone any chance to gaze in a rear mirror. The despair about appearance often seems so great that it is easier to stifle uneasiness and cover it in a general bad mood and partial blindness. Elegance and a certain dignity, however, are expressed in the way one looks – and is never combined with a fundamental denial. Sometimes it is almost a relief to see an older person who is not exhausted from a hopeless fight for youthfulness, but

---

[15] This quotation and some references to the language and literature in this chapter I owe to Dr. Ernst Beer, who many years ago gave a public paper in the Viennese Sigmund Freud Society about the 'Psychology of Age'.

who shows in another way – by care, by a realistic security in style and quality – a sense for aesthetics and serenity of the mind. This self-presentation conveys that the calculable distance from death, so far away in our youth, is not the only value that renders somebody attractive. There are aspects of age, which don't emphasize losses, but the inner richness of experiences and knowledge. There is wisdom of age that consists of innumerable links with what a human being has truly felt and experienced. Such a mind is still open to vibrant contact with the present. Of course, these good qualities cannot be expected as a rule, just as little so as the freshness and beauty attributed to youth. To confirm these two facts it is only necessary to stay for a while where plenty of old people are, and where young people are.

Considering looks, comparing with others plays an all-important role. Ageing is not just an individual process. As soon as one starts to compare, one finds envy, jealousy and greed arise in their destructive ways. Greed, and hostile rivalry ruin the capacity for love and pleasure. Envy is the angry feeling that somebody has and enjoys something desirable, which oneself lacks or cannot enjoy. Jealousy is based on envy but it includes a third person, who has taken away something desirable that one has had or that one should have according to one's own conviction. An important difference between envy and jealousy is the fact that envy intends to destroy the object hatefully while jealousy hates the rival, but can continue to love the desired object. If fear of losing the beloved object supports envy and makes jealousy grow to insatiable greed, the beloved object is destined for destruction, as we see in Shakespeare's Othello. Envy, jealousy and greed are closely linked and play prominent roles in the relations between the older and the younger generations.

4.1 The "duel of age": age and rivalry

> *'When he stood in front of me with his keen, young eye,*
> *I knew in this moment…he or me.'*
> *(Arthur Schnitzler: Das weite Land, 1972, 6th edition, 318)*

In everyday life one sometimes gets the distinct impression that there is far in the background a hidden grid measuring who is older and who is younger and thus further away from the reach of death. Newspapers and journals, for instance, offer the ages of prominent persons, although this might be totally irrelevant in the given context. Many readers might compare their own age with that of the person mentioned, as they look for assurance that they have a better chance to live longer. When we read about people aged 100, it is calming, and even those who died early can induce us to feel secretly triumphant, as if each year one outlasts somebody is a proof that one will not die: 'I have not died for 80 years, so why should it happen the next 80 years?' Other persons who survived heavy misfortune, dangerous activities or cosmetic surgery thereby seem to have guaranteed their immortality. Usually such a "duel of age" – as I call it – functions unconsciously; comparison with others and rivalry plays a main part in it. Envy and competition remain unconscious, and also the aim to overcome fear of death and other narcissistic violations regarding age and transience does not reach consciousness. Sometimes it might be appeasing if somebody's age is mentioned: this person perhaps has achieved a lot but there is no reason for envy, because he or she will die soon. *The age-duel is based on an unconscious screen of envy, checking whether others are in a better position.*

This perpetual comparison stirs endless speculation as to how dying could have been prevented or more exactly how *we* might hope to prevent it. So a surprising sudden death easily can be explained, for instance, because 'he smoked too much'. One immediately knows what somebody else should have done or avoided so that one might escape such a fate. This impulse even makes us ready to take responsibility, because being guilty includes the hope for mending a fault.

In such age-duels the other person also becomes the focus of aggressive fantasies and feelings. The plays of Arthur Schnitzler impressively disclose such tragic psychic processes. There is, above all, the illusion that by destroying the envied object one's own unbearable problems will be solved. But the death of an admirable young man cannot prolong the life of the older man who suffers from envy. That the young one no longer is to be envied is then the only destructive satisfaction. Usually guilt feelings, persecutory anxieties and the fear of revenge and punishment will hinder any satisfaction. The wish to annihilate an envied and hated person is even greater if somebody is extremely greedy due to his own unsatisfied life. Actually one's own life can be devastated by such negative feelings – a vicious circle that is difficult to escape without help. Somebody might like a vampire drain others of their life energy, if they appear more happy than he or she. Ruthless, violent and hostile intrusion into the life of others provokes the hateful reaction outside which is felt inside already for a long time because of internalized bad objects.

Rivalry works not in one direction but both ways. The elder generation often envies youth and all the happiness associated with it while the younger generation begrudges older people their position and real or imagined power.

In fairy tales we offer to children (and ourselves) the chance to discover their (and our) secret desires and forbidden wishes and to work them through on the neutral terrain of 'unreality'. Think of Snow-White: here the conflict between the good figure Little Snow-White and the bad queen is easily solved according to an old recipe: the queen is only the step-mother; the real mother has already died[16]. So it is not the real, without doubt good mother the one, who envies her daughter that she is 1000 times more beautiful and who does not even hesitate to

---

[16] Melanie Klein described the split in good and bad objects. We find such a split elaborated not only in fairy tales, but also in the famous stories of Harry Potter, who became a worldwide success: he, too, lived with silly, bad step-parents, while his own parents were wonderful magicians who unfortunately were killed. (Cf. Zwettler-Otte 2002, 2nd edition: Von Robinson bis Harry Potter, 155-167)

poison the girl! Little Snow-White is saved by Divine Providence, a Father in heaven, who loves the beautiful young girl more than the ageing woman with sagging self-confidence and compulsive need to check her appearance daily in the talking mirror? Psychoanalytic interpretation allows a more sophisticated idea: there are not only bad mothers persecuting beautiful daughters; there are also daughters, who wish to expel mothers whom they experience as ugly and bad, but since such death wishes are forbidden fantasies, they are projected onto the mothers, and so the criminal daughters become poor victims. So this fairy tale might seem simple, but actually is quite complicated, especially if we think of the fact, that Little Snow-White is the reason that her mother died during her birth.

Thus death wishes wander around, and often remain hidden, who is the object of all that deadly rivalry. There are innumerable elaborations of oedipal fights in literature. For instance in Don Carlos by Friedrich Schiller: King Philipp and his son love the same woman; originally the young queen was engaged with Don Carlos, but for political reasons had to marry his father, thus becoming Don Carlos' step-mother. Here to be the stepmother means not devaluation as bad mother, but an excuse for incest. She is only the stepmother. The king must recognize that the love of the young couple continues. In spite of all the confusions of this complicated love story the basic conflict is simple: the father envies the son because of his youth, the son envies the father because of his power. Schiller shows the complexity of these psychic processes by doubling the son with the figure of Carlos's friend Posa, who has won the heart of the queen by his masculine and clever character, thus representing the hidden, longing side of the relationship between father and son. Finally the king finds an excuse for declaring both young men as traitors and killing them. He himself is doubled, too, by the figure of the grand-inquisitor. The deadly paternal power of the old ones triumphs and persists to possess the desired woman. This drama has been successful over several centuries, because it permits expression to feelings, which dominate the rivalry between the elder and the younger generation. The young poet Schiller managed intuitively to comprehend the processes going on in the old men, using the detour of his own fear and aggression regarding the world of the fathers.

However, there are other kinds of relationships between young and old people than pure rivalry. There also are channels for constructive communication. The wish for immortality might turn not only to religion or to the care for one's own children; it might also search for satisfaction in devoting oneself to cooperation with the next generation. Based on an intrapsychic process we remain in some way alive and effective in the inner world of those who go on living, sometimes even longer than one generation. There is no doubt that this wish is involved in our creativity.

4.2   The threat of separation due to old age

Increasing age means an increase of separations – separation from the old parents, from the growing children, from the familiar work environment, from dying friends, partners and acquaintances. This process also has meaning for young people who might see more clearly than the elderly themselves that the latter are left alone and that they are in danger of extinction. This provokes fear and eventually guilt, if it is linked with hostile wishes. These reactions to confrontation with old people, for instance with parents, might be to a large extent unconscious or at least far from awareness. Nevertheless, they contribute to the difficulties of care for old people during the last years of life. Often grown-up children neither are able nor want to recognize that roles have switched and that now the parents are the ones for whom the children should care. The parents, however, often deny that they are no longer capable of living independently. Then the children may insist blindly that the parents go on indulging them, at least by providing an inheritance. The aggression and destructiveness connected with such an attitude cannot be ignored. Rolf D. Hirsch (in: Radebold, 1997, 103) points out that often it is a justified reaction if old people resist when challenged by the young people to be wise, ideal and ready to make sacrifices, for instance, taking care of the grandchildren. They might feel the greedy, angry or ruthless character of such demands, often underlined with a subtle reproach that they themselves never got enough from the parents or not in the right way. The sense that the parents will die soon is experienced as a threat to be left alone totally and finally. Sometimes not fear but anger might dominate; then even the death of the parents seems impudence, as if it was a malicious action done willingly in order to withdraw from obligations. The parents seemingly desert the child, not: the child might wish to let the parents down, because there is no chance anymore that they will be or become the good parents one would have needed. Often it is about 'unsettled bills', as already mentioned and as will also be an issue in chapter 4.6. Such bills are characterized by a discrepancy between the claims and the real possibilities. One can establish a sadomasochistic relationship if one persistently addresses angry demands to somebody who is incapable or unwilling to meet these claims, whether parent, a partner, fate or a heavenly power. The unconscious aim of such a behaviour can be a perverse pleasure to torture or/and to be tortured.
There is another menace: parents who become weak and frail, and all their substitutes in everyday life remind us of our own death we shall not be able to escape. Thus old people become a 'memento mori' one wishes to reject; to isolate them often seems to be the only way out. The unbearable sight of parents wasting away causes a most painful break-down of the infantile fantasies of omnipotent, kind and loving parents, the idealizations can no longer be sustained and fall, and the intolerable discrepancy between our longing and reality often leads to a flight. Sometimes weak parents might reactivate guilt feelings because of infantile death wishes, as if they would become now virulent after so many

years of delay with a magic power. Also such fantasies colour the ageing of parents in a threatening way and might suggest taking a flight.

We can imagine, how badly all persons involved in such a situation will feel, if the parents' fear of the physical decay is stressed by the psychic pain of being left alone by the children who want to flee; thus fear of annihilation might turn into fear of death. (Eissler, 1997, 201)

P. Kutter (in: Radebold, 1997, 54 ff.) described in detail, how the self-confidence is attacked by the vanishing strength of the body, the loss of an attractive look, the reduced capacity for competition, the feeling to have failed in relationships and the increasing dependence. The narcissistic violations become more and more, and the necessity to renounce grows.

It is evident that most of the problems, which might culminate in the last section of life, are not at all new: who could not deal with physical problems until now, usually is even more incapable to do so in age; who had difficulties in making contact, becomes even more lonely in his late years; who suffered until now from rivalry, will hardly tolerate to see younger people with less problems. In some people the profusion of narcissistic violations provokes impotent rage, they seem to clench their fists against the youth and emphasize their threat of separation with bad wishes: the world should sink together with them – a desperate, hateful, measureless overestimation of oneself.

A patient was extremely concerned by his father's feeling of impotence. The old man had a very successful life; now he was paralyzed, and could not cope with this awful change. His son had the idea that it would be necessary to introduce a very low limit of age for all politicians and powerful people in the world. He was convinced that otherwise mighty old persons would have no other wish than to tear all people with them into death by nuclear wars and mass-annihilation, as soon as they notice their own decay. The contrast between the idealized strong father and the helpless father made his fall from Olympic height appear even more tragic. At the same time the son saved his father's strength by drawing a terrible picture of him as somebody who is capable of destroying the world. In analysis it was possible to see the infantile roots of this ambivalent fantasy, which was mixed up with idealization, fear and guilt.

It is not always that such a horror scenario is constituted by the imminent death of old people. It happens that the announcements of the final parting are coming not as a wild menace, but as a soft-melancholic melody of separation. Such a tender reminder of transience might also include gratitude for all that one got from this person and a revalorization of all good experiences one could share. Then the wish to make the final period of this old person as comfortable and satisfying as possible will arise on its own. A conciliatory way of parting does not necessarily depend on an especially good relationship. There is the chance that somebody mourns what he has not got and also will not get, and this might give him the strength to renounce. This can be true for old people, who will not see all their wishes fulfilled in their children, as well as for their children.

A very famous psychoanalyst, who was more than 80 years old, took so much advantage of her life and her work, that she overcame also the hurdles of age with an unbelievable pleasure. She never saw any narcissistic violations, instead she reported with a feeling of triumph, how she took the sting out of this or that physical problem. She was perfectly equipped with technical aids like magnifying glasses and planned journeys with persons she liked, whom she paid the travel costs and who took care of her. It was, as if all her small and great diseases had nothing to do with her, but all the successes she made were hers; she fought against age like against an external enemy. She neither threatened her environment with separation nor did she deny it. So she organized, for instance, with which preface her publications should be published, if she was still alive, and with which preface, if this would unfortunately not be the case. Probably her creativity is her greatest support, and it guarantees her in some way that she will survive her death. For dealing so luckily with age seems to be decisive to have also such a highly developed sense of reality that allows to intend what is possible and to enjoy the achievements with pleasure.

The house of cards

For those contented ageing people who allow neither themselves nor others too dwell on feelings about approaching death, because the bond to life is stronger, the last period of life becomes a narcissistic reward, not a violation. They skilfully build their house of cards higher and higher, knowing very well it will collapse sooner or later. In fact, that they perhaps one day will wish that it does tumble down - we are reminded of the 'pleasure of extinction'. The stability of the house of cards depends on many factors: the broad base often was established by a happy childhood, but often also by a successful reparation (psychotherapy) and development of individual strength. Of course, this house of cards can be loaded less and less, the higher it grows. At the top the emotional distance from others becomes greater and greater. Nevertheless, it will not likely collapse without our final and unavoidable agreement.

There is the danger that a person becomes frightened and angry when the house of cards starts rocking, and that he prefers to destroy it quickly himself in order to sustain the illusion of omnipotence and control. But it usually seems much more desirable to concentrate on accepting reality as calmly as possible, of adapting to given circumstances in the most clever way and of keeping balance and enjoying it as long as possible. Such an attitude might also engage the younger people; they then hardly will interpret the looming separation as a malicious act of revenge, if there is so much serenity of mind, partly accepting the necessity of departing, partly ignoring it without denial.

4.3 Age – feelings of shame and guilt

One's own age usually is not seen very clearly, but is rather hazy and riddled with blind spots. We can recognize this when, for instance, old people complain that certain clothes make them look old – as if they were not old. Or say that they don't want to join those 'old people' who actually are the same age. The process of ageing will be viewed with even greater disapproval in others if it is unbearable to see in ourselves, and some cannot dissociate themselves far enough from it.

What we perceive as a result of our defences is just one side of the matter. The other side is that there always remains at least a notion of what it is that is being blurred. Sometimes signs of ageing make the melody of separation appear menacing, so that it becomes nagging background music one cannot ignore. For this dissonance old people sometimes feel guilt. The cosmetic appearance, which tries inadequately to conceal age, and the age itself, become a topic of shame, connected with a feeling of impotence.

The ability to hide wrinkles with make-up has limits, so for some women each glance in the mirror becomes a new narcissistic violation. Daily the bitter insight is acknowledged that the increase of cosmetic labour combines with a decrease of results regarding beauty. It is not only women who are concerned with these problems; some men look daily in the shaving-mirror with increasing reluctance or hate their toupee because of its unreliable grip. Actually all these problems are never the reasons, just the occasions of pain.

Shame and impotence refer to secret fears that one might already be inadequate as a love object. But the diminishing chance of putting aggressive impulses into action can cause feelings of shame, helplessness and rage. Often the shattering experience of loss concerns both at the same time, libidinal and aggressive wishes. So the loss of one's teeth has the meaning of no longer being capable of biting and defending oneself nor of seducing somebody by being attractive.

However it is strikingly clear that some people suffer a lot from ageing and others don't. Again it is evident that in ageing, problems come out more clearly, but they are not at all new.

Sonja was an analysand of about 60. She could not cope with her dental substitute and was ashamed to need it relatively early. She was especially unhappy because her pronunciation had been changed by the dental substitute. She was convinced she now had a terrible lisp. Slowly it became apparent in therapy that this was just the final link in a long chain of physical shortcomings, which troubled her. In kindergarten she had been embarrassed that she had to wear insoles and high shoes instead of sandals. In school she had to wear glasses and was called "cobra". Some years later a dentist fitted her with braces, which made her feel like Dracula. After a period of quick growth an orthopaedic doctor insisted that she wear a gypsum bodice. But her adolescent resistance was already so strong that finally a compromise was achieved: she wore the bodice only during night. When she went for the first time to a gynaecologist, she was upset because the doctor mentioned she had large labia of the vulva. She once had read that primitive tribeswomen had large labia. Her fight for a boyish-slim figure lasted decades, and since she did not succeed, she hid her body under large clothes. This problem escalated during her midlife-crisis, because her breasts became bigger too. And now she felt so tortured by her dental substitute that she could not enjoy anything: it was for her an abiding reminder of final decay. When memories of her braces arose, she laughed: "So I have already been in the same trap as now!" In puberty she also believed that nobody would like her because of her teeth, especially not the attractive boy in her class, whom she adored secretly. Actually the young man was not yet interested in girls and still preferred to stick with other boys.

Sonja's feelings of shame easily turned into guilt. Her need for insoles proved her inability to stand her ground. Her glasses were an inheritance of her father; they represented a forbidden link to him and she felt that her mother teased her because of this. Her braces were a punishment for her caustic remarks against her mother. The bodice was punishment for her haughty bearing. Sometimes she appeared arrogant when she actually was afraid of making contact. The great labia revealed her masturbation and were according to her fears the awkward proof that she was not the boy the parents would have preferred. Her big breasts, which her friends had admired, reminded her of her early decision that they were "unnecessary", since she had no children; they represented her "unlived life", of which she was deeply ashamed.

This self-representation in no way matched the impression that other people had of Sonja. They saw her as, if a bit reserved, an attractive and successful woman devoted to her academic profession and widely acknowledged by colleagues. It is no surprise that the discrepancy between her view and that of the others did not facilitate contact: Sonja always tried to withdraw before somebody might come closer to her and discover all her physical "shortcomings", which without doubt would lead to a rejection, as she believed. In order to avoid painful experiences she had steered clear of many bonds. That this attitude improved during her analysis seemed to her to be a wonderful development that she had not expected due to her age.

4.4 The irrational Crescendo of hope

> *"As it was a clear evening I got to Stonehenge and saw it by moonlight,*
> *I was alone and tremendously impressed. (Moonlight, as you know,*
> *enlarges everything, and the mysterious depths*
> *and distances made it seem enormous.)"*
> *(Henry Moore, 1921, 117)*

As the previous case vignette shows, one can try to suppress hope regarding the future fulfilment of desires, but this does not work. On the contrary, the smaller the probability of its realization becomes, the more hope increases. This inner economy seems to stem from the unconscious mechanism of the superego to allow more pleasure if reality itself restricts fulfilment of wishes. Of course this mechanism does not liquidate desires. "Dum spiro, spero – As long as I live, I hope" is a Latin proverb. In our inner world often the pleasure-principle prevails over reality.

With the discovery of the *pleasure-unpleasure-principle,* commonly called the *pleasure-principle,* Freud found the centre of regulation, of how our psyche functions. This principle says that all psychic activity searches for pleasure and avoids unpleasure. This rule sounds so simple that it appears banal but it is merely the base of a highly complex and difficult process incorporating a lot of conflicts. Most of the time we only observe the movements of the waves on the surface; the tempestuous struggles of the pleasure-principle are fought in the depths of our unconscious psychic life. This goes on where we repress what seems unbearable, and the act of repression itself is banished from conscious awareness. But there is a way to reconstruct these processes by the laborious work of excavation, which psychoanalysis pursues.

There we discover our incredible skill in *not* seeing what we actually do see. Already the Roman poet Catullus, who was unhappy in love, reproved himself for looking away from the infidelity of his beloved Lesbia, and angrily demanded of himself: "...et quod *vides* perisse perditum *ducas* – and *realize* that is lost, what you *see* to be lost (Carmen 8)." One feels the recurring disappointments that he could have been spared had he – damn it – been ready to accept that this woman never will be faithful. However, the wish to believe in her love was stronger. Did Catullus really want to accept reality and to renounce pleasure? Did the pleasure-principle fail? Not really, because the pain and unpleasure were greater than the pleasure. He wanted to stop this unhappy liaison, which caused him so much frustration. Then he might become free for another bond, which perhaps might be happier. Thus the idea was to avoid pain and to look for pleasure elsewhere, respecting reality and acknowledging the fact that Lesbia was incapable of faith. To introduce such reality, as we perceive it, into our desires is a mature psychic achievement; in psychoanalysis it is called "reality-principle" which is connected with the pleasure-principle and actually does nothing but protect the pleasure-principle and aid it in finding realistic ways of attainment.

However, another difficulty arises with the reality-principle. We can perceive reality only with our own eyes, which give us a picture of the "objective"[17] external facts from our individual point of view, which is coined by subjective experiences. This makes us highly sensitive to some events and "blind" to others, especially of what we unconsciously repress. Of course, this belongs to reality, our *inner reality,* which plays a role in working through the external reality.

---

[17] Cf. Zwettler-Otte, 2002.

There is a realm where we are less bound to the reality-principle than in everyday-life: it is the fantasy which Freud called "the reservation" of our soul. There the pleasure-principle reigns with omnipotence; there our wishes are free to unfold, and our striving for pleasure is less inhibited, and even prohibited wishes can be fulfilled in fantasy without being punished.

Often there is an abyss between reality and desire, and sometimes we do not even notice because as soon as we admit this split it becomes painful, and we might have to renounce the hope for pleasure. On the other hand, a skilful fusion of realistic and fantasy-loaded contents often makes the fulfilment of wishes appear so plausible that it is highly enjoyable. Some bestsellers like "Harry Potter" thereby thrive.

I illustrate the superiority of the pleasure-principle by the following case:

A lady asked for an appointment for a consultation. I realized from her voice at the phone that she was an older woman. She seemed quite active and decisive without being demanding. The first impression when I saw her 10 days later completed this picture; she was well-groomed, probably about 70 years old, elegantly dressed, with a very lively face and attentive eyes. She made herself comfortable in the armchair before me. I was curious what she wanted from me as psychoanalyst. She hesitated and then told me that a heart-specialist advised her to undergo bypass-operation, but she felt uncertain about doing so. Should she try to overcome her anxieties or should she take them as a sound warning. She asked me whether I would do anxiety-strategy-exercises with her; she had read about them. I answered, that we could try together to understand, what she meant with "her anxieties." A behaviour-therapist would perhaps assign exercise anxiety-strategies regarding the operation. She considered the matter and then decided to undergo regular sessions with me.

Martha gave me a thoughtful survey of her life. She has grown up in a small city. As a single child she was "a bit too much protected", she said. Her father worked in the municipality, her mother sometimes helped in the kindergarten. She was a "woman of enterprise", and Martha emulated this. Her father was a quiet man, but she still recalled his face was radiant with joy when she approached him. With a boy friend she planned to go to a foreign country after finishing school, but the relationship did not last. He got a good job here. She was disappointed and stubborn, but ultimately reasonable. She went for a year to England to work as an au-pair-girl. Back in Austria she found a job as a secretary in Vienna. After a few superficial contacts with young men she soon met a law student with whom she fell in love. They married, and when their son was born, she interrupted her work for several years to devote herself totally to the beloved child. The wish for a second child failed, and they gave it up after two miscarriages. Martha described her marriage as "happy enough", although she sometimes questioned whether there is an even greater happiness. At this point her narrative stopped for a moment, until she hesitantly said. "Somehow I still think of this question." She seemed ashamed, that she still, at age 70, had romantic fantasies and desires. It was touching. I remained silent to give her space for this feeling that she missed something she was longing for since such a long time. There was the rational knowledge that she was an old lady and would live perhaps 10 or 15 years, maybe much less. And still there was the yearning for a relationship full of love and happiness, as strong as in her youth. Reality might allow little chances for the fulfilment of her wishes, but something in her pushed her to expect something essential in her life: there were no clear, concrete ideas, but she clung to the vague contours of some great fulfilment.

Martha changed the topic. Her husband had a difficult professional life, he was not so good in fighting. But they both loved their son. It was their greatest pleasure to see him grow. It was, as if raising him was easy, in spite of their diligent efforts to meet all his needs. Only the times, when he suffered from the usual childhood diseases were a bit stressed. Later on, when he was an adolescent, there were struggles with the father, whom he now seemed to despise. But this phase passed when he himself studied law. Suddenly she had tears in her eyes and she told me about the fatal car-accident of her son, for which he was not responsible. Her husband survived this heavy blow less than a year and died of heart failure, and she herself hardly could cope with these incomprehensible losses. The family doctor no longer wished to give her tranquilizers and instead sent her to a psychologist. With his help she gradually became capable of mourning her son and her husband. It had taken a very long time, but then her will to live returned. She started again to care for her appearance, mainly when she had a session with her psychotherapist. This concerned her a bit, although her hopes or wishes remained blurred. However, she had to realize that in spite of the fact that she was 60 years old and in spite of all realistic expectations, she was hoping for something new that would fulfil her totally, maybe even more than all she had experienced till now. In therapy she herself called her vague hope a 'paradox.' She disapproved of it and tried in vain to find out whether the psychologist agreed. He only encouraged her to follow her inclinations and do whatever she liked, but she experienced his encouragement as rejection, and during a long summer break she decided to end therapy and to make a journey. She travelled to London and made many excursions from there. When she looked at the enormous monuments of Stonehenge, she felt that her desires too were immortal; not just her vague desires for happiness and pleasure seemed endless but also those of all human beings. Being in the dusk of her life, everything appeared bigger, stronger, more primitive and elementary. 'No surprise, that our imagination tries to stretch into eternity', she thought, and she envied those who were religious. She recalled a friend who had lost both breasts and uterus due to her cancer, and when further metastases were found, she had said with a strange, peaceful smile: 'I feel I am coming home.' Martha had not dared to ask whether she was thinking of her parents who had died long ago, or of religious ideas. However, she understood that the longing of the dying woman transgressed the end of her life and projected great shadows into the width of heaven. This day Martha managed to *return, after the flood of tourists receded, to the prehistoric temple of Stonehenge and contemplated this until it became dark. Her thoughts also wandered back to her father. She had been shocked by his death, which she had experienced as a scary release, a sudden vanishing of his will to live. What hurt her deeply was that he let her go, too. She felt the contradiction of two truths: the seemingly endless striving for pleasure, and the cessation of this striving in dying.*

Whatever dissolved in her after this event, she felt much better. She reorganized her life, worked in a library, enjoyed the contacts there and reactivated former friendships and acquaintances. What disturbed her during the last year was not only the weakening of her heart, but how she experienced the examinations and conversations with her cardiologist. When he examined her heart with the stethoscope, his big serious face was so near to her, and this closeness - she felt - made her heart beat quicker. She considered her reaction to be impertinent and hid it, but at the same time she did not want to restrict her desire for closeness. That was her unconscious conflict, which paralyzed her decision regarding the operation and made her state of health appear even more dangerous than it actually was.

Finally she agreed to the operation. In a session before she went to the hospital she asked me with an evident fear of my rejection, whether I would take her in analysis in spite of her age. She understood my answer that of course we would not be able to restore her previous life, but analysis might help her to see and comprehend it in a new light.

During her recovery she rang me and we arranged dates for her analysis. We worked four times a week over several years. She tried to find her encouraging mother in me. As a child she clung to her when she was frightened by her depressive father, which impaired her own will to live. Unconsciously she had chosen later on her partners according to him as a prototype. Thus she tried to find a new edition of her first love to a man, but hoping for greater liveliness than she had seen in her father. She also transferred to her partner the feeling that it was a forbidden, incestuous love wishing to supplant her mother, and this reduced her pleasure and provided just a "happy enough" relationship to the men who followed her father. After the losses of her son and husband, and the difficult process of mourning, she again fell in love with an unreachable love object, the psychotherapist, who either did not recognize the rising hopes of the older patient or tried to use only constructive aspects of her attachment for the therapeutic work. However, it could not become clarified and worked through, that Martha unconsciously repeated the oedipal pattern in transference love to the psychotherapist, and she broke off the therapy. In her analysis she succeeded in accepting that her search for "happiness" would last as long as she would live, disregarding how likely the realization would be. One might speak of a limited success of treatment because she achieved a greater pleasure for life and capacity for bonding only, as the real threat of the end of life neared. But this was due to the late start of her analysis. It doubtless helped her because Martha could enjoy her last period of life, which lasted another 17 years, with a wise mind mellowed by experience.

Sometimes *the pleasure-principle disconnects itself from the reality-principle in order to survive.* Supported by the usual denial "One is as old as one feels to be" we often manage to mobilize wishful thinking in our inner reality and ignore the objective reality. Then hope rises all the more, the smaller the chances for realization become – it is an *irrational crescendo of hope.* It is exactly this condition that makes the desire appear even greater and more elementary. *The seductive charm of what is impossible seems to be as great as the seductive charm of what is forbidden.*

Martha used what she experienced in analysis to understand herself better. She became calm and developed a way of being present and alive. It was, as if she had become now in old age finally able to enjoy her life fully. When she was 80 years old, she moved in a residency for old people on the countryside, a region she loved since childhood. At Christmas she usually sent me a card. She wrote about a close relationship to a widower of her age and her cordial relationship to his grown-up children whom she felt were like a new family. Her last Christmas-card was written with a trembling hand; she was now 87 years old. She closed with the following sentence: "I think I never was so fine like now. Maybe I only now enjoy every day, every contact so much, not although, but because it is too late…"

4.5 "Without net"

Our knowledge of transience is split into acknowledgement and denial. This balance oscillates in older age and the awareness of reality that our life is limited and can end any moment, might become overwhelming. It can be disturbing if somebody of the same age or younger dies or if we lose our parents and realize that we might be next. The denial of death is weakened by such identifications with those who died. The shock can be even greater if preceding denial was extremely strong.

Sometimes just a glance in the mirror triggers a breakdown of repression. Such a shift of the psychic balance is called in German 'midlife crisis,' but this shift into a foreign language should be reason enough to be wary. It really is about separation-anxiety, or more concretely, about fear of death and the fear of loss of the pleasures of life and persons we love too. It is not the middle of the life that is feared but its end. With the term 'midlife-crisis' we have already manufactured a delay and a compromise. We acknowledge the termination, but claim that we have reached only the middle of our life-span, still being far enough away from the end.

There is no doubt that clear moments of recognition of mortality can turn up early in life, even childhood, but it happens more often later in life due to the tenacity of reality.

A severe disease can bring the end of life to the fore in such an undeniable way that it shatters and moves us most deeply. Probably all of us know such a moment in the realm of art. The desperate cry of Violetta in Verdi's opera La Traviata: "È tardi!" – "It is too late!" – exactly at the moment, when her lover returned and the fulfilment of her love-wishes and the acknowledgement of their love would become possible. Here the melody of separation – like her life itself – is interrupted by the unbearable pain of separation.

We have seen a version of such a balancing between internal and external reality in the previous case-history. There hope escalated in a crescendo, as age reduced the possibility of fulfilment of the desire, which had been inhibited by an inner prohibition of oedipal wishes. Analysis helped. The pleasure-principle did not totally break down; instead the old balance was restored, and with even greater latitude.

There not only are great oscillations between the prohibition of wish-fulfilments and the allowance of wishes that no longer can become fulfilled in reality. Small fluctuations, hardly noticed, also show that we sometimes are able to desire something only if it is absent and unavailable. (See Chapter 2) These are compromises between pleasure and unpleasure, between instinctual wishes and prohibitions of the superego.

The tendency to keep a balance can start a fresh dynamic. If something is in danger of being lost, it can provoke strong counter-movements. To become aware that soon it will be too late to realize some plans can be shocking and might push somebody out of his daydreams. This might cause a new upturn and a recollection of forces. This can be a breakthrough of long delayed wishes due to the clear awareness: "Now or never!"

An example of such a development is a 50 years old woman, who decided to enter analysis when her partner, with whom she had lived 20 years, suddenly left her.

Marion was desperate. She was in no way prepared for the separation, although she had lived with Peter in a permanent power-struggle. They had never been, what usually is called "happy". This was also the reason why they never decided to make their relationship legal and why they had not planned to have children. About this they reproached to each other again and again in the last years. And now Peter had fallen in love with a much younger colleague, who was pregnant with his child. He left Marion after torturous discussions. "And this just now, after I have quit my job in school and wanted to devote myself totally to painting", she wept. It was not difficult to hear, that her main trouble was not sadness about the loss of the partner but her rage that the separation was none of her doing or at least a common decision. And she suffered from the narcissistic threat that she might fail in a career as an artist. She had hesitated a long time before giving up work as a teacher and now, alone, she felt forced to change her plans again. She probably would not be able to afford the big flat alone, especially if she needed money for analysis. (This was the first hint at the aggression she now directed against me. She needed me as an object that would survive her attacks.) She started to identify with me: she had already thought of studying psychology because she was touched by what she learned about Freud, about parapraxes in everyday life, the interpretation of dreams and the latent meaning of great art. But since she did not want to study medicine and since she was told that as a psychologist she would remain at the bottom of the hierarchy of psychoanalysts, she preferred to study Art and History. She had planned to devote herself to painting apart from the "half-day-job" at school. Until now she had shown in exhibitions, but she could not have one of her own. At school she was well liked by pupils, but had difficulties with the director, whose bureaucratic ambitions she neither shared nor supported. Thus her profession became more troublesome. In her view this was the main reason why she hadn't enough strength to live as an artist. Some months ago the problems at school had escalated because the schedule of the next years gave her even less elbowroom, and so she had decided to quit. There was a secret reproach she had made to Peter: he shared all costs for living with her, but he never encouraged her to establish her work as an artist or offered his financial help. She felt that it was not her fault, but that of her school and of Peter that she was not yet a well known artist. And now she considered also me guilty, because I charged a normal fee and did not make reductions, as for instance for students.

Analysis lasted quite a long time, until behind all the rage painful questions emerged: was she gifted enough anyway to earn her livings with painting? Why did she remain two decades in this relationship with Peter if there was really so little satisfaction? Behind the wall of reproaches to her environment there were plenty of doubts regarding herself, leading back into her childhood and echoing in the therapeutic situation. Just as in childhood, she felt totally disliked here and yet incapable of leaving. With her partner she had repeated this dilemma; at the same time there was a sadomasochistic pleasure, a perverse satisfaction to stick to a deep hopelessness. All her aggressions served the purpose of defending her depression and her despair that she met neither the wishes of her mother nor the expectations of her father. She felt that this was the reason why both had turned from her with disappointment. And she was quite sure that the same would happen if she exposed herself via her paintings in a single exhibition. But her sadness, which she experienced as her innermost core, was also a link to her depressive mother, who in her memories consisted only of diseases and fears. Only when Marion pretended to be helpless at learning did she get attention from both parents. She believed her father actually never had wanted to have children because he was so overworked. This his mother, her grandmother, once mentioned. It offended her deeply because she had been so happy with her father, for instance, if he – seldom enough! – went swimming or bicycling with her. One of her happiest memories concerned an event on the Old Danube: her father and she had rented a canoe and decided to rescue a bee, which was helplessly drifting on the water. The rescue was successful. The symbolic meaning of this memory slowly became visible: her father had remarked when she entered the boat, that she looked smart in her narrow red swimsuit - a compliment, which was rather unusual and grew in her mind to a sign of love. But her happiness was impaired by her guilt feelings that she was glad that her mother stayed home because of flu. Anyway, this time there was a solution: a wonderful compromise, connecting herself with her father by an acceptable action. They rescued the struggling "bee" representing the mother who was crying for help. Thus Marion could do both: repair the endangered relationship to her mother and reinforce closeness to her father.

Most of the time Marion seemed dissatisfied with me. She had expected comfort and encouragement, and above all, I should facilitate the breakthrough of her talent or confront her with the need to give up. Before and after holidays her complaints usually increased, as if she had to prove to me and to herself that I was useless. Thus she coped with interruptions in therapy: one cannot miss somebody so much, who is worthless. It was during a summer break that Marion decided to make important changes in her life. I should not believe that she would have needed me to do it. Some time later she told me that she had kept a diary, imagining that this hour was her session with me so she somehow had my help without me being aware. With the support of a friend she had found a small charming flat. She could go from the flat up winding stairs to the attic, and there she had a little studio. For the first time she shaped a home that provided space for her artistic work.

Slowly she recognized that she had to disparage me and our work, because she was tremendously afraid to lose me. If I knew how much she needed me, I might withdraw like her mother always did. She had to criticize me, so that I would not dare to leave her alone with so many problems unsolved. In a similar way she had obstructed any change in her relationship to Peter. Unconsciously she had made herself helpless in order not to lose him. Separation-anxiety covered her hidden wish for separation, paralyzing her totally over long periods. Now she had to manage her life alone – apart from me as her analyst. This gave her the feeling of having to perform "the most difficult trapeze-actions". This image derived from one of her dreams. The issue was her fear of taking any new step, but it also showed clearly her pleasure in enterprises she had not dared until now. Independence for her still meant a danger of losing all attachments, but at the same time her pleasure in her strength and creativity increased. For some time it seemed necessary that she felt the peril of not being capable of surviving alone. However, soon she recognized that she needed inner free space for her painting. She called 19 publishing houses, until she got an offer and a contract for illustrating children books. Thus she could paint according to her own schedule and earn her living. One and a half year later she had her first single exhibition and hardly could grasp her luck.

The first picture she painted in her new little attic-studio had the title: "Without a Net". She described it to me as a blurred figure on a trapeze looking down in the dark emptiness while the eye of the observer was attracted by a bright trapeze on the opposite side. To that side the figure should jump instead of scanning the black abyss for a net. In the background was a great sand-glass, in which two thirds already had sunk down through the narrow waist of the glass: the life-time is shortened, and so the pressure increased to form a life according one's own design. This is no longer the task for others who should catch her, hold her or guide her, it is her own. There will not be another chance, if she fails. It is jumping without a net. The separation from her partner, from her previous profession and from her inner attitude is not only important for her career as an artist, she has also to develop the capacity to be alone in order to take up new and more mature relationships – a new hold, to which she perhaps will no longer have to clasp with such a blind, desperate and angrily demanding exclusivity.

Marion's analysis already has made great progress. The picture "Without a Net" was bought at her exhibition but she wants to keep it because she loves it as a reminder of her breakthrough. The legal counsellor, whom she asked for advice, seems not only to understand her wish, but also seemed to be interested in her.

4.6   Looking young – a pleasant psychosomatic symptom

Our physical appearance depends to a large degree on what occurs in our inner world. Charles Darwin in 1872 published his thoughts about "the bodily expression of psychic movements', which he had elaborated over three decades with reference to many publications about this topic. What he had discovered ranged over six fields: the expressions of children; of mad people; of people whose face muscles became galvanized; of representations in paintings and sculptures; of different human races, and of domestic animals. Darwin emphasized that expression cannot be related only to what we want to show willingly or instinctively.
Darwin quotes Shakespeare to demonstrate, that even to simulate a movement of the mind causes a soft excitement in our soul:

"Is it not monstrous that this player here,
But in a fiction, in a dream of passion,
Could force his soul so to his own conceit
That from her working all his visage wan'd;
Tears in his eyes, distraction in's aspect,
A broken voice, and his whole function suiting
With forms to his conceit? And all for nothing!"
(Shakespeare, Hamlet, Act II, Scene II)

This phenomenon that took Shakespeare by surprise we can certainly understand from a psychoanalytic point of view. However, we would not speak of simulation but rather of identification with the figure the actor is representing. He puts himself in the place of that figure through empathy; he 'cathects' with psychic energy - his libido - the psychic processes in which the figures, guided by the poet, invest their libido. Usually it is – similar to actions in fantasy - a 'cathexis' with smaller quantities than would be the case in a real experience yet great enough to produce physical impact. Sometimes the cathexis is not small because on the firm ground of the stage-boards, which represent the world there is less need to repress painful feelings. Some actors can allow themselves to feel more on stage than in their private life. The certainty that they can switch off after two or three hours facilitates a lot of freed-up feeling. Often, for some time afterwards, an emptiness follows that gets filled slowly with rather shallow feelings.

Once an actor asked me to help him to acquire a better understanding of a difficult role. We found that there were roles with which he easily identified due to similarities to his personal experiences; and then there were other roles, which provoked in him very ambivalent feelings: deep reluctance on one side, strange attraction on the other side. If he succeeded in working through at least to some extent what he had to defend in approaching any of these difficult roles, he became brilliant.

What we feel is mirrored in our appearance and bodily expression, regardless whether an emotion is experienced briefly or whether it is a persistent mood. Whether these feelings are conscious or unconscious does not matter very much, though, at any rate, the latter seem to exert more effect.
Darwin wrote that involuntary and unconscious psychic impulses also are expressed, and he saw why feelings get reflected in our expression. Face and body send information to the environment, which is important for our wellbeing. (Darwin, 1986, 374) If we manage to elicit empathy in another person, our suffering is soothed and our joy is multiplied. Our expressions reveal our thoughts and intentions more truly than words, which can always be deceitful, as Darwin pointed out. Thus it was already known in his era that facial and bodily expression is a signal, communiqué, to our environment.

After one and a half centuries we know much more about the extent of our unconscious psychic life and its effects. We know that such signalling is more effective if it derives from unconscious intention. Thus the other person does not feel manipulated. It also is clear that feelings that are repressed and not put into action search for other forms of expression. Sometimes they find no other way out than to go inside and reshape the body.
One of the consequences may be an infantile appearance that originates from a fixation in an infantile world and a childlike way of experiencing life. This might look like infantilism, or it might produce a lucky mixture of youth and adaption in adult life. In the first case the person appears infantile in a negative way; in the second case, a 'juvenile charm' is attributed to that person. In our society a youthful appearance is highly valued. One reason is that looking young

is a counter-trend to the threat of separation due to old age. A person who looks young is not likely to disappear, but rather seems to promise immortality. What a comfort for separation-anxieties! Just as the feeling for beauty also contains the possibility of its destruction (Meltzer, 1988, 6), the taste for youth comprehends (and controls) the idea of its opposite, the idea of its loss. The more weight lies on youth, the more certain seems the distance to the end of life.

Thus it can happen that juvenile appearance is highly esteemed, even if it is caused by psychic immaturity. It depends a lot on the dosage of childishness. In a low dose it can convey freshness, but if it dominates and is in contrast to the reality of the whole appearance, it can create a scurrile and somehow uncanny image. For instance a film actress, who played charming girl figures, might later on have difficulties letting these roles go in her professional as well as in her private life. It can reveal in a shocking way her inner stagnation. Sometimes the horror of such discrepancies between the real age and the false impression becomes a topic for jokes, as for instance:
"From behind: Lycée,
From the front: oh je!"
The infantile nucleus lies not always in appearance; it can also be expressed by the voice, which can sound like that of a whiny child, contrasting with the whole person and possibly hinting at an infantile fixation.
In these striking disharmonies of appearance, the bodily connections with early phases of life are without doubt a disadvantage. It is too obvious that there an emergency-brake has been pulled in the development.
It seems more often that there is a balance between being rooted in an infantile inner world and adaption to the mature age. The result might be pleasant: a juvenile, fresh look, not at all in a grotesque contrast to reality, but still in accordance. It can be a fluid balance, and sometimes there are just moments that let appear a face childlike or flash up juvenile features. They might provoke thoughts like: "This woman must have been once a beautiful girl" or: "That man still has a smile like a boy."
Keeping contact with our early years is a trait that belongs to the plasticity that fosters psychic health. Only a rigid exclusive fixation on early ways of experiencing, and on unconscious conflicts that cannot be mastered, render a pleasant bodily effect of psychic life into a psychosomatic symptom.

In the process of ageing there seems to exist a psychic current flowing back and reactivating whatever was important to us at the beginning. Early memories seem to be more easily available. A male patient, age 48, was teased during his academic career because of his boyish appearance. In a session he said with a smile: "Now it's time that we solve my stagnation in development, because if my psychic retardation will meet with infantilism of higher age, it might be an unsolvable intensification like that of a adhesive substance with two components."

4.7 Pleasure in old age

> *"She went slowly and kept her eyes on the ground.*
> *She looked in the old border beds and among the grass,*
> *and after she had gone round, trying to miss nothing,*
> *she had found ever so many more sharp, pale green points,*
> *and she became quite excited again.*
> *'It is not a quite dead garden' she cried out softly to herself.*
> *'Even if the roses are dead,*
> *There are other things alive.' "*
> *(Kellaway, 1996, 4)*

When we consider old age we mostly dread the threat of loss of pleasure: the possibilities of pleasant satisfaction change and are reduced, and they seem to vanish slowly but surely. Unpleasant prospects dominate the field.

Recapping and completing what we have started to elaborate in the second chapter we can sum up that *there is no psychic activity without a tendency either to search for pleasure or to avoid unpleasure.* The search for pleasure emphasises the final aspect, the avoidance of unpleasure focuses the causal aspect. Both aspects concern the same principle of psychic processes. Freud named this principle *pleasure-unpleasure-principle,* later on just *pleasure-principle.* In the 22nd introductory lecture he explains that "our total mental activity is directed towards achieving pleasure and avoiding unpleasure", that it is automatically regulated by the *pleasure principle*; pleasure seems to be in some way connected with a diminution of the amounts of stimulus, unpleasure with their increase. "An examination of the most intense pleasure, which is accessible to human beings, the pleasure of accomplishing the sexual act, leaves little doubt about this point." (Freud, 1917, S.E. 16, 356)

In a similar way Freud stated in 1900 in 'The Interpretation of Dreams' "that the accumulation of excitation (brought about in various ways that need not concern us) is felt as unpleasure and that it sets the apparatus in action with a view to repeating the experience of satisfaction, which involved a diminution of excitation and was felt as pleasure. A current of this kind in the apparatus, starting from unpleasure and aiming at pleasure, we have termed a 'wish'; and we have asserted that only a wish is able to set the apparatus in motion." (Freud, 1900, S.E. 5, 597)

Reality often does not allow satisfaction of our wishes immediately; we have to accept delays and even renunciation. This so-called reality-principle has no other aim than pleasure, but it does take into account reality in order to avoid unpleasure. It prefers delayed or reduced pleasure to taking the risk of unpleasure. When education and experience manage to put the reality-principle in the place of the pleasure-principle, it is not an abandonment of the pleasure-principle so much as its safeguard.

We also test in our imagination how the persons we consider important react to the satisfaction of our wishes. Part of our attention turns to internalized relationships. A feeling of wellbeing and self-esteem confirms that it is okay with our inner reality too, as we have learned regarding the safety-principle, a term coined by Joseph Sandler.

The precondition for balancing internal and external reality is that both are consciously perceived. This is the task of the part of the psychic apparatus named the ego. The ego tries to mediate between the drive-wishes of the *id* and the orders of the *super-ego*. Due to the defences of the ego some instinctual wishes are repressed, and even more so if the super-ego threatens severe punishments, such as withdrawal of love or castration. These struggles belong to the process of repression. Thus, it becomes an *unconscious conflict*.

To repress a conflict does not solve it, just like a fight in a room is not necessarily ended if somebody switches off the light. Unconscious conflict remains the core of psychoanalytic theory, as Cordelia Schmidt-Hellerau pointed out in her revision of Freud's theory of the drives. From a meta-psychological point of view contradictions between the id, the ego and the super-ego are based on the fact that pleasure for one system entails unpleasure for the other system. Thus the ego has no choice but to allow compromises, which manifest in parapraxes, screen memories, day dreams and in those phenomena, which bring the patients to therapy: the so-called symptoms.

Freud illustrates such a compromise in a slip of the tongue in "The Psychopathology of Everyday life" (1904, S.E. 6, 53 ff.). A man invites his colleagues: "I call on you to *hiccough (in German: 'aufstoßen")* to* the health of our Principal" instead of *'drink to'* (in German: 'anstoßen'). The similarity of the two German words facilitated the slip so that the repressed aggressive drive-wish was stronger than the politeness the super-ego demanded. The forbidden, unpalatable expression has the real feelings that the principal provokes: the impulse to spew. If the Ego is momentarily distracted, the Id allows itself a joke and gives the Super-ego a slap. In the audience a very severe Super-ego might make that the slip of the tongue goes unheard. Another person might burst into laughter thus recognizing the sudden reduction of tension and the pleasure this embarrassing scene evokes.

With these concepts we can explain many psychic phenomena. But there are other important ones too, which are more difficult to understand. In "Analysis Terminable and Interminable" Freud wrote:

"If we take into consideration the total picture made up of the phenomena of masochism immanent in so many people, the negative therapeutic reaction and the sense of guilt found in so many neurotics, we shall no longer be able to adhere to the belief that mental events are exclusively governed by the desire for pleasure. These phenomena are unmistakable indications of the presence of a power in mental life, which we call the instinct of aggression or of destruction according to its aims, and which we trace back to the original death instinct of living matter. It is not a question of an antithesis between an optimistic and a pessimistic theory of life. Only by the concurrent or mutually opposing action of the two primal instincts

– Eros and the death-instinct – , never by one or the other alone, can we explain the rich multiplicity of the phenomena of life" (Freud, 1937b, S.E. 23, 242).

The recall of painful experiences in the transference-situations and in traumatic neuroses also suggested that there exists a compulsion to repeat, which contradicts the pleasure-principle and is a major tendency in psychic life. In "Beyond the Pleasure Principle" (1920) Freud formulated a definitive version of his drive theory based on life- and death-drives. Schmidt-Hellerau showed in her revision of Freud's drive-theory that Freud was correct with his idea of a compulsion to repeat, but she pointed out that this does not necessarily mean that the pleasure-principle is lifted, being "beyond" the pleasure-principle. One rather might regard it as an expression of the pleasure- and regulation-principle (Schmidt-Hellerau, 1995, 289). In accord with this view is Freud's fundamental remark in "The Economic Problem of Masochism" that "even the subject's destruction of himself cannot take place without libidinal satisfaction." (Freud, 1924, S.E. 19, 170)

This confirms the phenomenon I termed the "pleasure of extinction".[18] It seems that even the destruction of oneself is cathected with libido. In other words, destruction cannot work without libidinal cathexis. *Thus the pleasure-principle, which represents the basic dualism of drives even more clearly with the old term 'pleasure-unpleasure-principle', remains the central principle of regulation regarding psychic processes,* in spite of the impression that masochism and the compulsion to repeat are incompatible with the pleasure-principle.

One more remark about the word *pleasure* (in German: *Lust*): Lust is derived etymologically from the Latin adjective *lascivus – which means lascivious, lustful, boisterous, loose* with its Indo-Germanic root l(a)s – desire and the Old-Indian lásati – spielen. In "Three Essays on the Theory of Sexuality" (1905, S.E. 7, 135 and 212) Freud regrets that there is in German everyday language no word for sexual need that serves as counterpart to the word 'hunger' expressing the need for nutrition. The language of science uses 'libido' for this purpose. In normal language there is only one appropriate word, Lust, to denote both of a need and a gratification; thus it can have the meaning either of desire or pleasure. An example:

I would like to have a glass of water = Ich habe Lust auf ein Glas Wasser = need.
I enjoy living = Es bereitet mir Lust zu leben = gratification.

Here is a rare case where the English translation provides clarification to the original: Freud said that unfortunately "Lust" is "vieldeutig," i.e., has several meanings. Freud speaks about lust in a double sense, and so "vieldeutig' is

---

[18] „Extinction" is here used in a medial way: it has an active as well as a passive sense, because it concerns the process of becoming extinguished – thus being passive –, but at the same time it is about the act of extinction initiated by the individual itself, though normally neither willingly nor consciously.

translated correctly as "ambiguous". It seems worth noting that Freud wrote in the same year an article entitled "The antithetical meaning of primal words". There Freud referred to a book by the linguist Karl Abel, who showed that in ancient languages there are words that contain opposite meanings, because they originally marked two extreme points. In any case, we can state that 'pleasure/Lust' includes a need, on one hand, and satisfaction of a want, on the other.

In earlier eras there was a verb, derived from the substantive Lust, used only in a reflexive form. Thus we find at the time of Martin Luther the phrase "Es lüstet mich" meaning "I feel the desire". But it is expressed reflexively, in an impersonal way, of not taking the responsibility, unlike "I wish..., I want..." Language itself, reflecting unconscious intentions, incorporated a tendency to reject the authorship of one's own wishes. We also find this inclination toward irresponsible passivity in the phrase "falling in love", thus emphasizing the unconscious, incontrollable aspect of this psychic event.

In the state of being in love fantasy plays a potent role, but this is the case in many other circumstances too. For instance, when somebody experiences the environment as dissatisfying he may withdraw. The search for pleasure then shifts into the realm of fantasy, which Freud called 'Naturschutzpark' ('nature reservation' or 'young plantation'). There satisfaction can be imagined to a large extent without protest of the reality-principle. Yet even here absolute freedom does not exist. Even fantasy depends on building stones of external reality and on conditions ruling the internal world. Thus Freud's metaphor of nature reservation fits also regarding the limitations there. If we page through leaflets of national parks, Yellowstone Park for instance, which Freud mentioned, we see beside the praise of the beauties of nature a lot of rules aiming at protection of this paradise. The warnings of dangers, the extensive rules of conduct, and the passages about patrolling supervisors (with or without broad Stetsons) attest that freedom is limited there as in the realm of fantasy.

However, there are other ways of finding pleasure besides escaping into fantasy. For instance, instinctual aims can be shifted. In "Civilization and its Discontents" Freud identifies sublimation as another technique for fending off suffering. Sublimation is "the employment of the displacements of the libido which our mental apparatus permits of and through which its function gains so much in flexibility" (1930, S.E. 21, 79). The instinctual aims are displaced so that they don't encounter the prohibitions of the external world. Every mother will try to discourage her baby from the pleasures to smear around his faeces, but if the baby does the same with colours, parental hope arises that this is the launch of a creative genius. Similarly, if an old person regresses to the anal phase and plays with excrement, it is disgusting. If this person paints instead, it is considered a self-therapeutic act, even if the artistic execution is rather modest. Under certain circumstances, the pleasure gained from psychic, intellectual or artistic work can rise to a point that one feels invulnerable. The gratifying sense of greater independence is offset by the lessened intensity of this pleasure and more difficult access to it. Not everybody can aspire to this level of pleasure.

Another form of displacement uses the screen of time. Pleasure can be acquired in the past, thus evading historic reality and creating a personal myth by idealisations centred around the heroic self. In the search for pleasure truth and fantasy become blurred.

Focusing on future pleasure is another path. This route can be the basis for great enterprises in which excitement and fantasizing makes for elaborate planning as well as accompanying energy to realize those plans. Conscious reality testing at every step might halt some plans before they begin. The dream of a house of one's own seems to include a fantasy that harmony, love, respect and space for the development of all one's capacities will thereby be enabled. Sometimes preparations are made for a life for which the persons involved are in no way ready due to their inner obstacles. Then the search for pleasure hits an impasse.

It might be that plans devised during the whole life are contemplated again and again without coming closer to realization. As in Arthur Schnitzler's 'Comedy of Words', Dr. Eckhold complains: 'I'm the sort of person who never gets beyond the wishing stage.' (Schnitzler, 1892, 482) In this play enormous aggression, dammed up for years, is exposed all at once in relation to his wife, who once betrayed him. One feels that Eckhold had long been looking forward to this outburst, expecting the greatest pleasure after such delay, and one can see that there is a connection between his restraint of realizations and his fear of his own destruction. But to vent one's aggression in a controlled way can indeed be enjoyable.

Let us look now at the role and kinds of pleasure in old age, taking acutely into account that all pleasure threatens to vanish.

A key concern regarding age is the fear of being separated from most activities that provided our everyday pleasures. On closer look it turns out that the problem often is not the loss of pleasure, but the narcissistic violation that we no longer may be capable of satisfying those pleasures, which the social environment acknowledges, and even demands. This concealed concern makes some people speak and joke about sexuality in order to keep up the appearance of partaking in it. The prudery of Victorian age switched to its opposite long ago, resulting grotesquely in the same disgust and control of pleasure, now not due to prohibitions but to claims raised by society or one's own narcissistic demands.

A good example is Hermann Bahr's comedy 'The Concert', mentioned earlier, where a famous pianist longs for the comforts experienced in his long marriage. But the adulations of a determined female fan seduced him into pretending sexual desire. For reasons of self-esteem he tried hard to act as if he was an attractive lover full of desire, untouched by age. Actually, after a concert he wished nothing but to get his slippers and rest his legs high. This conflict led only at the beginning to a triumph of the fake.

Inge Merkel's novel 'A quite normal marriage' explores the reunion of Odysseus and Penelope, and paints a touching picture of human passions. Penelope suffered from sexual dissatisfaction for more than a decade. The return of Odysseus stirs touching and tragic-comical scenes over a long emotional night. She accedes with relief to his request to douse the light because she thinks that although she might still be attractive in make-up and beautiful dress, now he would only see her grey hairs and wrinkles. And Odysseus was not only afraid of impotence; he was conscious of his own emaciated body and wished it covered by merciful darkness. Only in his nocturnal narrations of his adventures does closeness re-emerge. When he was in danger of slipping away again from Penelope, it was, as if he was not suffering from homesickness, but craved distance: 'He slipped away from her towards inside [...] This strange homesickness that pressed in his bones and his cooled down blood, had nothing to do with a cheerful sailing and the pleasure of enterprise [...] He was curious to know death' (Merkel, 1994, 415). Later, at his deathbed Penelope speaks to him for a long time in a highly ambivalent way: should she mourn a dying mate or hate a rambler? 'Today I am old enough to know that love is more than being blinded and feeling desire for a beautiful body; furthermore, that it does not depend on the few upswings in bed or in the grass, but that it is about the backing one gives each other against life and death.' (422 f.)

Here it is clear that the main problem is the narcissistic violation due to age and that the emotional bond is needed as protection against impending death. That this concerns the *internalized* bond Penelope has proved by waiting so long for the absent Odysseus. This love – in theoretical language: the cathexis of an object with libidinal energy – accords with the wider conception of sexuality used in psychoanalysis. It is not reducible to sexual intercourse, but comprehends the whole psychic activity we call "love".

The source of the instinct is somatic; its object is exchangeable and renders our capacity to love flexible. It can refer to people, animals, plants, things or abstract values. The instinctual aim is the activity to which the drive urges, guided by our fantasies.

The sexual drive itself is composed of partial instincts and is bound to different erotogenic zones, which can be stimulated and which alternate. Thus, a sucking baby experiences pleasure in the oral erotogenic zone; in the anal phase expelling or retaining faeces provides satisfying control of physical functions and a way to express or refuse love by this "present"; in the urethral eroticism urinating becomes a pleasurable act of ambition and aggression. Only when the genitals became the prime zone of satisfaction do we speak of genital sexuality.

When this mature form of sexuality recedes during old age, the previous erotogenic zones may regain importance. Oral pleasure, eating or smoking, might prevail and become the centre of interest. The wish to control, stemming from the anal phase, has numerous forms of expression, such as a passion for collecting things (retaining a precious possession). Such a hobby is approved by society. It is a regression to earlier means of pleasure, if during old age mature ways of satisfaction are achieved. If this was not the case, it is a fixation upon earlier phases. Many acts in which we take pleasure seem unrelated to sexuality because they are shifted to another level by sublimation, and usually only in analysis is the link to the original instinctual satisfaction discovered. The anal component of pleasure in exercising power, for instance, normally is not conscious.

If the needs for sexual satisfaction declines at the same time as do physiological forces, there is no special painful tension. But if the feeling that one has missed too much pleasure dominates and that it is impossible to catch up, then the question arises – as in any separation – whether what is lost can be mourned, even if it might not be really lost because it was never possessed in the first place. Once more we can detect the linear development of difficulties. If somebody could not develop his capacity for love, it has serious psychic reasons; and these same reasons, which limited or prohibited mature sexuality, will also make the process of mourning more difficult. It is hard to drop something one never had. In the next chapter we will look at some vicissitudes of loss and separation.

At any age there is always the option of retreat into fantasy during adverse external circumstances. Thus in old age any reductions in the scope of physical satisfaction might be compensated by a rich fantasy life. Sometimes, a concentration on inner reality becomes excessive and can be linked to a diminished testing of external reality. Sometimes, however, this refocusing of one's attention on the inner world leads to recognition of new aspects of external reality that were not so accessible before. Such wisdom was attributed in earlier times and in other cultures to elderly people. This turn inward often was marked by blindness, which symbolized a looking away from superficial observation of external reality. In classical antiquity prophets often were represented as blind men.

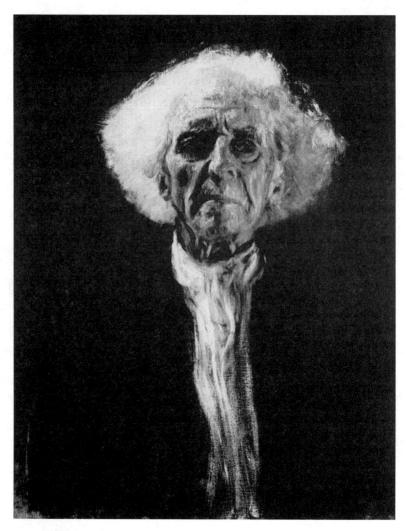

Figure 3
Gustav Klimt: Blind Man, Collection Leopold, Vienna
In old age our focus on the past and on the inner world often intensifies.
Blindness symbolizes this turning inward. An inner richness can offset the
trials of the present and the diminishing of the future.

A striking displacement due to age concerns time. The past seems to come to the foreground, especially experiences long ago. To relive the past can be very pleasurable: one enjoys the richness of experiences that young people cannot be sure they will ever achieve. Age is also a time of alterations and shadings of memories according to one's wishes. In personal narratives memory is often not about attaining as true a representation as possible, but about strengthening one's self-esteem. This tendency also aims at compensating us for the narcissistic violation of ageing.

Another route of displacement of interest is a shift from the present to the future. Religions urge an orientation towards a life beyond that on earth, but it is not religions alone that can be reproached for denying transience. A focus on ideals and values, which are expected to outlive mortal lives, can be a consoling distraction from reality and cover the denial that when our life ends so too will our awareness of such qualities. Still, it is not always denial in a clinical sense if we feel bound to lasting values that we practice. A devotion to ideals is connected to a bond to the next generation, for whom a better future based on their inheritance is envisioned.

If such an altruistic attitude, relatively free of envy, proves impossible, greed may dominate the scene. It is not by chance that one speaks about the greed of old age. Sometimes elderly people, who feel that fate, god or whatever had withheld fulfilments from them, wish to hold tight onto as many goods as possible before their ultimate loss in death.

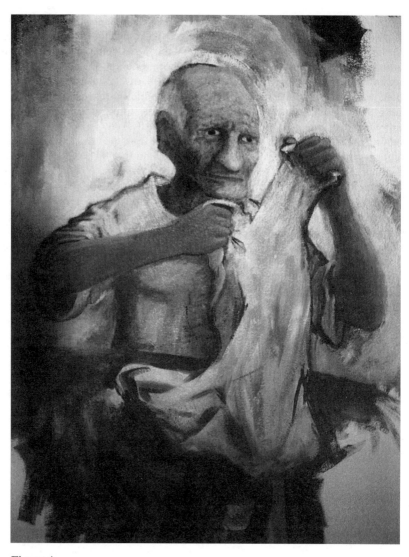

Figure 4
Johannes Schweichhart: Picture of complaints, Salzburg
As the end of life approaches, hate, envy, greed and destructiveness may
increase and we strive to defend our anxieties.

Certainly, what Franz Kafka wrote in a letter to his father is true: 'Greed is one of the most reliable signs of deep unhappiness.' (Kafka, 1975, 37)

We can see that pleasure does not really end in old age, rather, the form of it changes. So it may return to older physical sources, or it may choose other objects and other aims. The choice is not a fully conscious one; it is guided by conscious and unconscious fantasies. It can emphasize inner reality instead of the external, where the competition is ever more fierce. It might turn towards the past, or it might try to eschew the turbulent present in favour of gossamer fantasies of the future. Despite all these variations of emphasis a certain degree of relatedness to reality is necessary in order to remain capable of living and relating. In old age the capacity for enjoyment evidently depends on a certain balance between wish and reality, and on the capacity to turn to the external as well as to the internal world. If the pains of the past can be accepted, enough energy is available for participating in the present. Within this movable frame the pleasure principle can continue to function and regulate the psychic processes, until eventually the poles are changed in the "pleasure of extinction" and the return from the organic to the inorganic realm takes place. It seems to be important to die *one's own* death; and it is important at all times regarding the smooth functioning of the pleasure-principle whether a real individual need is perceived and experienced as *one's own* desire and satisfaction.

5.1 Mourning or depression

The first chapter addressed the two fundamental modes of coping with separation – mourning or depression. One may understand these modes as extremes between which there are many graduations and shades. In mourning and depression the melody of separation is slowed down, as if this might delay the painful process of separation.

In mourning, the bond to a lost object is loosened slowly, painfully and to a great degree unconsciously and uncontrollably. It might be introjected and it might continue to exist in memories, but there is no denying that in the living present a vital relationship is no longer possible. After a successful process of mourning the ability to make new bonds is no longer blocked, and the world that seemed to be empty for so long becomes alive again.

In depression, however, the object that is no longer available in the external world, becomes internalized unconsciously: "Thus the shadow of the object fell upon the ego." (Freud, 1917a, S.E. 14, 249) The subject has fetched the object inside by identification with it and put it in the place of the ego. The loss of the object is denied; the separation does not felt really happen. But the high price to be paid is that of the loss of the ego, which appears as an ongoing disinterest and incapacity to love and to work. It is not always the real loss of an object that triggers such a pathological process; a severe slight, a radical rejection or a implicit turning away can have the same result without even being noticed.

While the work of mourning usually is considered to be a healthy psychic development and depression as a pathological stagnation, Winnicott saw in depression a chance of a recovery too. He called depression "a healing mechanism; it covers the battleground as with a mist, allowing for a sorting out at reduced rate, giving time for all possible defences to be brought into play, and for a working through, so that eventually there can be a spontaneous recovery" (Winnicott, 1987, 275). I think this insight Winnicott's is important because it hints at our ability – probably a preconscious process – to establish facilitating conditions for further development, in this case for developing the capacity of mourning. The loss of an object *is* traumatic, and sometimes the ensuing depression has the function *to freeze* a situation so that it might perhaps become thawed up later when one might overcome the loss in a slower mode and with a more tolerable degree of pain. Winnicott spoke about "a freezing of the failure situation" (1987, 281) regarding failures of the environment.

Out of a wide variety of parting situations some separations and their vicissitudes will now be looked at more closely, starting from the extreme pole of refusing separation altogether.

5.2 Symbiosis and denial of separation

> *"With you in the aeroplane I fear no longer the danger.*
> *One dies only, if one is alone."*
> *(Marguerite Yourcenar: Fire, 1967, 25)*

Separation and the danger of separation can be kept from consciousness. If somebody is routed into a symbiosis, a change of the situation is unimaginable. So there is no occasion to fear separation. But sooner or later an exclusive concentration on a single bond causes problems. Relationships are always ambivalent, and the development of two individuals usually does not progress synchronically. There is the 'danger' that one of the pair develops further and can no longer bear to be confined by a symbiotic bond. This reaction might stir hate on one side or, often, both sides partly due to suffocating control, and to fear that the control might fail. Separation wishes get projected to and fro. If a notion to escape arises, it is felt to be a forbidden wish, and a vicious cycle of clinging and wishing to flee is activated.
The illusion of feeling absolutely secure can only be attained for a very short time.

A very successful actress suffered from fear of flying. But she was not ready to let this symptom inhibit her career and she had found a way to cope with her fear. As soon as the aeroplane was about to take off or to land or when there were turbulences she asked the person next to her – whomever it was – whether she could hold his or her hand. As soon as she felt contact, she was relieved immediately and felt out of danger. She had discovered a kind of behaviouristic coping-strategy against separation-anxiety by creating the illusion of a bond to a protective, omnipotent object. When her analysis progressed to the point that her symptom vanished, she complained partly seriously, partly jokingly that analysis had spoiled her aerial flirtations. Actually her inclination to indulge in quick, superficial relationships diminished in favour of a deeper relationship, which was not possible for her before.

Here it was the quickly established superficial but physical contact to a person; in other cases it is a mascot – a figure expected to bring luck –, especially if given by somebody whom one loves. This figure serves as a "transitional object" and supports, as in children, a feeling of a strong bond that triumphs over danger. Jewellery and clothes too can become a guarantor of protection due to magic thinking. On journeys one patient always wore her friend's scarf as a symbolic pledge of her safe return. If this scarf clashed with her wardrobe, it had to be rolled up in her handbag, which she considered already a bit of increased risk.

The most reassuring idea of a bond that overcomes everything is offered to believers by religions. There are, of course, a lot of variations. Religious ideas can concentrate on fantasies about fusion in a Nirvana-imagination, or else they might suggest eternal (re-)union with a godlike figure. This religious imagination can be characterized by a severe superego-aspect with fixed laws, so that protection is achieved by conducting oneself strictly according to these laws. Another religion-oriented assumption focuses on the ideal of a purely loving, forgiving, rewarding and protecting attitude. In Christian religion, there is also a ranking of saints who may be selected as advocates and companions in life, if one wishes not to rely on direct appeal to a distant God the father or God the son. Whatever happens, can be reckoned as the will of God, and with "Thy will be done!" the bond becomes divine.

There is perhaps no more beautiful representation of how our perceptions of transience succumb to the seduction of transcendence than the poem 'Autumn' by Rainer Maria Rilke:

'The leaves are falling, falling like from far,
as if in heavens wilted distant gardens;
with a denying gesture they are falling.

And in the nights the heavy earth falls down
from all the stars into the loneliness.

We all are falling and this hand here falls.
And have a look at those: it is in all.

Yet there is One, who holds this falling down
with endless softness in his hands.'

Once more the unbearable apprehension over separation and parting is contained by an idea of an infinitely good, holding object, god, with whom one will be united forever.

The feeling of an absolutely certain bond is incompatible with separation-anxiety and 'absorbs' fear of death, as Winnicott put it. But it also is incompatible with development. This is the unpleasant flip side of the comforting illusion. In the process of development it is unavoidable that the child loosens and modifies the earliest relationship to the mother, especially regarding the extension of it to a third person. Later, in new editions of the symbiotic relationship it is the appearance of a third object – whether another person or other interests – that forms a fracture line, where relationships may break.

Some separation-anxieties are summarized as "castration-anxiety", concerning a part of the body that is missing or can be removed, like a penis, faeces or a baby.

These forms of anxiety cannot be overcome if for unconscious reasons the search for a total symbiosis and the resistance against change and separation become dominant.

The capacity to tolerate separation is a precondition for further development and for any shift to something new. Without this readiness we experience stagnation and a drying up of productivity and creativity.

If the threat of a possible separation leads the person to fixate on a particular bond, such a symbiosis, based on denial, may freeze the psychical life temporarily or even permanently.

The denial of separation differs from depression. The latter refuses to let an object go; rather it is sunk into the unconscious where the internalized object is re-established without the subject knowing it and without stopping the complaints about the loss. The symbiotic denial that there is any need for separations can be conscious too. At one end of the spectrum there is serious delusional clinging to a counterfeit unity; at the other end, there is the mascot that we take with a wink while joking that, of course, we do not believe in magical thinking since we are enlightened and rational human beings.

5.3   Conflict and compromise

There are innumerable steps between bond and separation; but to speak of steps does not mean that there is any great stability. There are two opposed forces in a lively process, which might arise as a dominating tendency, but not as a final stop. The struggle of contradictory tendencies often can be seen in patients' conflicts. Even the outcomes of such struggles aren't always unambiguous, but can be full of compromises. Some examples follow.

5.3.1 External separation, internal fixation

Consider divorces where no internal separation follows the legal one. A couple 'gets' a divorce without really parting. The divorce can be delegated to the outside, but this might only be a protest against mutual dependence, against all the disappointments and 'unsettled bills', which indicate the discrepancy between the wishful fantasies and reality. The aroused emotions subside again and there is not much change at all. Often these contacts – even intimate ones – continue; the struggles, especially concerning the children, go on, now referring to the decision of an external authority. Thus little energy remains for forming new bonds.

While in such cases the contradictory tendencies – separation on one hand and the retained bond on the other – can be observed on the surface, it might be the case too that only the separation is indeed visible but the ongoing bond remains invisible and unconscious. The following case of a 38 years old man, who was very successful in his profession, demonstrates such an unconscious conflict:

Severe sleeping disorders and the failure of several psychotherapy attempts were the occasion why Peter fulfilled a wish he had felt since his school days: to undergo an analysis. This idea had rather a narcissistic thrust. He considered psychoanalysis as the most sophisticated psychotherapeutic treatment in which only a superior few can engage. With this elitist attitude he concealed his despair over needing help because he felt so near a breakdown. He was afraid of ruining his career and also his private life because he was sure that his wife would not remain with a failure such as he. In the initial interview I noticed his lofty language and his distinct articulation, which reminded me of a trained manner of speaking, which one usually hears from an actor or a broadcaster. It sounded fluent, but it did not really fit a man who came from the countryside and who had made a remarkable career. In the first year of treatment it became evident that his affected manner of speaking was a way to differentiate himself from his parents. He hated it if somebody spoke in a dialect, like his father, with whom he had hardly any contact since his mother died 10 years ago. Yet he had loved his father very much when he was a child, even more than his depressive mother. Whenever she had withdrawn, his father had taken over care for Peter. When Peter entered school, he felt superior to anybody else because his father already had taught him a great deal. Both of his parents were ready to support Peter if he wanted to go to university. Nevertheless, he felt like a traitor when he decided to move to the city and seldom visited home. He was ashamed of his parents although he did not know why. Slowly it became clear that he was not only ashamed that they were plain people, but also felt guilty because he distanced himself from them. Before his sleeping problems had started, he had been very touched by the support of his boss, who held him in high esteem, and who now recommended him – earlier than expected – for a leading post. This promotion reminded him unconsciously of his abandoned good relationship to his father. There were several indications that after the death of his mother Peter feared his relationship to his father might become too close, and so he stayed away. He even feared – and secretly wished – that the relationship to his paternal boss might become too close, thus revealing a latent homosexuality. Only when Peter recognized how much he suffered because of the withdrawal of his depressive mother did he come to understand, that he had escaped his mother's depression by fleeing to his father, and now he was fleeing from having too strong feelings for me. During puberty he felt so uncomfortable because of his closeness to his father that he tried hard to differ from him, especially in his manner of speaking. He listened many hours to audiobooks read by a famous actor – without noticing that by this he had chosen a new, nobler 'father'. Soon he had met a girl, whom he married, when he was 22 years old. But this marriage did not last. He had concentrated on a search for a woman who would be "always funny", as a contrast to his depressive mother. His wife, however, was "funny" also with other men so that he could not bear it and sought a divorce. After this he had several longer relationships. Only a few years ago he married again – to the daughter of his boss. Desperate and confused he had wondered whether he had really been attracted by this woman or by her father. It was quite a long time until the confusion was solved by analyzing his transference, which was dominated by his deep disappointment that he failed in conquering me, just as he felt he had been incapable of cheering up his mother. Slowly, he began to experience his marriage "like a totally new relationship".

A radical separation of this patient from his parents hid the inner fixation on his father caused by serious unconscious conflicts. The psychic illness of his mother, who repeatedly collapsed into depression, moved him to intensify his bond to his father, but this bond had provoked problems regarding his sexual identity.

5.3.2 Inner separation, external fixation

Physical separation does not guarantee that there will be paralleled internally, and that the individual therefore is in a psychic balance. Conversely, the same is true: outward stability of a relationship does not prove there is not disintegration under the surface. A minor external influence might trigger a breakdown of a relationship, similar to an undermined sand castle, which can collapse with one stroke. In Arthur Schnitzler's 'Comedy of Words' there is a dramatic representation of a secret schism in a marriage that outwardly seemed solid (refer also chapter 4.7):

Dr. Eckhold and his wife Clara are visited by Prof. Ormin, who wants to say good-bye before he leaves for the war in Japan with an ambulance-unit. Eckhold envies him and regrets that he himself has never done such an adventurous thing. Quickly it turns out that his envy does not really concern the enterprise, but he is reliving the old jealousy, initiated 10 years before by a short affair of his wife with Ormin at a time when Eckhold had become estranged from her. When Ormin departs, all the welled-up hate bursts out. Triumphantly, Eckhold informs Clara that he had known about her affair, but that he remained silent for the sake of their common interests and their children. But this reticence did not prevent him from 'keeping apart in the depth of my soul my existence from yours and to look forward to the hour, which now finally has come.' He suggests divorce, since now their daughter was leaving in order to marry. Desperate Clara resists the destruction of their marriage. She accuses: 'You have had the right – perhaps – to chase me away, maybe even to kill me. But you did not have the right to withhold from me the punishment you had decided to impose on me.' (Schnitzler, 1892, 488) Finally she gives up the futile struggle. She rejects the notion of writing a farewell letter too: 'Words are lies' (491) and leaves.

Implying a likelihood of suicide Schnitzler shows the desperation generated by a separation that cannot be undone because it was enacted secretly and in the past. Like a bolt from the blue the woman is confronted with the fact that her efforts, despite her one lapse, to be a good wife for her husband had failed. She had not built up a "false self". Instead her husband declared false everything that she had built. The marriage needed just a tiny stimulus – the farewell visit of the rival – and an avalanche of destruction was unleashed.

What is conveyed in dramatic terms here happens in an everyday form in many relationships. Secretly nursed resentments, which one cannot overcome, result in an inner retreat that goes unnoticed by the partner and is reflected in a vague feeling of alienation, emptiness and loneliness. Thus the source cannot be traced or comprehended; the separation is internal, hidden by a firm façade.

In this literary example the concealing of an inner separation is an existential falsehood. Lies function to permit the individual to enjoy a feeling of inner freedom and independence by denying actual dependence. In children and adolescents it can be a first attempt at autonomy even though the environment will hardly acknowledge it. A case vignette of a young man, who was considered a chronic liar, demonstrates such an inner separation:

Whenever Jack, 17 years old, told a lie, he felt he had reality under control. Thus he created, for himself, controllable objects with which he could cope better than with the persons in his environment – stepparents and teachers, who criticized him and made nothing but demands. By lying he escaped feelings of powerlessness, of being locked up and endangered. These feelings had arisen in his lonely early childhood. He repeated these traumatic early experiences with stepparents whom he felt to be cold and exploiting, in spite of all their efforts, and whom he hated because he was dependent on them. Actually he hated his own parents, who had neglected him due to their personal difficulties and agreed that he be adopted. He became ruthless, as he felt he was left in the lurch ruthlessly. In analysis I often did not know whether he spoke the truth or not. Thus he conveyed to me the experience of how one feels if one is no longer sure what is true and what is false. When I interpreted that he had to make me feel, how lonely and confused he had been, he reacted with deep emotion, and a long working through of such experiences started. Jack thought that it was impossible to like him the way he really was, and so he was always under pressure to invent something, anything, which he thought would make him appear more acceptable and more interesting. His lying was a function of his false self, as described by Winnicott: it hid the true self that was vulnerable, and obsessed by impotent rage and aggression. He fantasized that his parents had given him away, because he was such a little monster. Thus he made himself responsible and thereby got everything again under his control. He hated his stepparents, but his hate had roots in his dependence on severely disturbed parents, who were unable to hold him and who let all his impulses run wild. When he was lying, it was revenge. Now all the others would be left in the cold, for he created a 'reality' in which the others had to believe. Later on, when it was no longer necessary to separate from his first objects, he slowly developed – after a lot of failures – the capacity for authentic bonds.

5.3.3 "The dead mother" or "frozen love"

A special version of separation is the constellation that Andrè Green described through the concept, "the dead mother". The distinctiveness of this constellation is that the child experiences loss of the mother even though she is still physically present. But she is no longer devoted to the child because she is distracted by something else, a loss, a worry or a severe violation (for instance if she believes that her husband betrays her); something she suffers and that causes a loss of interest in her child. She seems to be 'dead', psychically dead, because she can no longer cathect her child with libido as she did before. But she is 'dead' for a second reason too: the child itself – also unconsciously – withdraws his libido, his love from her. This de-cathexis is a kind of emotional murder, but one which happens without hate. The love "has been frozen by the decathexis, a form of love which keeps the object in hibernation." (Kohon, 1999b, 4) In the unconscious there opens a gaping hole in the place where the mother has been the primary love object, a "psychic hole". Some children manage to cover this hole by developing extraordinary intellectual achievements or artistic gifts: thus sublimation might be successful, but the capacity for love may nevertheless remain impaired.

The concept of the "dead mother" became the best known of the innumerable publications of Andrè Green, although it is difficult, rich and complex, as Gregorio Kohon noted in his dialogue with Green (Kohon, 1999b, 51 f.). This unusual reception is caused – according to Green himself – by the confluence of personal experiences with clinical observations in analyses with patients, who underwent such a "dead-mother syndrome", and augmented by theoretical studies of such experiences.

A combination of these three components – personal, clinical and theoretical experiences – is not unusual, at least not regarding the first and the third component. We often devote ourselves to those issues to which we feel for one reason or another curiously attracted. Green himself cites this fact when he writes, that we choose our theories according the pleasure-principle, not according the reality-principle (Green, 2005a, 283). I think that the success of a concept is mainly a result of the *secret attractiveness, the allure* of some of its psychoanalytic contents (Zwettler-Otte, 2004, 78-88). This allure becomes most potent when personal unconscious material meets with psychoanalytic thoughts and is touched by them. This can serve in a way similar to an interpretation: unconscious repressed contents pressing towards the surface emerge for a moment. There, less strength needs to be invested in repression, and this results in a temporary reduction of tension, providing a relaxation experienced as pleasure. The concept of the "dead mother" fulfils this condition of secret attraction. Who would not at some time identify with the sentence: "I have not (or never) been loved < well enough >" – and to connect with this scientifically legitimated complaint the hope and the claim for compensation? It is not only a valid concept but a seductive one, and it opens outlets for our ambivalence. The mother, who is present and yet absent, calls forth love for the early mother who is selflessly devoted but she also seems to justify hateful feelings because of her loveless indifference. Thus the "dead mother" represents a conflict between separating and binding and elaborates a compromise between the mother's and the child's love and frozen love.

5.4   Separation and distance

Whenever two individuals separate the question arises: how far they really retreat from one another. Separation is about inner distance as well as external space. Both may move synchronically, thus producing a compensating effect. Often distance stimulates the longing for closeness and makes the absent love object appear more desirable than it was when it was present. Distance becomes filled with fantasies of desire. Conversely, given a permanent real presence, one might very well take the other for granted so that he hardly is noticed.

The continuum of separation extends from temporary distancing to eternal loss. While in symbiosis two people merge without allowing any room for independent action, there is, on the other hand, the possibility that the external and/or inner distance stretch out infinitely. Then the other person is 'forgotten', his inner representation sinks into the unconscious and becomes extinguished. However, to 'forget' or to 'extinguish' is an active, dynamic process of destruction, even if it goes on unconsciously. We have seen this destructive form of silent decathexis at work during our considerations about the death-drive. Such a separation from an object can be initiated by hostility, but also by the need for relief and for more space regarding new relationships.

A similar unconscious process is recognizable in alienation. In analyses one usually can find that whenever somebody or something is experienced to be 'strange', there is an unconscious rejection, which puts the 'bad' object in a greater distance.

If one posits concentric circles of closeness, one might imagine a close love-bond growing more distant. Love can change to friendship or to a more aim-orientated relationship where strong mutual feelings no longer dominate, except, for instance, for ongoing care for the children. A development in the other direction is possible too, from outside to inside. Then an acquaintance might shift into a relationship centred on common interests. It might become a friendship, and sometimes even love.

Problems usually arise because of confusions of these concentric circles, which easily become shifted and disturbed. Many difficulties arise out of contradictory wishes: for instance, when someone avoids closeness and wants "just a friendship" while the partner is dissatisfied with it.

In aim-oriented relationships a third aspect occurs; triangulation cannot be avoided. This can be experienced as a relief because it is not the feelings for each other that are central but a common task. However, this situation does not often work. Rivalry can come to dominate the scene and distract attention from the main purpose. The function of a third party is lost if it is mainly about provoking and expressing emotions.

In frightening situations a plummet into regression can occur. The originally aim-oriented relationship changes; the regressed person fantasizes and attributes power and strength to the partner according to their own needs. If the partner accepts this role he will see primarily the helplessness and incapacity of the other one. This creates an unnecessary and unrealistic imbalance of authority and infantilism that impedes the common task. Many patients will regress during brief contact with medical doctors, and many parents feel like small pupils if they stand before a teacher whom they experience as omnipotent or as a strict paternal or maternal authority. If this authority figure shows a reserved attitude, this might accord with the objective aim of the contact, but it may be wrongly understood as coldness or a demonstration of power because a need for closeness has arisen. Hence, separation and distance cannot be tolerated.

In many situations of adult life a capacity for flexibility is required in order to allow movement between the concentric circles of closeness and to accept temporary increases of distance without feeling compelled to break off the relationship. To cease contact is destructive and can be stirred not only by a wish to destroy the other person but also to retain or to be retained by him or to dominate him. Even a slipper thrown at somebody is meant to reach him, and the obvious repudiation is often nothing but a (often unconscious) attempt to make the partner run after oneself or to provoke whatever reaction. It is often a helpless effort to separate without really dissociating.

In Goethe's play "Iphigenie" we witness an excruciating process of separation that succeeds only because Iphigenie and king Thoas part through a benign agreement. Iphigenie is filled with gratitude to Thoas, who saved her from death and wished to marry her. Nevertheless, she experiences life in a foreign country as a 'second death'. Thoas allows her to leave but this permission is not enough for her:

'Not this way, my king! Without blessing,
Against your will, I do not part with you.
Don't banish us! A kind right of hospitality
Ought to rule between you and us; thus we are not
Separated for ever and secluded.'

Iphigenie is striving – in spite of desired separation – to save the continuation of the relationship to the man, whom she esteems, though she does not love him. Only in this way can she consider an external separation to be possible:

'You are dear and worthy to me like my father,
And this impression remains in my soul.
If the most unimportant one of your people
Ever will bring to me back the sound of your voice,
Which I was used to hear from you
And if I see your costume on this poorest;
I'll receive him like a god
I'll myself prepare his couch,
Invite him to the fire
And ask him nothing but your fate
And you.'

Iphigenie is connecting her father, who is not only taboo due to incest but was willing to sacrifice her, with Thoas to whom she might have transferred similar feelings of "strangeness". She connects Thoas with anybody who reminds her of him. Gratitude, and guilt that she cannot respond to his love, open the way for generalisation and idealization. Every one of Thoas' people will be honoured.

'O the gods should reward your deeds
And your mildness. Fare well!
O turn to us and speak a soft word of good-bye!
Then the wind will crowd the sails softer
And tears will flow more gently from the eye
of the one, who is parting. Fare well,
and give me your right hand as a sign
of our old friendship'.

Thoas: 'Fare well!'

Iphigenie cannot give Thoas the love he is longing for, so she delegates his reward to the gods. Thoas' forgiveness and renunciation becomes the precondition of a gentle separation and entry into a process of mourning. The inner securing of the bond against revenge and hate makes it possible for a real parting to happen, which allows the suspending of distance at any time to reactivate the bond.

5.5   Projected wishes for separation

Separation anxieties often are disguised wishes for separation. The disguise is due to the feeling that separation is not only awful, if one experiences it passively, but is forbidden too. Thus one is not allowed to think about it, much less to do it. This mechanism is at play in symbiotic relationships. It is not only fear of separation that cannot be tolerated; even the idea of being alone cannot be imagined. It seems unbearable that two individuals are separate entities. Therefore any border that separates individuals is denied, as is any possibility that distance between them might grow. Whatever impulses are stirred for greater room to move freely are banished and projected outside, so that it is spotted and attacked in the other person only. Feelings of omnipotence, of envy and fantasies of dominating the partner play a great role and defend against the dreaded fate of being separated, of loneliness and of divorce. The wish for separation is not recognized as one's own inner need for change but is felt to be an external persecuting danger. One's own activity is denied and turned into passivity so that one is utterly innocent. The "beloved" object is embraced tightly to pre-empt its efforts to be relieved. Such behaviour has a magical, importunate feature. Nevertheless, it usually is useless. There is no consolation because the real cause of the fear is neither recognized nor abolished. It is as if one would clean a disturbing spot on the outside of the window, although the dirt is actually inside. All efforts are in vain. All reassurances of the partner are met with mistrust since secretly one's own wishes for separation remain and continue to be projected onto the other one.

However, the underside of the effort to control everything is sadness. Julia Kristeva (1989, 64) called it the negative of omnipotence. It is a first sign of a removal of that for which one is fighting and a last filter of aggression. If the grip of the object is in danger, violence and terror might follow.

5.6 Aggression and terror

Whether it is separation-anxieties, which are projected wishes for separation, or about mad jealousy imagining the loss of the love-object, or about real separations, which are intended by a partner or forced by circumstances, the threat of the slipping away of the other can provoke impotent rage. A deeply rooted conviction that one will be left alone forever can mobilize all one' forces to regain control and to prevent loss by aggression, terror and violence. The partner becomes confined and treated like a dependent marionette. If he protests, this is proof that he has plans of flight in mind. If he does not protest, it is a confirming resignation. Thus the "beloved" living object becomes suffocated because it appears a bad object that deserves hate. Fear of separation turns into fear of annihilation so that any defence seems justified. The horror of impending catastrophe is reflected in the terrorist's face who wants to destroy the bad object before it would destroy him. In destruction still lies the hope to possess and control the object better than when it was alive. So Shakespeare's Othello in his madness considered the murder of faithful Desdemona the only chance to prevent her loss and the triumph of the rival. What a fallacious victory attends the deed.

5.7 Emptiness

'A single human being that one misses,
and everything is devoid of people.'
(Alphonse de Lamartine: L'insolement)

The loss of a love object often is followed by emptiness. It is as if the only lovable person has vanished from psychic space. Loneliness spreads. A demonstrative loneliness erupts with the intention to insist on the extinction of the other objects because this desired object is missing. Emptiness becomes the space of suction on the lost object in order to bring it back.

The destruction of a hated object also produces emptiness. "When a person's hate is destructive of his internal objects, we know that the emptiness he feels is due to his destructive activity. With his internal objects mangled or useless, there is nothing of value left, and he will feel only the deadness of the annihilated objects or the emptiness of an evacuated space" (Bollas, 1987, 130). An atmosphere of triumph can be spoiled by guilt and fear of revenge. In analysis, the feeling of emptiness often turns out to be a veil that covers the wider view and hides a lot. The complaint "I am so alone" raises the question: "Alone with whom?" Sometimes this question raises the veil and lets then see the destroyed objects. The destruction does not necessarily happen violently; it might have chosen a silent form that consists of a barely noticed detachment of libidinal investment. The feeling of emptiness is in such cases a consequence of a radical separation whose process and result were repressed.

For a student of art my office had great symbolic meaning during her analysis. First she had experienced it as "comfortably empty": it was a room, where she had enough space. This lasted some time, until she recognized that it was analysis and I, who in her mind created this space. "Only in the museum had I felt so free" occurred to her. Her associations passed on to Etruscan sarcophagi, and slowly the emptiness was filled with the corpses of female rivals, starting with her sisters. She triumphed over them whenever she felt well in a roomy place and liberated from the narrow struggles with siblings. Emptiness meant happiness in the beginnings of her analysis. Finally, she had an interested object for her own. Finally, she was no longer reminded of sharing with others and having to take care of them. Emptiness had the meaning of a liberating separation from her sisters and later on from other women, whom she unconsciously envied because of capacities that she missed in herself. These memories of "all the lost battles of rivalry" occurred to her, when she could no longer deny her envy towards me. She was convinced that I gave papers on every journey I made and that I deserted her in favour of my career success, while she was lying at home in a depressive mood, incapable of writing her essay about art. In a dream, she saw my office burning, so that it became empty and black. She expected me to be angry and feared my revenge. Since this did not happen, she asked me with a smile whether we might use the burning coal in her dream to light a pipe of peace. This way she expressed her wish for a ritualised reconciliation after her destructive fantasies against me and analysis. This dream came up again in her associations later and introduced new ideas, which had been unconscious until now. She wished not only to destroy me as an envied object, she also wanted to make me yearn for her. I should be full of desire to see her, just as she longed for me, especially during breaks, at weekends and during holidays. Now my office reminded her of a church, due to the indirect light. As a child she had to wait in the last row of the church because she was evangelical and not allowed to participate in Catholic ceremonies. She remembered that she spent these hours in melancholy desire and had gazed at the great golden mosaics on the ceiling representing God the Father. Other class mates were allowed to approach him, not her. Only in her fantasies did the priest invite her into the very first row. The silence and emptiness of the church was for her a desired space, and she invented a comforting solution for her slight, which was connected with oedipal feelings of being excluded. In the transference, my role oscillated between that of the desired, idealized object and that of a mother, whom she sometimes persecuted with envy, and multiplied by the sisters.

Thus a feeling of emptiness can hint at opposed vicissitudes of separation: at a separation that was (unconsciously) intended by murder of a hated object, or longing for an absent object whose presence, attention and love is deeply missed.

The latter reason for feelings of emptiness opens a larger field where imagination, symbolisation, fantasy and creativity flourish. If separation and loss do not exceed a tolerable degree, they trigger the development of the individual, especially during the first years of life. Nevertheless, separations remain from a subjective point of view frightening and painful events. Often a separation is a shock. Due to horrific fantasies, it is experienced as a terminal loss, even if in reality it is temporary and short. For a small child a separation from the mother, who went into the next room, might seem endless and irreparable. What the child experiences as a chasm, might be just a small crack. Without such experiences the capacity for symbolisation could not develop. The child, who is alarmed by separation from the mother, starts to call her and to look for symbolic equivalents for the missed object.

In adult life also the awareness of what is missed is decisive. If a lack becomes conscious, it provokes desire and longing, and so fantasy, imagination and creativity are conjured up.

Thus the experience of emptiness contains the polarities of destructive as well as of creative fantasies. It can be connected with (unconscious) guilt because of destructiveness and with fear of revenge; and it can be a prelude to great happiness if the separation from a love-object can be overcome by an act of creativity, thus providing a feeling of greater independence from external reality.

5.8 Psychosomatic impasses

If love and hate are too subtle to be verbalized, if there is no capacity to speak or if there is nobody to listen, then conflicts which might be raised by strong feelings cannot be verbalized either. They hardly will become conscious and cannot be worked through and conveyed to others. They are not filtered and sink down, unconscious and unarticulated, to a physical level where expression occurs in symptoms and dysfunctions. Therefore, for the psychoanalyst symptoms are not wrong tracks, but "truths of the speaking subject, even if to cool judgement they seem to be delusions". They are taken seriously as hints to the past, reactivated in the therapy revealing wishes and desires to the analyst and giving them "access to the powers of speech and at the same time bring the powers of speech into ostensibly nameless recesses of meaning" (Kristeva, 1987, 6 f.).

However, the capacity of verbalisation is not enough to produce change and cure. It is also necessary that somebody understands and picks up the hidden, unconscious meaning of the words (Zwettler-Otte, 2011, 128 ff.). Sometimes this "translation" is so difficult that it needs an intense commitment of attention and time, as provided in the psychoanalytic cure.

Valli, a 20 years old student, did not protest when the general practiser sent her to me with the diagnosis: bulimic anorexia. Three years earlier, she had been in a dangerous physical state due to anorexia and now she suffered from the opposite; she was tortured by voracious hunger. She hated herself for lack of discipline and for an inability to think of anything but food. Looking back, she considered her anorexia to be a heroic period in her life, when she still could control herself and was proud of her "wasp-waist". She believed that it was only for her slim figure that Stefan had fallen in love with her. Now she was sure that she would lose his love. Nevertheless even this threat could not stop her gluttony. On the contrary, she seemed to aim at the danger like a bicyclist who steers exactly onto the rocks he wants to avoid. It was not difficult to see that she unconsciously intended to provoke a separation, which she consciously feared so much, and that she repeated in this way a conflict that had been virulent many years ago, when her parents divorced and her father moved to another country. Her two years older brother, however, stayed with the father. Valli had not wanted to go to another country and lose her classmates, but living alone with her mother confused her. On one hand she pitied her mother, but on the other hand she thought that it was her fault that her father was gone, because she lost her attractiveness and did not pay attention to her appearance. For her it was more important to participate in charity activities of a society than to care for her family. Valli thrived at lessons even when she was ill, but she felt that nobody noticed. She felt ignored. Also just before her final exams she mentioned that she wished to become an actress. Her father dismissed her wish as crazy, her mother discouraged it; her brother mocked her. With resignation

Valli compromised by studying dramaturgy. She felt forbidden to try as many female roles as possible, to experience different facets of femininity, to be looked at on the stage and to be admired and loved. "Once more" she was not allowed to join in the play, once more she was excluded. At best she was an observer. The wording "once more" opened the way for memories of her time in the kindergarten. She had been allowed to go with her friend into a ballet-school and knew that she would become a ballet-dancer. Actually, it was less the pleasure of movement that fascinated her but the appeal of the wonderful ballet-costumes. Hesitating she told me about the light-green glowworm costume of her friend. The skirt of tulle was very short and one could see the tiny green panties whenever she moved or bent down. Valli became aware now of her sexual curiosity and of the meaning of her fascination. To slip into a ballet-costume meant reparation, a beautiful metamorphosis of the frightening sight of the genitals, which she liked to touch, because it caused such a strange feeling of pleasure. She was afraid to have ruined herself, "kaputt" (broken) by masturbation. The little green silk-panties, however belonged to a most beautiful, dainty, attractive part of the body. It was a partly successful effort to overcome the shock that her body looked so different from that of her brother, and it calmed down her fear to have seriously harmed her body. Her love to ballet escalated, when she and her friend once danced in a performance; her parents were in the audience, and afterwards her father said that dancing the czardas she had thrown her legs higher than her friend. She was so delighted about this praise, but she felt also uneasy and guilty to have "seduced" her father. This created such a conflict that she was ill the next day. When her friend gave up the ballet-school to learn singing, Valli's ballet-career ended. Until now the mother of her friend had driven the girls there, Valli's mother could not manage it without a car. Valli did not fight; she allowed the circumstances to stop it. Her resignation was due also to the slight that the ballet-master had not given her a desirable role in the ballet "Die Puppenfee". He planned to use her only as an extra. Nobody noticed a connection between these changes in Valli's life and her serious eating disturbances, which started soon after the end of the ballet lessons. Valli had lost – it would be more correct to say: left – the field, where she had been able to work through oedipal wishes and fears. She regressed to the oral level and expressed her protest by ceasing to eat. It was the same track she entered later during her puberty when her father left the family and she was diagnosed anorexic. When both parents criticized her ambition to become an actress she felt that the prohibition of her exhibitionistic wishes was repeated. She switched to bulimia. She could no longer control her impulses, which shifted to the oral level, and again and again gave herself up to an "oral orgasm". (Ermann, 2004, 284) This obsession was stronger than the real possibilities of sexual satisfaction with her boy friend, who probably had chosen such a "difficult" and unstable girl friend due to his own inner problems. When he had first met her during her anorectic phase, he was fascinated by her slim waist. He fell in love with her. Once, he drew her figure on a big paper and studied with excitement the contours of her body: "Once your body is there, then it is gone", he said to her, pointing to his preoccupation with parts of the body that were there or were missed. This somehow fit his incapacity to decide whether he should study psychology or sculpture. Now he was shocked by the transformation of Valli into a "shapeless monster without waist". Sometimes he joked that he would "chisel" her former beautiful form out again of her fat body.

In the meantime, Valli progressed in her analysis. At the beginning she had been suspicious whether I would be capable of helping her since she saw me as a "not unattractive woman, but not enough devoted to slimness". Nevertheless, she expected me to be as hostile to pleasure as her mother, but also as unfaithful as her father. She also heard me mocking at her like her brother, who did not like her and joined the father, mainly in order to climb up the mountains with him every weekend. This was a sport, Valli was not interested in because she felt even less gifted for it than for ballet. She is now finishing her study, and for half a year, she has been involved in the production of a play in a small theatre. She lost weight "nearly without noticing it", because her insatiable appetite vanished, and she is now content with her appearance. Her friend has – encouraged by her – started psychotherapy, which she considers sceptically, because it is not a psychoanalysis. But she appreciates their relationship enough to share his wish to give it a chance for further development. However, even more valuable than these external proofs of her improvement is her new capacity to articulate feelings and to face and discuss conflicts with her friend, her parents and her brother. She is now in contact with what is going on in her inner reality and is no longer forced to express problems on a somatic level.

6 Separation-anxiety in the psychotherapeutic process

6.1 Psychoanalysis and psychotherapy

Whether one starts psychotherapeutic training as a candidate or one is interested in psychotherapeutic treatment as a patient, at some point the question arises as to which method one should choose. It is a choice that is made primarily emotionally although it will be elaborated with rational criteria. The same is true for the choice of the psychoanalyst or psychotherapist. Very often one learns to value a method through some impressive person who represents this method. One might be touched by something he said and one continues to be interested. Thus the path to a psychoanalyst or psychotherapist starts with an emotional contact, even if we rationalize our "interest" – a very rational term for a very emotional process.

The topic of the apt form of psychotherapy cannot be discussed further here and is anyway very controversial. We only shall look at it regarding decision-making. *Decision means always separation from another or several other alternative(s). The prerequisite is the capacity to differentiate between the possibilities – one of the most important results of the capacity to separate.* If one has opted for a certain kind of therapy, other kinds of therapy with different assumptions and premises are excluded, and one parts with those possibilities. To come to a reasonable decision, one would have to know quite a lot about the theory and the clinical practice of all these kinds of psychotherapy. But the comparative research about psychotherapies has not developed very far. However, the theory and technique of psychoanalysis, is quite well elaborated. Many therapies are missing a theoretical base of their method; they form a "dark continent" (Green, 2005a, 30), of which we lack reliable maps. It would be our task as psychoanalysts to study this realm with our instruments so far as we are capable of clarifying and defending our capacities and limits within this vast jungle.

There still is not a sufficient understanding that linking differing basic assumptions of various therapies can lead to incompatibilities and confusions. It is not possible to work to reveal unconscious conflicts and to suppress them at the same time. A family therapist may consider it a good idea to send a patient, who is in a crisis, to a general practitioner, while in many cases a psychoanalyst would call it an acting out. Another example: if a patient does not pay the fee according to the agreements made at the launch of the treatment, some therapists don't mention it though secretly their aggression rises. They feel obliged to protect the 'positive relationship'. The psychoanalyst interprets the patient's hostile acting of aggression in order to work out together with him the reason for it. This can be a hidden wish for love resulting in reluctance to pay for it, or it might imply the contrary motive of a devaluing of the therapist, who is not worth his money.

Pointing at the possibility of incompatibilities does not mean rejection of other kinds of psychotherapy. It would rather be advisable for all kinds of therapies to act on the advice of Gotthold Ephraim Lessing's play of the wise Nathan. This wise man was consulted by three sons whose father left one of them a ring that would make the owner agreeable to God and men. But the father, who loved them all, had given all three a similar ring and no one knew which was the valuable one. Nathan advised that each of them should try to prove that his ring was the right one. Thus, each kind of therapy might try to prove that it is – according to clear theoretical and technical considerations – the right treatment for the specific case.

"Psychoanalysis" and "depth-psychology" are often used synonymously. Freud used the term "Tiefenpsychologie" (= depth-psychology), when he noted the fact that psychoanalytic conclusions were valid not only regarding psychopathology, but also in general, for instance regarding our dreams (cf. Freud, 1923, GW 13, 228; S.E. 18, 252).

If a psychotherapy claims to be depth-psychology but does not work with repressed material, and instead uses suggestion, encouragement, support and counselling, than it is a deception (see Zwettler-Otte 1995, 23-26 and 2009). Sometimes, therapies with one session per week are called "analysis" in order to feign psychoanalytic depth, so why should a patient be eager to invest four times as much time and money?

So incompatibilities among therapies remain problematic, although it would be helpful for patients to have a clear explication of different treatments, as far as possible. It is interesting that many therapeutic schools claim to be based on psychoanalysis or depth-psychology without taking on the basic assumptions of psychoanalysis – the existence of unconscious conflicts, of resistance and transference. The reasons for such unjustified claims are – beside all the well-publicized hostility against psychoanalysis - connected with the other side of the coin, the secret allure of psychoanalysis, which I mentioned earlier, and with the narcissistic motivation to be close to this controversial kind of psychotherapy, which is the most intensive and demanding one.

The lack of clarity among the therapists of diverse psychotherapeutic schools is of course reflected in patients. They feel attracted to kinds of psychotherapy that portray themselves as psychoanalytic or depth-psychological for the same reasons, but they hope that they will not have to make the same sacrifices of time and money as a proper psychoanalysis demands. This is an understandable but mostly unrealizable wish that is as old as psychoanalysis itself. Freud compared a half-hearted commitment to psychoanalysis with a serious, intensive one: "I am well aware that it is one thing to give utterance to an idea once or twice in the form of a passing aperçu, and quite another to mean it seriously – to take it literally and pursue it in the face of every contradictory detail, and to win it a place among accepted truths. It is the difference between a casual flirtation and a legal marriage with all its duties and difficulties." (Freud, 1914, S.E. 14, 15)

Some patients claim that psychoanalysis has to be free of charge, disregarding the fact that acquiring this knowledge demands from the analyst-to-be about 10 years of training including one's own analysis. The same patients usually don't mind spending an enormous amount of money for beauty care, journeys, car etc. However, some psychoanalysts themselves often feel under pressure to gratify such expectations and wishful thinking. This point has nothing to do with the obligation that we have to provide free places in psychoanalytic out-door-clinics for those who actually need social benefits. Many psychoanalytic societies of the IPA (International Psychoanalytic Society)[19] have already such departments. For prospective patients and for those who consider becoming psychoanalyst it might be helpful to know whether an analyst they address belongs to the IPA. Psychoanalysts of the IPA have careful and extensive training based on their own analysis, theoretical seminars over years and close supervision during their start as analysts. Thus if an analyst belongs to the IPA, it is, of course, no guarantee but still a much better chance that it is not one of those therapists who call themselves analysts without proper training.

6.2   The choice of an analyst

The title of this chapter may raise doubts whether it deals with problems faced by a prospective patient looking for an analyst, or the decision of an analyst as to offer analysis to a particular patient. This uncertainty is what I want. I am in fact dealing with both aspects, which are closely interlinked. My focus will be some of the components that enable or prevent an analytic couple - patient and analyst – coming into existence.

There are different opinions among psychoanalysts about the components facilitating or inhibiting the start of an analysis.

It is clear that from an extreme drive-theoretical standpoint the psychoanalyst is more or less an exchangeable object. The prospective patient has neither a great chance nor a great need for a choice. He will establish his transference according to his own inner reality without much regard to the real person of the analyst.

---

[19] The IPA was created in 1910 and owes its origin to Sigmund Freud, who believed an international organisation was essential to advance and safeguard his thinking and ideas. It was preceded by the Viennese Psychoanalytic Society ("Wiener Psychoanalytische Vereinigung" = WPV), which was first an unofficial group, the so-called psychological Wednesday-society ("psychologische Mittwoch Gesellschaft") of doctors gathering around Freud from 1902 on with the expressed intention of learning, practising and spreading the knowledge of psycho-analysis. On 15.4.1908 the name of the group was changed to "Wiener Psychoanalytische Vereinigung", and on 13.4.1910 it became an official society, attached to the "International Psychoanalytic Society", which has now institutes all over the world.

Other colleagues focus on the object-relation. Considered from an extreme object-theoretical viewpoint, the influence of the analyst's personality will be more decisive. Not every analyst provokes the same pattern of transference in every patient. Apparently small, superficial similarities with persons who were important in the patient's earlier life or echoes of former emotional atmospheres trigger specific experiences in the patient. With another analyst these memories might emerge less quickly or with less intensity. Often a patient is not really un-analysable, but just not analysable by this specific analyst. "It is no less serious for the analyst to be mistaken about his own capabilities than about the patient's." (Green, 1993, 36)

In my view, only the combination of a drive-theoretical and an object-relational aspect makes sense. The choice of an analyst (regarding the patient as well as the psychoanalyst) offers us an essential example of the fact that intra- and inter-psychic together form such a dense web that touching one side moves the whole web, disturbing the whole structure. We cannot pick just one element. There is nothing to make us decide in favour of one or the other extreme position – indeed, any attempt to do so is a misleading oversimplification. Following a famous wording of D.W. Winnicott – "There's no such thing as a baby" –, underlining the close interdependence of mother and child (Winnicott 1991, 127 ff.), we might say:

There is no such a thing as an object...

(which is not cathected by drives).

It was Freud who first showed the interdependence of drive and object in 'Beyond the Pleasure Principle' (S.E. 18, 63), saying that the binding of these is a preparatory act which introduces and assures the dominance of the pleasure principle.

This point has been reworked recently by André Green, who follows Freud's conviction that pre-eminence should be given to the drives. Green points out: "Transference is, above all, bound; that is, the analyst offers a relationship at the beginning of the treatment, the threads of which are woven together in the course of the analytic experience, leading to its final denouement and making way for new relationships with other objects." (Green, 2002, 131)
With regard to the role of the person of the analyst, we have to recognize that "[...] intersubjectivity is related to the respective intrapsychic dimensions which enter into the composition of intersubjective relations. In fact, the two dimensions, intersubjective and intrapsychic, are interdependent." (Green, 2002, 58) The question, then, of having to choose either an intra- or an interpsychic orientation compounds an artificial split whose justification lies only in the fact that it was necessary to complete Freud's view in some aspects. Green

continues, "[...] the experience of transference and the comparison between the transference of transference neuropsychoses and that of patients presenting non-neurotic structures (borderline, narcissistic personalities, patients suffering from psychosomatic phenomena) helps us to realise that Freud greatly underestimated the role of the object." (163). And Green states clearly: "We can now understand, better than ever before, that it is not a case of choosing between drive and object, but of thinking about how they are coupled." (125) To conclude a never-ending discussion about either drive or object he reminds us, in "The Chains of Eros": "Psychoanalysis has exhausted itself for too long in opposing the theory of drives to that of object relations. The time has come to grasp that the solution lies in the theorisation of the *drive-object pairing. There is no sexuality without an object, but there is no object which is not cathected by drives and which does not respond to the cathexis by introducing the effect of its own drives there.*" *(Green, 2001, 136).*

My considerations regarding the choice of an analyst are based on the assumption that neither the drive-structure of the patient nor the personality of the psychoanalyst are alone decisive for the question whether they make up their mind to start an analysis, but that both factors are already at work during the start of an analysis.

The choice of an analyst is the choice of an object. Again, this is true for both sides, although we may assume that it is only the patient who is driven by some need to search a new object. If things work well the analyst will succeed in understanding together with the patient what kind of object the patient unconsciously intends to make of the analyst, following old models of his relationships because they are usually unconscious. Thus, it is the function of the analyst to be a very special object, which is only partly a real one and partly allows to be transformed in the patient's mind into different figures. The analyst recognizes and responds to this role of the patient (cf. Sandler & Sandler, 1998, 47 ff.) prescripts, without taking it over. Instead, he will interpret what is going on so that the patient can escape the compulsion to repeat. *Thus, the choice of an analyst is also a separation from old objects. The patient often seems to realize this with some fear.* Like Janus, the analyst might display two faces from the patient's point of view: that of the real object and that of the transference object. This double role is without doubt decisive in the first interview. However, it will be necessary during the whole treatment that the analyst cleaves to the psychoanalytic attitude regarding the unconscious transference, especially when for the patient both roles inevitably get blurred. And the patient will again and again come to a critical moment of choice during the analytic cure when he has to decide whether he can bear and make use of this special form of relationship. It is for both sides a demanding form of a relationship, characterized by the priority of understanding over satisfaction. However, instinctual wishes don't have such sublime aims as knowledge and insight. Therefore the fallacious idea will often, secretly or openly, prevail that only the satisfaction of the patient's longing for love will provide his cure. It is a decision, which arises one way or another in every session, and, it is, again, a matter for both analyst and patient. Because the *choice of an analyst (in his function as a very special object) is not only a starting point, but an ongoing process. One partner of the analytic couple has to fight for remaining an analyst, while the other partner will have to fight to accept this – even against his wishes.*

This struggle for both analyst and patient is between insight and resistances aiming to avoid painful feelings and for easier satisfactions. Gregorio Kohon described how the form of love Freud called „*Wissenstrieb"(drive for knowledge)* must win the battle: "The impulse for knowledge does not exclude the desire to ignore. This is fully demonstrated in every session, every day, by the patient on the couch: after all, it is the patient's unconscious resistance to knowledge, which allows psychoanalytic treatment to happen. This is not a limitation of psychoanalysis; on the contrary, it is what gives psychoanalysis its creative edge." (Kohon, 1999a, 156 f.)

To this, I would add – in relation to the analytic couple – that it is not only the patient, who struggles between the impulse for knowledge and the impulse for ignorance. Sometimes the analyst too becomes involved in this conflict, and at times is in danger of giving in to the patient's wishes for a different form of care and comfort, instead of interpreting what he sees. D.W. Winnicott wrote in his paper "The Aims of Psycho-Analytical Treatment" about this issue. He described his usually economical interpretations and demonstrated how he has sometimes to fight against the wish to relax: "I never use long sentences unless I am very tired. If I am near exhaustion point I begin teaching." (Winnicott, 1990, 167) Here fatigue stirs a stab at compensation. In other cases, the waning of concentration might occur and weaken the capacity to work analytically. Oscillations of attention are unavoidable and no reason to seriously reproach the analyst. It simply shows that the psychoanalytic cure is not only trying for the patient but also for the analyst. The latter, too, has to struggle to do his job, and there are for him moments of choice whether he lets things go or whether he interferes, interpreting. A phrase of a rider comes to mind: "It is not the question, whether one loses control over the horse or not, but how quickly one gets back control, if it is lost."

There are many roads to a *first contact with psychoanalysis.* Some of my patients heard about it at school; some came across psychoanalytic literature "by chance"; some felt nudged in its direction by colleagues working in a hospital; some had a friend in analysis; some heard a public lecture, and so on. However, they discovered it, each became curious about it because of a feeling of having been touched in a very personal way. This feeling was sometimes very vague, and sometimes struck like a lightning flash. One student, in his first interview with me, explained that reading Freud's 'Interpretation of Dreams', he was reminded of classical tragedies that provoke in the audience the sense of "TUA RES AGITUR" ("its deals with *your* concerns"). What is important for our subject is that, even in this preliminary realm, we can see the involvement of drive-derivates: the development of curiosity, the arousal of preconscious conflicts and wishes that create a feeling of *being touched* and often also *envy that a psychoanalyst might have a hidden knowledge that makes him win in competition.* All these feelings motivate a return of interest to psychoanalytic issues over and over again. *If personal and familiar thoughts are touched, this means bound. Thus the first contact with psychoanalysis addresses the issue of binding and separating.*

Very often, there is *a lot of ambivalence,* which reflects a pre-existing inner struggle between the drive for knowledge and the passion for ignorance. Depending on which of these is pre-eminent, the prospective analysand's perception will be heightened for the confirming or denying the value of psychoanalysis.

Some people remain locked in such a struggle, maintaining a discrete distance from analysis. For others, the decision to contact an analyst takes a very long time, often many years. Some, indeed, wait for so long before finally discovering the solution for their defence in that they might now be too old for analysis, an excuse, which nowadays has less likely to be shared by an analyst than in Freud's time (cf. Junkers, 2002). Here it becomes evident that it is a choice for both the analyst and the potential patient to make, a choice determined by conscious, preconscious and unconscious factors, as to whether analysis will be considered useful or not.

I think that beside all hostilities against psychoanalytic treatment – which have not changed so much during the last 100 years –, and beside all efforts to substitute for it cheaper and less demanding forms of psychotherapy, there is the *secret allure* of psychoanalysis that is greatly underestimated in comparison to the animosity it invokes. *This attraction is, in my opinion, principally aroused when personal unconscious material (with all its drive-theoretical implications), and unconscious conflicts, comes into contact with psychoanalytic ideas. During this encounter "repressed material which struggles for freedom" – as Freud said in 'Psycho-Analysis Terminable and Interminable' (Freud, 1937b, S.E. 23, 209) – is able to emerge briefly and consequently places less of a demand upon the exercise of repression. This temporary unburdening reduces tension and can be experienced as pleasure. Naturally, without the analyst as an object, this relief usually cannot last long, and the defences may become even stronger afterwards. On the surface, what we can see is a high degree of ambivalence. Such ambivalence has characterized, from the very beginning, the way psychoanalysis is received by the public as well as by the individual.*

A positive reception of psychoanalysis seems to me to have two prerequisites:
1. that psychoanalysis is represented by psychoanalysts in the right way,
2. that the feeling of being touched, curious and relieved is perceived, by the psychoanalysts as well as by the recipients.

What is needed is work on the part of the transmitter and on the side of the receiver. The term 'work' is fitting, since it is about overcoming resistances. 'Work' is an important word in psychoanalytic theory. We speak of dream-work, the work of mourning, of working through etc. (cf. Green, 1999, VII). 'Work' is a strenuous process that deals with the change of a balance and thus with destabilisation. I think that we have not done our part very well; we rather left everything to chance. If we call the consequences of this neglect "crisis", it sounds like "fate" and not like willingness to take responsibility for this work. That is why I would not speak of 'crisis' but prefer to speak about *the work of reception*. It needs two partners, similar to other professional relationships, like that of doctor and patient, teacher and student, businessman and customer etc.

In this preliminary area too, psychoanalysts – both as individuals and/or as members of a professional group – have some influence as to whether they make themselves available. I refer to the way psychoanalysis is represented in the public sphere. Sometimes, indeed, there is no representation, which has its own unfortunate implications for the profession. The representation – or lack of it, as a negative form – is influenced by unconscious factors and by the conviction – or lack of conviction – that analysts themselves have concerning the value of analysis. Janice de Saussure stated in a paper about 'Dilemmas and challenge of the psychoanalyst today' that, in her opinion, "the crisis we have to face as psychoanalysts comes from our own loss of trust in the psychoanalytical process" (Saussure, 1996, 135), and she recommends that we strengthen our enthusiasm by deepening our understanding. She does not go into details, but we can assume that this deepening of our understanding of the psychoanalytic process is linked to our own inner state. Are we still in a position to *live from the forces that were liberated in our own analysis?* And were we capable of *transforming it into an analysis interminable?* Or have so many years passed since we concluded our training analysis that our experience will appear to us like a madness of youth, because we have no idea what is going on in our present unconscious? Do we have in the back of our mind the awareness that we might at some occasion need to refresh our psychoanalytic capacities for understanding?

Freud pointed to this possibility: "It would not be surprising, if the effect of a constant preoccupation with all the repressed material which struggles for freedom in the human mind were to stir up in the analyst as well all the instinctual demands which he is otherwise able to keep under suppression. These, too, are 'dangers of analysis', […] and we ought not to neglect to meet them. There is no doubt how this is to be done. Every analyst should periodically – at intervals of five years or so – submit himself to analysis once more, without feeling ashamed of taking this step." (Freud, 1937b, S.E. 23, 249) Maybe this recommendation of Freud's is not put into action often enough. I would like to connect it with two considerations of analysts nowadays. A. Green as well as A. Sandler questioned whether analyses should last so long. This problem includes the capacity of separation on both sides. Both, analyst and patient or candidate, are in danger of being lazy and inclined to delay this uncomfortable work of parting. Green refers to Freud's advice and speaks about a "military service": returning every few years for a short period to the couch to keep the contact to one's own unconscious alive in a psychoanalytic relationship, which would be preferable to extended analyses (Green, 2002, 46).

A third reference to this issue was made in a discussion of analysts belonging to the group of Melanie Klein. Somebody asked whether it was possible to learn a special analytic technique only by supervision, without one's own analysis in this technique. The answer after a lot of consideration was positive.

Thus, the analyst repeatedly has to make a choice, whether he is ready *to care for an optimal maintenance of his psychoanalytic capacity and if he is ready, in which way does he want to achieve it, by another tranche of psychoanalysis, or by supervision.*

If an analyst needs psychoanalytic help without admitting this to himself, envy might prevent him recommending analytic treatment to someone else. Also if an analyst looking back on his own analysis is dissatisfied with the experience, he might be tempted to suggest to potential patients less demanding forms of psychotherapy. *Envy and disappointment* influence the choice of an analyst, whether he recommends entering analysis or not; this is especially the case, when these feelings are unconscious.

I have mentioned that having studied the public reception of psychoanalysis from its beginnings I am convinced that we should not speak about a *"crisis" of psychoanalysis*. This word means a decisive moment, whereas the "crisis" of analysis is a permanent condition. The ambivalence psychoanalysis always met has lasted for more than one hundred years, because analysis was decreed dead and buried from the start it belongs to the core of psychoanalysis to attract and push away at the same time.

With such an oscillation between attraction and rejection many potential patients approach an analyst for their first interview. Anyone interested will be able to find in *external reality* arguments for or against the analytic enterprise, and supports and obstacles galore for the decision, which has probably been made already inside and which only needs confirmation.

To prevent misunderstanding: my interest here is a vision of inner reality in confrontation with external reality. I don't deny that sometimes there are real external difficulties involved in arranging a psychoanalysis. But if it really concerns external obstacles, we are led back to the poor representation of psychoanalysis in the public arena, and to the challenge to make psychoanalytic treatment available in public institutions such as outpatients' departments. Whatever the facilities are, they belong to the possibilities on offer. By the way, it was customary in the first generation of psychoanalysts that each analyst took a patient who could pay very little or nothing at all, although especially the latter situation entailed a lot of technical problems.

Prompted by ambivalence, the frequent choice made by prospective patients is a compromise. Instead of psychoanalysis, psychoanalytical psychotherapy is requested or a psychotherapeutic method that presents itself as based on 'depth-psychology' – which sounds to some people a bit less daunting than 'psychoanalysis'. Daniel Widlöcher, a former president of the International Psychoanalytic Association points out our own contribution to misleading the public when psychoanalysts neglect to make it clear that there does not exist a "psychoanalysis lite", along the lines of a "Cola light"; nothing that contains all the advantages and none of the disadvantages of long-term treatment. He stressed that it is the complexity of the transference, which is absent in more easily available psychotherapies (Widlöcher, 1996, 327).

I think that we have neither conducted sufficient research nor adequately taught others about the difference between psychoanalysis and psychoanalytic psychotherapy. Therefore, we are not clear enough in our intent. In this context, a paper of Johannes Ranefeld (2003) seems interesting, claiming that psychoanalytic psychotherapy is not a diluted variant, a deficient form of psychoanalysis. It is psychoanalysis, and especially demanding in regard to the analyst's ability.

In spite of many psychotherapeutic alternatives patients still come to psychoanalysts. Some believe that they should try proper analysis because of their impression that psychoanalysts make fewer promises than other psychotherapists. A student, recalling his first contact with psychoanalysis, said: "I had the feeling that there was a greater honesty in this psychoanalyst giving a public lecture; he stated that he himself did not know what might be the outcome of an analysis he had started with somebody, he only knew that he was ready to work with this patient and that this patient was ready too." Although the lack of diagnosis and scientific proofs was a concern for this potential patient, he decided to follow his feelings. What touched him were the honesty and the renunciation of the temptation to manipulate. It was the *space created by uncertainty* which, for this person, paved the way for new development.
In *making contact with a psychoanalyst* we can be sure that it is not only conscious arguments that underlie the decision as to whom to approach. Someone looking for an analyst tries to make a rational judgement, but emotional factors play a greater role. The patient mentioned above, for instance, did not choose the analyst whose lecture he admired. He chose me "due to sympathy" as he said. The unconscious libidinal impulses towards me and the contempt he had felt towards this "weak" male analyst, beside the admiration, he would discover only after years of analysis. The choice of a specific analyst has undoubtedly *not only to do with the conscious wish to have an analysis, but at the same time also with unconscious wishes to avoid one.* Behind the "sympathy" of this patient was – as we found out thanks to a dream – a fantasy

to become my "favourite son". He also hoped I would not treat him too harshly, as eventually the male analyst would do, who may have covered with his "weakness" an underlying tendency to cruelty. In the choice of an analyst there always is involved an element of resistance and pathology.

Another patient had been proud of her careful selection of the right analyst. She changed her mind in the third year of analysis: "I can no longer say that I really have chosen you out of reasonable arguments; somehow I only managed to bring myself here like a severely injured person might bring herself to a hospital before breaking down" – and reverting somewhat to her former conviction she added, laughing – "but a carefully chosen hospital!" This reminded me of Winnicott's True and False Self: "It is as if a nurse brings a child, and at first the analyst discusses the child's problem, and the child is not directly contacted. Analysis does not start until the nurse has left the child with the analyst." (Winnicott, 1990, 151) Later on this young woman was able to see that not only libidinal wishes for my help were key motives but also an intent to prove me wrong and make me fail in her treatment.

To summarize: *the "choice" of an analyst is not a primarily conscious decision but is mainly based on unconscious impulses, wishes and fears.* The student tried to escape his castration-anxieties by avoiding an analyst who might really be fierce (like his father) behind a façade of weakness. The female patient imagined that behind my empathy would be a flaw that would allow her to thwart me – which she had not managed with her mother and her elder sister. Can we ever speak of a "choice" of an analyst if consciousness plays such a small role? A psychoanalytic initial interview leaves free space for the unconscious to unfold. Thus the patient may realise that here something important can be *continued*, which leads to a decision to enter analysis. This *continuation* we call in our theoretical language *transference*. In the first interview the unconscious fantasies form invisible hooks, which delve deeply in the past and upon which the present hangs. (Cf. Sandler & Sandler, 1983 and 1986, who dealt with the present and the past unconscious.)

There is another aspect that is important in connection with beginning an analysis. Freud spoke about the *narcissistic wound* mankind endured on learning that "the ego is not master in its own house" (Freud, 1917, S.E. 17, 143), since the unconscious rules there. The possibility of learning to decipher messages from the unconscious, though they will be incomplete and untrustworthy, promises at least some control over the power of the unconscious. Thus, the narcissistic wound might eventuate in a *narcissistic triumph*. There is also another source of narcissistic supply in the rapt attention that the patient receives from the analyst. This is often recognized clearly at the end of the analysis. One patient, hesitating about ending his analysis, said: "Now I know, why analyses last so long: because it is so nice to have one." And more seriously he added: "Although, I now have a very good relationship with my wife, I feel a big loss about the end of our work: this is the only place I have the right to demand full attention just for me." And it was a long time before he could value his independence more highly than the narcissistic rewards of psychoanalysis.

There is no doubt that Freud's saying in "The question of lay analysis" (Freud, 1926, S.E. 20, 183-250) about the connection between research and cure („Junktim von Forschen und Heilen"), meets the need of many analysands to be considered a companion on a journey into unknown territory rather than as a dependent patient. This portrayal of being the analyst's companion is an important narcissistic reward, as opposed to the authoritarian attitude usually expected from medical doctors. It introduces a "therapeutic split" (Sterba, 1932, 53 ff.) in the Ego of the patient and contains an essential nucleus of truth that provides a compensation for the experience of becoming dependent again. It is interesting that Freud uttered this thought about the connection between research and cure as early as 1895 in a paper about hysteria („Über Hysterie"), which was summarized in a medical journal: „The method of research, which has to be applied to hysteria, coincides with the cure." („Die Untersuchungsmethode, die bei der Hysterie anzuwenden ist, fällt zusammen mit der Therapie." – Tichy, Zwettler-Otte, 1999, 39)

No matter which symptoms, disturbances, inhibitions or inabilities somebody is suffering – maybe a pressure from the past that needs to re-emerge – the patient needs a new event (the present of the transference situation) for events of his past to really become history. The new experience of transference is the necessary condition for the past to *become*", Gregorio Kohon wrote in his book "No lost certainties to be recovered" (Kohon, 1999a, 162).

Returning to the choice of the analyst, who recommends entry to analysis in the initial interview, we have to consider the role that *the personality of the analyst* plays. In 'Analysis terminable and interminable' Freud stated that not only the quality of the patient's Ego, but also the particularity of the analyst, influences the outcome of the analytical cure and will make it more or less difficult to deal with the resistances of the patient (Freud, 1937, S.E. 23, 247). Here again we find an important hint that Freud did not elaborate in detail. The importance of the characteristic features of an object only became clear later on and was to be emphasized by analysts working out object relations theory.

Winnicott, for instance, did take into consideration the *differences amongst analysts*, as well as the fact that *the analyst himself changes*. He wrote "[...] analysts are not alike. I am not like I was twenty or thirty years ago. Some analysts undoubtedly work best in the simplest and most dynamic area where conflict between love and hate, with all its ramifications in conscious and unconscious fantasy, constitutes the main problem. Other analysts work as well or better when they are able to deal with more primitive mental mechanisms in the transference neurosis or transference psychosis. In this way [...] they extend the field of operation and the range of the cases they can tackle. This is research analysis, and the danger is only that the patient's needs in terms of infantile dependence may be lost in the course of the analyst's performance." (Winnicott,

1990, 169) Winnicott not only stresses the importance of the particular analyst as an object interested in the particularities of a specific patient, but also the narcissistic reward the analyst may gain. If the analyst takes a greater distance from the patient, he may regard him as an interesting being to be studied and cured with skill, having more in mind the narcissistic rewards of such an approach. "The assumption of the cure position is also an illness, only it is the other side of the coin. We need our patients as much as they need us", Winnicott stated (Winnicott, 1986, 116 ff.). He described two extreme positions: the "care-curer" and the "technicians", who are in danger of forgetting that care also belongs to medical practice (113); Winnicott tries to return to a holistic approach, arguing that an analyst has to provide both care *and* technical skill. We can find a similar idea in Michael Parson's "The Dove that Returns", "The Dove that Vanishes": Parsons points out that it would be wrong to compare an analyst *either* with a healer *or* with a non-attached, technically competent repairman, because the essence of psychoanalysis includes both.

All these factors – summarized as the analyst's particularity – contribute to the decision whether one wants and needs an object with which to form an analytic pair and to acknowledge that libidinal, aggressive and narcissistic aspects are involved in this choice for both participants. It is to be hoped, however, that the analyst's choice is a good deal more conscious one than that of the patient. The analyst might, for instance, think: "This is a nice person, and after a few years of psychoanalysis he/she might be less inhibited and incapable of making decisions and enjoying his/her life." Such a view contains a mixture of drive-aspects. The libidinal aspect is seen in the sympathy that appears carefully measured. The aggressive aspect aims at the pathology. The narcissistic aspect lies in the pleasing vision of how this person might improve thanks to the analyst. There are dangers everywhere. When analyst and patient fit too well they may become a couple who bolster each other's defences, "normalizing pathology" (Kohon, 1999a, 52). An example would be a prominent analyst and a patient who is very successful in his profession. They might become a narcissistic couple, allying against the rest of the world instead of engaging in analysing the patient's social fears, his megalomaniac ideas and his hidden bleeding wounds.

In order to weigh both possibilities, we must consider that the patient as well as the analyst might act against the common task of analysis. The patient might be aware from the first interview that he is not ready to invest so much time and money. He might become conscious of his fears, or he might feel that he does not wish to start this enterprise with this psychoanalyst. The analyst also might decide against taking someone into treatment. Many reasons for such a choice spring to mind: some will be rooted in the analyst's preferences and dislikes, whether he is aware of their inner vicissitudes or not. Others will be connected with concerns about the potential patient's resistances, which might seem too powerful; or concerns about the patient's circumstances, as, for instance, in the case of a brilliant façade that would be endangered by a successful analysis, so that the cost might exceed the profit. Another reason might be that the analyst realizes that his capacities will be inhibited by counter-transference regarding the fact that this patient is involved in relationships unbearable for the analyst, as for instance, criminality or fascist ideas. Not every patient provokes in the analyst the urge to provide a holding-function. One might label the opposite reaction as a *"dropping-function": a recognition of one's own limits at the right moment. Both choices – the holding and the dropping – can be the result of professional reliability and a sense of responsibility, based on the awareness that analysing means to intervene seriously in another individual's inner and external life.*

The decision of a potential patient to start analysis and the analyst's decision to take this patient into treatment is a dense network of factors. The most important factors are usually unconscious at the time of the decision.

The role of the analyst is not as transferable as it might appear from an extreme drive-theoretical point of view. The personality of the psychoanalyst is very important, although it might be distorted and misinterpreted by the patient's inner reality. This process is about the combination of intra- and interpsychic processes, not about the priority of any one of them.

The analyst takes a double role as real object and as transference object. The choice of analyst and patient to enter this special and demanding relationship is a decision that has to be made not only at the beginning but again and again during the psychoanalytic cure.

The first contact with psychoanalytic ideas causes in most future patients a feeling of being touched in some resonant personal way. This is the core of the *secret allure of psychoanalysis* and has in my view been neglected in comparison with the outright hostility psychoanalysis has encountered. *Attraction and rejection result in an image of strong ambivalence that characterized the reception of psychoanalysis from its beginning until now.* That is why I suggest we do not speak of a "crisis" of psychoanalysis, but rather of an enduring facet regarding the reception of psychoanalysis (cf. Zwettler-Otte, 2006b and 2009).

Ambivalence influences not only potential patients but also psychoanalysts themselves. They have to decide how they portray psychoanalysis to the public, whether they care to test the extent of their psychoanalytic capacities, whether they respond to the compromises that other forms of psychotherapy offer, and how to respond to those who are looking for psychoanalysis and need it. If in the first contact between analyst and potential patient curiosity arises on both sides regarding possible new, positive developments, the choice can be made in favour of a psychoanalytic enterprise.

Five aspects of the first interview

Focusing on the *initial interview* I would like to draw attention to five aspects which seem to me crucial for the patient's and the analyst's choices and for bringing an analytical pair into existence:

1. The drive for knowledge might be activated.

The patient must have an idea about why *it might be helpful for him to understand his own Unconscious (cf. Eckstaedt, 1991, 14).* He might become aware that the analyst will refrain from giving information or advice, because it is not a lack of knowledge that is pathogenic, but rather the reasons for this lack, the inner resistances that create and sustain this lack, as Freud pointed out in "On 'wild' psychoanalysis".

2. The priority of feelings

The diminished respect for rational knowledge is paired with an intensified acknowledgment of feelings. The patient's transference will have begun to burgeon during the call to fix an appointment (cf. Argelander, „Vorfeld-Phänomene", 16); and what seems to me to be equally important is that the patient will already have an impression about how the analyst will react to his demands. Eckstaedt is right that often the decision about analysis is made during the first sentences spoken on the phone (Eckstaedt, 1991, 38). This decision is an emotional one and has a lot to do with transference love. Julia Kristeva asks at the end of "In the Beginning Was Love": "Is it not true that analysis begins with something comparable to faith, namely transferential love? 'I trust you, and I expect something in return'." (Kristeva, 1987, 52). This remains true even in the case of someone declaring that he or she does not trust either analysis or the analyst. A new patient said at the end of the first appointment, rejecting my offer of a second, intended to make sure she would not feel pressured in her decision: "No, I want to fix it right now. It does not matter *whom* I won't be trusting." She did not realize that behind her contempt there was (amongst other things) hope - and trust, moving her to start analysis with me before I might recognize her hate and withdraw my offer.

3. The connection of the present and the past.

During the initial interview the inner reality of the patient usually appears closely intertwined with external reality. Old relationships to former and present objects will demand to be re-established in "the architecture of the present" (Eckstaedt, 1991, 13). "The unconscious of the past intrudes into the unconscious of the present" (Sandler & Sandler, 1983, 423). A slight sense of this movement may be felt during the first interview with the patient. In the best case the choice for analysis will be supported by experience of an *atmosphere of tolerance* generated by the analyst. This tolerance will turn out, during the actual analysis, to be an attitude of acceptance towards repressed infantile, perverse or ridiculous wishes, enabling the patient to integrate an understanding of these aspects of himself. It is easy to see that such tolerance is incompatible with a diagnostic interview which a patient may experience as intrusive, and which, instead of guiding him into treatment, would make shy him away (Leupold-Löwenthal, 1985, 38).

4. The analyst's capacity to bear uncertainties.

Even if the analyst feels ready to sketch a first draft of the (re-)construction of the patient's past, the most important experience for the patient will be the cautious attitude of the analyst, the admission that these are now only conjectures waiting for confirmation or abandonment, as Freud put it in "constructions in analysis" (1937). Again – as mentioned earlier – the analyst will renounce to pretend certainties where there are none, and he will provide a space for *re-experiencing* (cf. Kohon, 1999a, 160) that really matters. A touching example of such an attitude occurs in a case-vignette Andreas Giannakoulas gave. There the analyst's hesitation about holding a picture of the patient's father, which the patient had offered him hesitantly himself, kept "a sense of distance" which could contain the patient's loving and aggressive feelings and his teetering between fusion and separateness; (Giannakoulas 2001, 157).

5. The special analytic situation as a serious play.

While there may be the danger for a suffering individual to get lost in the inner reality, addressing an analyst is a step into the opposite direction, into external reality. This impulse, which seems to be a 'healthy' reaction against regression, we might call "hunger for reality" (Zwettler-Otte, 1996, 237); making an analysis will not mean turning away from inner reality, but providing a space where it will be less dangerous to look at it. Taking into account what David Tuckett added to the "Construction of the Potential Space" (loc. cit. 161 f.), warning about the use of concepts like "play", I would nevertheless like to maintain that it can be helpful if the patient, in the first encounter with the analyst, can get at least a vague idea about "*the unnatural and contradictory*" in psychoanalysis (Loewald, 1980, 364 f). While the patient is entering a psychoanalytic relationship to gain a deeper understanding of human relationships, there is at the same time, and from the very beginning, a movement in the opposite direction: one towards the denial of "real" relationship, one that makes psychoanalysis into a kind of "*dramatic play*" which the analyst and the analysand are enacting. In this play the history of the individual will be revived and structured, and through this new meanings will be found and old ones re-found. But this relationship itself is not to become real, having the essence and transitoriness of a theatre-performance and being like the play of a child. Even if the patient forgets about this impression as soon as he is "well-settled into the timelessness of the treatment" (Green, 2001, 45) it may be that, several years later, he can return to this point, terminating his analysis "with the renewed desire to question all received truths [...] capable once again of acting like a child, of playing" (Kristeva, 1987, XI).

6.3   The setting and the frequency of sessions

We shall restrict our considerations here to the normal psychoanalytic setting of an analysis that takes place several times a week (three to five times, 45 to 50 minutes, the patient lying on the couch). In some analyses, the patient sits opposite the analyst. The external arrangement alone is not enough for determining whether it is an analysis or psychotherapy. This fact can also be used to blur the borders: many treatments are unjustifiably called "analysis". What is important is that the analyst arranges the optimal schedule of sessions according to the analyst's experience and to the need of the patient regarding his structure, his resistances, his demands and his unconscious and manifest transference (Green, 2005a, 29).

If the analysand arrives daily and free-associates on the couch, this is not only a way to flush unconscious material to the surface. It is also a caesura, a *separation* and differentiation from a normal conversation. The psychoanalytic setting embodies the inner structure (Parsons, 1999, 64 ff.) and represents the mind in a dream-like state. This historic offspring from hypnosis provided a link between the psychoanalytic setting and the dream, the censorship and the resistance from the start onward. Free association has some similarities with the state just before falling asleep and so it facilitates the activity of the unconscious. Thus, unconscious material is brought to the surface and allows the intrapsychic conflict to be examined. This process occurs in front of an observer, the psychoanalyst, who cannot remain a non-participant. His attention bridges the abyss between latent and manifest material. In a manner of speaking, he takes over the role of the ego of the patient and tries to sort out the unconscious wishes that are obscured by the patient's defences. But the analyst also plays a double role. He offers through his special setting a peaceful, reliable environment that invites regression via the resting position and the encouragement to say, whatever comes to the mind. R*egression* is also fostered by the regular rhythm of the sessions, the silence and the benevolent attitude of the analyst, who is outside the patient's sight line and who does not convey his own reactions. All these regression-facilitating elements *separate* the psychoanalytic situation from normal everyday life, where not everything that comes to mind is spoken and where it is not always quiet and reliable.

However, the psychoanalytic setting includes elements opposed to a freedom granting function. The patient is invited to say whatever occurs to him, but to do nothing about it. This means he should verbalize all his feelings and wishes, but he should not act out anything. He should tolerate the situation that his wishes are understood, but not fulfilled. His sessions are fixed and obligatory, whether he uses them or not. Also these restrictions *separate* the psychoanalytic situation from a normal one where activity and flexibility is mostly welcome. The analysand often feels disappointed or confused by this polarity of freedom and restriction. Thus, the psychoanalyst represents two kinds of objects. The patient wants to separate the objects and to keep contact with just one of them (Parsons,

1999, 66). That is exactly the split that the patient should not be able to make; otherwise he would lose his analyst.

Andrè Green demonstrated how the psychoanalytic situation is stretched between three poles: a dream-like narcissistic state, the maternal-caring attitude by the analyst, and an incest-prohibiting attitude (Green, 1984). The psychoanalytic frame creates a triangulation redolent of the oedipal situation and the unconscious structure of the Oedipus-complex, and similar to the inner state of the dreaming individual in whom wish and prohibition fighting one other.

Comparing the psychoanalytic setting with other psychotherapies one will recognize in the latter that there is less tension between opposed attitudes, between allowance and restriction. The therapist takes mainly the role of a "good" object. This renders psychotherapies more comfortable, as also regarding arrangements concerning fees and the cancellation of sessions.

The correct frequency of sessions for psychoanalysis is often debated by psychoanalysts. Colleagues, who wish to take pressures of reality more into consideration are opposed by those concerned about a tendency to adapt to less demanding psychotherapies and to neglect our psychoanalytic method. I agree with the provisional decision to await further results of psychoanalytic research regarding analyses conducted with three and five sessions per week before formulating new "minimal standards" for candidates. However, it might be necessary to do more public work to explain clearly to potential candidates, patients and funding institutions the conditions that psychoanalysis needs for functioning and why so much work and time is necessary. This is not the only way our method differs from other psychotherapies. We are pleased that our results attest to our efficiency, which is acknowledged even by representatives of health insurance schemes. They notice, for instance, that in certain diseases there are shorter stays in hospital after a patient starts analysis, so that ultimately psychoanalytic treatment is cheaper.

However, it is not only because pressure of financial situations that the frequency of sessions is an important theoretical and technical issue. A tight density of sessions emphasizes the *presence* of the analyst – a conviction we find in the British school of psychoanalysis. Lower frequency, as the French psychoanalytic school suggest, stresses the analyst's *absence*. The arguments in favour of five sessions per week rest on the greater intensity of the transference obtained thereby. Colleagues, who favour three sessions per week, argue that it is not about a therapeutic activity of healing and "repairing" but about propelling an unconscious process that continues during the analyst's absence.

The dialectic of presence and absence is linked to our topic of separation. It becomes an issue in analysis, as often as weekends and holidays provoke reactions in the patient. These reactions have to be understood as rooted in the regressive state and in the return of early traumatic experiences of separation with their connection to unconscious conflicts revolving around wishes of love and murderous hate that might make the real presence of the analyst even more needed.

6.4 Weekends and holidays

Patients often are surprised in the first year by the interpretations of the analyst that show to them that the changes in their mood coincide with separations from the analyst. This happens usually after long breaks, like holidays. Gradually, also the oscillations on weekends are recognized. The surprise reveals that the patient has not been aware of the intensity of the bond to the analyst until now. Some patients, especially if they are candidates, defend such feelings, rationalising with their theoretical knowledge that this belongs to the "transference" and a new edition of childlike wishes and fears. Others are less concerned with the separation than with their envy and jealousy regarding the analyst whom they imagine to be enjoying perpetual delight in a paradise, while they feel left alone with awakened, but unfulfilled needs for closeness. However, becoming aware of inner dependence is painful and engenders rage. Thus holidays often are critical phases. At these times shortly before, during or after the breaks, wild acting out might happen that can be self-destructive and can break off the analysis. Therefore, the early signs of separation-anxiety have to be watched and interpreted carefully in analysis.

Separation-anxieties often dominate because they belong to the symptoms of borderline-cases that we see so nowadays often in our consulting rooms. Sometimes separation-anxiety is coupled with a complementary fear, the fear of intrusion (Green, 2005a, 68). This is the female counterpart to male castration-anxiety. Thus separation-anxiety and fear of intrusion on the level of the ego have parallels on the libidinal-genital level in castration-anxiety and penetration-anxiety.

Independent of the clinical diagnosis one sometimes has the impression that these two kinds of anxieties defend each other: separation-anxiety can be smoothed by the fear of too much intimacy. Fear of intrusion or penetration might make the distance from an object more tolerable. *The dilemma is that often the absence of the analyst is not bearable* (due to separation-anxiety) *nor his presence* (due to intrusion-anxiety, which can escalate to fear of a break-down).

Such a dynamic can be the real reason why somebody might reject on principle an analysis with a high frequency of sessions. It is an effort to nip the conflict between the wish for and fear of closeness and dependence in the bud.

However, even if an analysis is not dominated by the struggle of contradictory wishes, the absence and presence of the analyst are turning points in the relationship. It is similar to the experience of a baby who feels satisfaction and love for the "good" object that is there, but uneasiness and fear, if it is missed and therefore turns quickly from a "good" object into a "bad" one.

"...the good breast is never just good: the appearance itself of desire denotes the absence of what is missing. The relationship with the breast entails the ongoing process of comings and goings, of the mother's presence and absence. "With each absence (if it is not too prolonged) the desire for her presence is established more clearly." (Kohon, 2005, 65) This dynamics of absence and presence, of "Fort" and "Da" inevitably causes ambivalence. The same is true for the analyst, who satisfies and restricts needs.

During the long years of an analysis other unavoidable breaks, apart from holidays, happen, planned or not, if the profession of the patient demands travel, or if he or the analyst needs to stay in hospital. How these breaks are experienced by the patient can be understood only based upon the whole psychoanalytic process. Sometimes behind professional tasks the patient hides his hostile and tyrannical impulses for acting out and wishes to force the analyst to adapt according his intentions. Nevertheless, such separations do not happen very often.

6.5   Transference love and the "limited" love of the analyst

If one wants to demonstrate the impressive development of psychoanalysis from the start of the 20th century to the 21st century, the chapter about transference love would be an eminently suitable one. Freud first considered transference love to be a mere disturbance of psychoanalytic work, and this was without doubt correct insofar as this form of "love" always serves as resistance and aims at the suggestion to the analyst: "Let us do something else, not analysis!" Soon Freud recognized more clearly the central role of the transference as the battlefield, where analysis wins or loses the battle against the patient's psychic illness. After Freud these considerations continued to be refined. Of special importance was a paper by Paula Heimann, who acknowledged the analyst's countertransference to be a valuable instrument of analysis. The school of Melanie Klein concentrated during the second half of the 20th century on the interpretation of the transference. Some psychoanalysts think that this "had a crippling effect; it has created a tunnel vision", which, although profound, has also led to the belief that transference could sum up all psychic activity (Kohon, 1999a, 158). Nevertheless, the careful attention for the movements in the transference remains important, but nowadays the view broadens again in developments in modern psychoanalytic theory and technique. After the Freudian and the Kleinian model Antonino Ferro constructed the "bipersonal field", based on the concept of Wilfred R. Bion. This opened a wider perspective that contains the whole analytic relationship including the setting and the arrangements, encompassing also the unconscious fantasies of the analyst and the lively interaction between the psychic functioning of the analyst and the patient (Ferro, 2003, 42 f.).

Freud wrote in "Observations on Transference Love" "that anything that interferes with the continuation of the treatment may be an expression of resistance" (Freud, 1915, S.E. 12, 162). But to try to suppress these instincts would be "not an analytic way of dealing with them, but a senseless one. It would be just as though, after summoning up a spirit from the underworld by cunning spells, one were to send him down again without having asked him a single question. One would have brought the repressed into consciousness, only to repress it once more in a fright." (164 f.) The patient's demands for love should not be satisfied. "The treatment must be carried out in abstinence", but "the patient's need and longing should be allowed to persist in her, in order that they may serve as forces impelling her to do work and make changes". The analyst will "keep firm hold of the transference love, but treat it as something unreal", so that the most deeply hidden erotic life will be brought into her consciousness and under her control. There are, Freud wrote, "woman of elemental passionateness, [...] children of nature", who cannot afford this achievement because they – free according a wording of Heinrich Heine – are accessible only to "the logic of soup, with dumplings for arguments". In such cases of missing capacity or readiness for sublimation the analyst would have to withdraw without success, wondering "how it is that a capacity for neurosis is joined with such an intractable need for love" (167). If this love would not be resistance, but be genuine, the readiness to do analytic work would be increased and one could continue to work with a moderated and transformed love and uncover the patient's infantile object-choice and the fantasies woven round it. Transference love and love in ordinary life are similar but transference has a lower degree of freedom since it is evoked by the analytic situation, pushed forward by resistance and disregards reality. For the analyst transference love is "an unavoidable consequence of a medical situation, like the exposure of a patient's body or the imparting of a vital secret". That's why he must not take any advantage of it: "The patient's willingness makes no difference; it merely throws the whole responsibility on the analyst himself." The ethical motives unite with the technical ones. If the demands for love would be satisfied, the patient's capacity for love would remain impaired by infantile fixations – instead of becoming free for real life. This would be like the scene of a dog-race, which a humorist spoiled by throwing a single sausage on to the track, thus making the dogs rushing to the sausage and forgetting "all about the race and about the garland (of sausages) that was luring them to victory in the far distance"(169).

Freud sketched here the transference love of a female patient for her analyst, but all his statements are valid for male patients too. This is demonstrated in an impressive way by Gregorio Kohon's description of an analysis of a psychotic young man "Love in a time of madness" (Kohon, 2005, 43 ff.) "Strange love, this, the patient's transference-love towards a stranger" (72). It erupts "into the consulting room with uncanny strength", increases due to the asymmetry of the relationship and creates by idealization a state that allows even intense feelings of hostility to emerge. By this psychotic young man they were expressed in letters to the analyst that were overloaded with hateful feelings. However, this hate was somehow dampened by his giving letters to his analyst instead of speaking. "To write the words, instead of speaking them, created a transitional space that could be used by both of us. The emotional impact of the communication was mediated by the act of writing, by the paper, by the silenced words" (51).

Freud and many psychoanalysts of the first generation believed that non-neurotic patients were not capable of transference and therefore not analyzable. Today we know that borderline-patients, for instance, establish quick and strong transferences: "A patient who suffers from separation anxiety at the first weekend of analysis – as if he had been coming for treatment for years – would lead me indeed to consider this reaction pathognomonic of serious borderline pathology." (Kohon, 2005, 90)

The development of transference love means establishing a new boundary that from its inception is orientated to end with a separation. Of course, the patient need not be consciously aware of it. Very often, however, at the start of the analysis he is conscious of it, but as soon as he sinks into the subjective timelessness of the unconscious the awareness vanishes that a therapeutic relationship is a limited one and is dissolved when its aim is achieved.

In another sense, transference love is shadowed by the ultimate fate of separation. This love is a new version of early infantile passions. Separation from those old objects of buried loves of childhood is unavoidable, although this happens in a variety of forms. There may arise a new understanding of persons who have been loved, feared or hated in one's early years. They might become rediscovered while the old views of them can be dismissed or changed. Analysis fosters the capacity for love and bonding and therefore the appearance of new objects. However, it also facilitates "a new discovery of objects" (Loewald, 1960, 225) – a new discovery of objects who were there all the time.

The old bonds cause the 'pressure of suffering,' stimulating the patients to seek therapeutic help to find a way out of the familiar prison of the psychic disease. Thus every start of psychotherapy includes a dose of humility, a narcissistic injury, containing the confession that the one's lonely struggles have failed. "Far from being a mere intellectual exercise, or at the opposite end a purely cathartic one, psychoanalysis demands from the patient, first, *a certain capacity for humility,* which enables the subject to acknowledge having known so little about himself. This occurs apart from the presenting complaints, the degree of pathological disturbance, or the social circumstances. In the second place, psychoanalysis demands the existence of *a conflict of suffering"* (Kohon, 2005, 84). Freud used the words "conflict of suffering" (in German "Leidenskonflikt") in a letter to Eduardo Weiss. This term encompasses in my view more than the usual notion "pressure of suffering" ("Leidensdruck"). It hints at the vitality of the individual caught in a struggle of contradictory forces. This is different from a rigid, dull suffering, as tough as it might still be.

The analyst, as an object of transference-love, enters more or less voluntarily into inheritance of old relationships. This provokes reactions in him, in his countertransference, which he learned to recognize, tolerate and use during his long training in order to understand the patient and to make helpful interpretations. There is an unavoidable transference of the analyst onto the patient because the analyst too is not "a blank sheet" and reacts with different feelings about specific patients. The question whether an analyst likes or dislikes a patient, has been often discussed as a key factor, but it is not often elaborated in literature. Liking a patient is not a prerequisite, but it might "affect the analyst's level of tolerance for the patient's regressive behaviour and destructiveness." (Kohon, 2005, 80) It remains important that the analyst's love for his patient is a limited one so that there are clear limits. This ensures the patient that analysis will continue, whatever happens within these limits. Thus, the limitations imposed by the setting provide a double assurance. They protect and hold the patient, and they prevent the analytic frame from being swept away. Due to this vital guarantee madness and delusion may emerge and be worked through. These limits protect the analyst as well as the patient. It is the analyst's task to take care of them. He is able to do so, because his love is a very special one. Kohon names it a "detached" love (Kohon, 2005, 81): a love from which paradoxically the attachment has been withdrawn. This enables the analyst to bear the persecutory anxieties and the hate of the patient and to understand the absurdity of his passionate wishes. The libidinal energy withdrawn from the patient has another destination: it belongs to the psychoanalytic task and the ideas offered by the psychoanalytic theory. This is the passion of the analyst, which has to be combined with his love for the patient, so that he remains lively, real and good enough for his patient.

The greatest intimacy between analyst and patient comes about "whenever the latter allows the former to *analyse* him; that is when the insight offered by the analyst is accepted, taken in, and used by the patient for his own benefit – not just to please the analyst" (Kohon, 2005, 82).

Perhaps these foregoing consideration may succeed in conveying to the inexperienced just how complex and complicated the analytic process is. Psychoanalysis is not a therapy that meets the ancient ideal, formulated by Asklepias, that a treatment should be "tuto, cito et iucunde", safe, quick and pleasant. Instead, it is uncertain as a cure, demands a great deal of time and is therefore expensive. It is painful and laborious for the analyst and for the patient. However, there are very few therapies in the whole realm of medicine that comply with our wish for absolutely reliable and quick positive results without burdensome side effects.

Otto Rank, who was mentioned earlier in connection with birth as a „model" of separation-anxiety, compared the psychoanalytic situation with the unrolling of a thread from the spool of infantile fixations, winding it round the analytic spool, and from there to the spool of reality. Thus, he illustrated the transference and the development of libido during analysis (Rank, Ferenczi, 1924, 23). This metaphor reflects the laborious process and suggests that one would not start such an operation if there is just a little knot or one insignificant thread lying about. For this, smaller interventions may suffice. Freud was open-minded regarding other psychotherapeutic methods, as shown on December 12th 1904, when he gave a paper "About Psychotherapy" in the Viennese medical college of doctors. He said: "There are many ways and means of practising psychotherapy. All that lead to recovery are good." But then he reaffirms his conviction "that the analytic method of psychotherapy is the one that penetrates most deeply and carries farthest, the one by means of which the most extensive transformations can be effected in patients". And he adds: "I may also say of it that it is the most interesting method, the only one which informs us at all about the origin and inter-relation of morbid phenomena." (Freud, 1905, S.E. 7, 259 f.) A century later most of the more than 11 000 members of the International Psychoanalytic Association probably agree.

6.6   The role of the third in regard to separation

Many patients feel that there is no escape when they swing back and forth between contradictory wishes for intimacy and distance. They search for the right 'other' and yet at the same time they sabotage any close and satisfying relationship. Hermann Lang wrote a paper about Franz Kafka entitled "Fort-Da. 'I cannot live with her, and I cannot live without her'." He called the dialectic of intimacy and distance a "claustro-agoraphobic dilemma" and explained how the anxiety-neurotic life stretches torturously between the poles of claustrophobia and agoraphobia (Lang, 2003,115 f.). To free oneself from such a dyadic relationship is only possible if a subject can establish some distance from the primary object and form a nucleus of independent identity. To do so, a third structural moment is needed that offers a form of relationship other than this dual-union. Usually the father represents this third moment but other things also can serve as substitute. Even language and symbolisation can take on this function. Then the society, the community of communication, asserts the prohibition of incest and dissolves this dyad. Deep ambivalence is important too, for it characterizes the relationship between human subject and primary object: *the desire for being held regressively in symbiotic fusion is opposed by the fear of being devoured and annihilated.* When the symbolic function intervenes the symbol substitutes its presence for the primary object. This substitution is a third moment and makes the experience of absence, loss and mourning unavoidable. That is why symbolisation belongs to the depressive position. Hanna Segal compared the symbol with "a precipitate of the mourning for the object" (Segal, 1991, 40).

In psychoanalytic treatment the arrangement of the setting and the use of language together constitute a third element mediating between analyst and patient. The setting provides a demarcation as well as a means of connection, which are favourable preconditions for solving the basic conflict between autonomy and fusion. Focussing only on the two-person-relationship analyst and patient would bring us to an impasse. This plight has been neglected in psychoanalytic literature, especially regarding separation anxiety. However, when elaborating the "tertiary process" (Green, 2005a, 188) it became clear that there is a primitive triangular structure in the early mother-child-relationship, in which the real father plays an important role in the mother's mind long before he is recognized as such by the child. This experience indirectly exerts a strong influence on her relationship with the child. Hence, many phenomena in psychoanalytic treatment should be considered from a triangular point of view. Green summarizes the tertiary structure "comprising the subject, the object and the other of the object, this other not being the subject. Thus the child's relationship to the mother would refer to one of the mother's other objects, a sibling, or an object of the mother's desire other than the father, sustaining this or that passion. The *other of the object* could also concern another object of the mother's own childhood: her own mother, her own father, or one of her brothers or sisters, a wet-nurse or housekeeper. It is not difficult to grasp then, the multiple possible applications of thirdness." (Green, 2005a, 200 f.)

Winnicott's statement that there is no baby without the mother has been cited. However, it is equally true that there is no mother and no baby without a father. "Mother and baby can only exist in the context of a third term, which does not need to be physically present in order to be *there.*" (Green, Kohon, 2005, 92)

The appearance of the third element in analysis intensifies conflicts and separation-anxieties. As soon as the patient forms a bond to the analyst and feels the need for his presence, his absence – during weekends, holidays or due to other events – becomes threatening. The patient cannot deny for long that he misses the analyst, and with increasing anxiety he becomes aware that his analyst is not only away but probably with someone else in these periods outside analytic sessions. Jealousy, envy, impotence and rage erupt and mix with different forms of separation-anxiety. This spectrum encompasses anxiety attacks, physical complaints and innumerable kinds of acting out. Jean-Michel Quinodoz illustrates his book about 'the tamed loneliness'[20] with apt examples. He shows that some patients are acting out separation-anxiety by arriving late or forgetting their session; it is, as if they acquire comfort by controlling the separations. Or they make errors regarding the fee as an unconscious "revenge" for the analyst's absence. Quinodoz describes in detail how his patient Olivia suddenly started to spend weekends working in intensive care wards. The analysis of this surprising behaviour revealed a double projective identification. On one hand, she shifted her intense emotional engagement from the analyst to other persons on whom she projected her own helplessness. By providing care she tried not only to soothe the pain of others but also her own. On the other hand, by acting out in this way she identified with her analyst as idealized caretaker (Quinodoz, 2004, 35 f.). However, I believe that her identification with her analyst as an omnipotent, idealized object devoted to the needs of other people includes another aspect, too: the patient demonstrated to her analyst

---

[20] It is certainly not by chance, that also Quinodoz's book-title „La solitude apprivoisée" – like "The melody of separation" – dares to approach to this issue of separation only in the context with a term of binding: "apprivoiser" (to tame) means to establish a close bond; "melody" forms an unit.

through her devoted care for persons in need what he ought to do – instead of leaving her in the lurch. And it seems to me that the fact that he did not do what, according to the patient's view, he should have done provoked aggression in her. The good object easily turns into a bad one if it absents itself. The threat escalates if the object is experienced as a part of the subject's ego that he might lose together with the object. Thus, Olivia's flight from her separation-anxiety to her charitable actions may have hidden also her negative feelings and her reproach against her analyst.

In general, separation-anxiety decreases during the psychoanalytic process. Sometimes, however, progress arouses separation-anxiety because it makes the conclusion of analysis seem more real and imminent. There is, of course, a countercurrent that Quinodoz calls a feeling of "buoyancy" (in French "portance"). He describes it as the feeling of being able for the first time to fly due to one's own strength and to find a dynamic psychic equilibrium achieved mainly by disidealisation of the object and renunciation of omnipotence. Quinodoz characterizes this feeling of "portance" as awareness by the patient of how little stability the internal and external world, which are impermanent, have to offer. Still, he employs a metaphor of sovereign superiority and describes the new balance: 'One not only becomes master of the movement, but one also plays with it like a surfer, who takes his swing out of the wave.' (Quinodoz, 2004, 249) Sometimes pictures are so seductively beautiful that one is inclined not to examine carefully how much they accord with the processes they illustrate. According to Quinodoz the patient acquires by dissolution of separation-anxiety "la portance", a strength that implies carrying power as well as elation. Due to such an inner stability the patient becomes, after analysis, more capable of bearing loneliness and separation, and to feel an "élan de vivre" (13). Even if one takes into account that sometimes it might be manic defence of separation-anxiety, which looks similar: the value of Quinodoz' metaphor is that he emphasizes the natural, healthy power of drives and shows that it is better to recognize and use them than suppress and fight against them.

6.7 "Analysis terminable and interminable"

This is the title of one of Freud's last papers. There in 1937 he discussed the limits and difficulties of psychoanalysis. He also was sceptical as to whether analysis really had a prophylactic effect. In regard to ending an analysis he starts with an obvious statement: "An analysis is ended when the analyst and the patient cease to meet each other for the analytic session" (Freud, 1937b, S.E. 23, 219 ff.) This usually happens when the patient no longer suffers from symptoms, anxieties and inhibitions; and when the analyst judges that enough unconscious material has become conscious that repetition of the pathological process need not be feared. Of course this depends also on favourable external circumstances. A shortening of the duration of analysis cannot be expected since our therapeutic demands have increased so much. Freud also tries to lower expectations, hinting that such therapeutic processes are usually incomplete. He quotes the Austrian satirist Johann Nestroy: "Every step forward is only half as big as it looks at first." Negative therapeutic reactions and guilt feelings of the patient often hinder success and suggest that there exists not only striving for pleasure but also a death drive resulting in aggression and destruction. "Only by the concurrent or mutually opposing action of the two primal instincts – Eros and the death-instinct – never by one or the other alone, can we explain the rich multiplicity[21] of the phenomena of life" (243). Due to the difficulty of the analyst's work and his preoccupation with repressed material that can have as disagreeable an effect as X-rays, Freud suggests that the analyst should "periodically – at intervals of five years or so – submit himself to analysis once more, without feeling ashamed of taking this step." Freud emphasized that this does *not* mean "that analysis is altogether an endless business". He ends with a clear statement: "The business of the analysis is to secure the best possible psychological conditions for the functions of the ego; with that it has discharged its task." Finally, Freud considers two prominent themes in analyses: *female envy for the penis,* and *masculine protest,* which is a struggle against his passive or feminine attitude to another male. Both problems can arouse the strongest resistance, preventing change from taking place, giving the analyst the impression of having "reached bedrock, and that thus our activities are at an end" (252).

All these thoughts are valid today, more than 70 years later. However, there have been some changes:

- During Freud's era analyses lasted often only a few months or few years. Today there are analyses that last more than a decade and a half, until they finish.
- This is caused by the expansion of the spectrum of psychic illnesses and disturbances which are treated psychoanalytically.
- The calls on analysis have increased a lot: not only the elimination of symptoms is intended. Otherwise, in many cases one might use less demanding psychotherapies.
- Analysis instead aims at structural changes that facilitate the development of the personality.
- All these changes are connected with the development of psychoanalytic theory and technique, especially regarding the differentiated understanding of transference and counter-transference as important factors.

Soon it became acknowledged that the therapeutic impact of analysis cannot be compared with reparation, which repairs damage once and for all. The result of an analysis – even if very successful – is a revitalizing one and is therefore

---

[21] Since Freud wrote in the German original „die *Buntheit* der Lebenserscheinungen" I would like to suggest to translate: „the *colourful* mulitiplicity of the phenomena of life".

changeable, subject to oscillations and shifts. Like the acquisition of special capacities this contact with one's own unconscious has to be "exercised", if we want to prevent repression from recapturing terrain we have lately conquered. In this sense every successful analysis becomes interminable, if we want to maintain the progress we achieved and are ready for a lifelong struggle.

Thus notions about obtaining a simple straightforward cure by analysis are an illusion. Wilfried R. Bion also stated: "The whole of psychoanalysis seems to me to be shot through with a certain optimism – these ideas of "cure", that there is a good time coming. What do we know about what is coming? What do we know about this universe in which we live? It is possible that the patient needs to be stronger and more disciplined in order to be ready for whatever happens – not just prepared for heaven, a cure which is heaven on earth" (Bion, 2005, 42).

7 Separation and creativity – experiencing and creating art

Without the awareness of actual and prospective separations there would be no creativity. The emphasis may lie on differentiations, as these are necessary on the level of sublimation as, for instance, in scientific tasks. Or on the emotional level, if a desire for an absent elusive object results in the wish to (re)create it in a piece of art, realistically embodied or symbolically represented.

This last chapter is devoted to examples of successful mourning and reparation achieved either by creating or experiencing art in the manner of an artist.

7.1 The capacity of mourning – an aspect of Arthur Schnitzler's novel "Dying"

Arthur Schnitzler often has been called Freud's double. In a novel, he wrote a year after his father's death he dealt with the most basic and most painful kind of separation and entitled it "Dying". It is the story of a young man, Felix, who is told by a physician that he has a fatal illness. Hesitatingly he informs his fiancée Marie. The novel starts with the shock of Felix, who learned this terrible news a few hours before, and with Marie's horror at this news. The description of the following months demonstrates with acute artistry the psychic elaboration of this experience for both individuals, in the dying man and his love-object. On her I'll focus because she develops through an extremely painful and mostly unconscious process the capacity of mourning. Of course, both are deeply upset by the impending involuntary separation. But in Felix the process of dying consumes him and the death-drive gains superiority over the life-drive. In Marie, however, the death-drive's antagonist, the life-drive will triumph.

In Marie we don't see the preceding trembling over the impending misfortune, oscillating between reality and denial. We meet her in the moment of the diagnosis of her lover. Her rejection of the information is abrupt and determined: 'No, this is not true.' She sticks to this disavowal during her time with Felix, though it becomes weaker and weaker. Nevertheless, she joins in when he stakes all his hopes in a change of location or an exotic medicine.

As her denial fades, so also does her pain. The latter was overpowering in the moment she faced the shattering of all her expectations for her life and her love[22], and this agony wells up again and again. Nevertheless, slowly it will subside. "She felt so sore at heart, so infinitely sore! She would have liked to weep, but in her emotion there was something dry, something wilted" (Schnitzler, 1915, 153).

---

[22] Cf. Green 2001 b, 108 f.

The countercurrent commences and Felix notices it with the bitter thought: 'She loves living too much.' This countercurrent power unconsciously *fights against the entanglement with death, it limits identification with the dangerously ill partner,* and Marie recognizes with bewilderment and guilt that she is moving away from him. 'She discovered how her gift of empathy slowly vanished. Her compassion was a state of being nervously overwrought, and her pain has become a mixture of fear and indifference' (119).

For some time she did not allow herself to go outside. But what she resists with severe self-reproach succeeds a few days later 'without any inner struggle, so natural, as if it would happen every day' (149). Here again in a literary masterpiece the inner fight is mentioned by using a negation; "without", and it actually happens under the surface of consciousness, unconsciously, as a stream might flow a long way under the earth.

This intense psychic process going on underground is masked by a 'infinite weariness' (161), which does not leave her for several days, although she sometimes feels refreshed: The contradiction in her state of health reflects an unconscious conflict between mourning and a wish to hold onto Felix, on one hand, and the urge to free herself and to prepare for a new start, on the other hand. Again, the poet resorts to a negation, following Marie's view: 'It is certainly not a lack of sympathy.'

Like Felix, she fought with all her strength against separation, and in the first shock, she vowed that she would not continue living without him. But she can neither stick to her vow nor to her dying lover. While his desire for eternal union with her escalates in his last moments to selfish fantasies of fusion, she is growing more afraid of his clinging and of his demand that she should honour her vow.

At the beginnings Felix announced clearly and simply what was going to happen: 'I have to go and you have to stay.' But neither could he stick to this realistic view nor was Marie able to hold her illusory, romantic wish to die with him. For her, separation ultimately means rescue; for him, death. Both have to go their way, and Marie cannot help but desperately shout 'Let me alone!', when he wants to force her to join him in death.

We see Marie's development in a direction opposite that of Felix: from initial denial of the painful reality she will arrive after a difficult inner and unconscious conflict, at a phase of detachment, of mourning and thus to acceptance of reality. The dying individual is removed further and further from the reality principle and can only escape to the comfort of fantasies to fulfil his wishes for intimacy. In Felix the response to inevitable separation is characterized by introversion of the death-drive, which manifests itself by decathexis of the objects of the external world. It is no longer Marie with all her sorrows and desires as a real person to whom he clings. He is no longer able to see her due to his own enveloping need. The spontaneous decathexis results in gradual repeal of a differentiated and individual relation to Marie. Of course, she cannot adequately be replaced by a nurse. He needs the familiar primary object around, just like a child needs his mother who, too, is ruthlessly exploited. Due to regression caused by fatal illness Felix loses this 'capacity for concern' for a beloved object, which Winnicott has described. Felix notices that Marie has become interchangeable. He now sees her as 'a sweet girl' and thinks that he might like another girl equally. 'Her character was now nearly indifferent for him.' (132 f.) The dissolution of the object-relationship is characteristic of the death-drive; Andrè Green called this tendency "disobjectalisation" (2001a, 874).

In Felix we see him turning inexorably away from the external world and his sinking into the world of fantasies. Marie, however, turns – though with guilt – more and more to the real external world, which will exist after the death of her lover. Thus both are separating: the dying individual by retreat into his inner world, and Marie by dissolving her bond to him. Both processes of separation are to a large extent unconscious and cannot be influenced by sheer will. This is a clear indication that separation and mourning cannot be "learned". At best they can become partly conscious in their meaning, so that they can be tolerated better by our understanding.

Marie's wish to survive is expressed even in small gestures. For instance, if Felix reaches for her hand, she gives it, 'but so that hers rests on his'. Growing already is her fear that he wishes to draw her into death. Her wish to survive has to gain the upper hand (164). 'She was healthy, she was young, and like out of 1000 sources her pleasure of living was running out' (150), as soon as she was out in the open air and among people. To see him sick wasting away, however, was like a chain of "cumulative traumata" – a term coined by Masud Khan, who argued that the accumulation of small injuries is not much less traumatic than a single great trauma. A healthy mind tries spontaneously to defend itself against such damage, an infection with death.

In accord with this point is the wish that the terrible phase of being forced to watch the beloved person suffer and die should end quickly. Marie 'no longer shrank back from the idea, the malicious word occurred to her that renders the most horrible wish into a hypocritical compassion: 'Oh may he be released!' (170). Correctly this thought is: "Oh may I be released!" But this confession would be heavily burdened with guilt so that the wish for release can only become vocal as projection onto the other one. The other one would be freed, not oneself. What is not allowed to become verbal Schnitzler has indicated with an image of freedom: Marie, pale and with tear-stained eyes sank into her daydreams; suddenly she sees 'the figure that was herself getting up, going out to the street and walking away slowly. Because now she could go wherever she wanted to.' The poet describes psychic change not with words, but with a vivid picture. This coincides with the fact that the psychic process is at that moment preconscious and not ready for verbalisation. The wish for release is identical with the death-wish regarding the other, and it is so great a taboo that it has to be shifted to the other. Thus the imagined murder that frees oneself from a bond that has become unbearable, is converted into a death that is a release for the dying individual. How much our society struggles with such forbidden thoughts, we can see in the issue of euthanasia.

There are many indications that Marie is deeply engaged in her work of mourning and that at a certain point this process will conclude. We have watched her spontaneously turn to external reality, to life outside the depressing sick-room. We recognize that in spite of her deep psychic pain she denied reality only during the first shock of the news. She is on the healing path that a deeply troubled but healthy person can travel.

It would be different, if she was unable to forgive herself for longing for life, if she, like her dying beau, stuck tenaciously to the illusion that separation can be avoided by mutual deaths, or if she blamed herself for leaving him even for short times, or failed to recognize the more malevolent symptoms of his illness. However, considering all these possibilities we can see how easily all these reproaches could be directed against her lover: that he left her, that he might have had a chance for cure if he had been treated earlier.

A similar pathological development might be expressed in somatisation that often starts when unconscious impulses are barred access to consciousness. In this case Marie might display symptoms of illness similar to her partner, due to unconscious identification with him.

However, we do not see these reactions in Marie.

Thus we can infer that the capacity to retain sight of reality, to heed the reality principle and not just the pleasure principle, determines whether separation can be coped with or not. In mourning the search for solutions proceeds unconsciously, as in depression. But unlike the latter there are no obstacles that cannot be overcome, so that the way to the preconscious and then to consciousness is open.

7.2   The metaphor of petrification

Petrification is an effort to stop time, to halt a process and to prevent a feared catastrophe, especially a separation that cannot be undone.

Animation of a dead object is a process running in the opposite direction. It symbolizes the return of a (dead, destroyed, petrified) object and the reparation of a loss.

Both processes have common roots, but also an interesting asymmetry. This I'll show in regard to mythological figures Medusa and Niobe, who became petrified by horror and mourning, and Pygmalion, who animated a statue he created.

7.2.1 Converted to stone

Medusa

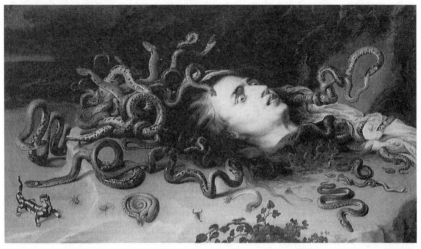

Figure 5
Peter Paul Rubens: Head of Medusa, Vienna
The horrifying head of Medusa is linked to the terror of castration, and can be
generalized to the fear of losing any part of the body.
Ruben's painting remained hidden away for many years in the archive of the
Museum of Art in order not to frighten visitors.

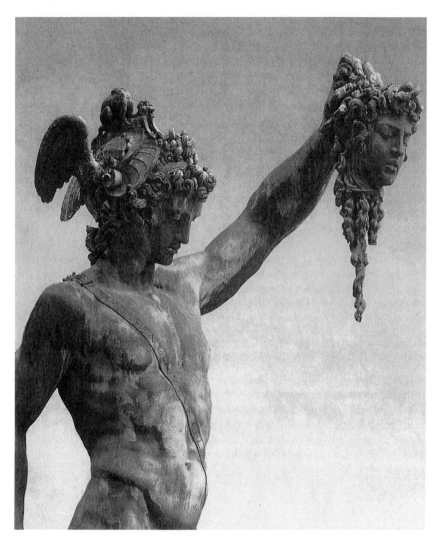

Figure 6
Benvenuto Cellini: Perseus with Medusa's Head, Florence.
Beauty tries to control horror.

We probably all know the feeling of being surprised, astonished, taken aback, even of being shocked. At such moments, it can feel as if something inside comes to an abrupt halt. The body then seems to take over, only to shut down as well. It stops moving, stops breathing, apparently stops being alive. To be "turned to stone", to be "petrified", is an evocative image of such a process, which combines an external experience and an internal movement, an affect which leads to a standstill. Sometimes, however, the familiar brief cessation doesn't stop. Instead it becomes a perpetual petrification. When this occurs it means something has happened that is so traumatizing that it cannot be experienced on a conscious level and cannot be coped with.

This affective response of 'petrification' has its opposite in the affective reaction of 'animation', or the creation of liveliness.

There is no better way to explore these phenomena than by recruiting classical mythology, which was familiar with petrification and animation. I restrict myself to the Roman poet Ovid and his metamorphoses. In 1911 Karl Abraham, who wrote about "Dream and Myth" – a contribution highly regarded by Freud –, a acknowledged that Ovid recognized the meanings of symbols accurately. Abraham was astonished to discover how much Ovid shared ways of seeing things that seemed remarkably modern (Abraham, 1911, 235).

Petrification is usually caused by the sight of something terrifying. In 1922 Freud wrote a short article about the myth of Medusa:

MEDUSA'S HEAD

Freud took for granted that the myth of Medusa was known and that the mechanism at work in dreams, where often the genital is displaced to the head. Freud proposed the psychical equation: "To decapitate = to castrate. The terror of Medusa is a terror of castration that is linked to the sight of something." Such a shock is often reported in analyses: it occurs when the female genital is seen the first time, which is experienced as a confirmation that the threat of castration must be true. There actually are genitals without a penis. The snakes on Medusa's head, "however frightening they may be in themselves", serve nevertheless as "a mitigation of the horror, for they replace the penis, the absence of which is the cause of the horror". And Freud explains the technical rule that a multiplication of penis symbols signifies castration. The sight of Medusa's head turns the spectator to stone. Beside the snakes as multiplied penis symbols there is one consolation: becoming stiff means an erection, and so the spectator converted to stone clings to the conviction that "he is still in possession of a penis, and the stiffening reassures him of the fact". So Medusa's head takes the place of a representation of the female genitals, isolating their horrifying effects from their pleasure-giving ones. The erect male organ has also an apotropaic effect; to display the penis (or its surrogates) is an effort to prove that one is not afraid (Freud, 1922, S.E. 18, 273 f.).

One year later, in 1923, Sandor Ferenczi dealt with the same topic in a very short note adding: "The fearful and alarming staring eyes of the Medusa head have also the secondary meaning of erection." He points out that, just as in

153

dreams and fantasies, we can see displacement "from below upwards", and that "the absence of a penis" is signified by the "representation of the opposite". Ferenczi mentions that this "phantom itself is the frightful impression made on the child by the penis-less (castrated) genital." (Ferenczi, 1923, 366)

Ferenczi is not only speaking of the horror the (immature) spectator experiences when confronted by female genitalia, he also seems to be drawing attention to the horror expressed on the face of Medusa herself. What has she seen that makes her so aghast? Is it connected with the snakes around her head? Is it because she sees the man who is going to behead her? What could cause such fear in the woman who terrifies men? Ovid[23] has some answers. Medusa, one of the three sisters called the Gorgons, had been a great beauty, being especially attractive because of her beautiful hair. We understand her horrified facial expression through the story of her abuse by Neptune, who raped her in the temple of Minerva. As a punishment to the God for his attack (and perhaps too as a punishment to Medusa herself) Minerva, the virgin goddess, (who was placed on a par with Athene by the Romans) transformed Medusa's wonderful hair into terrifying snakes. Whoever now looked at Medusa would be petrified.

In the myth, Perseus finally manages to decapitate Medusa:
"narrat ... eripuisse caput collo."
'he tells... that he snatched the head from the neck.'

In doing so, Perseus himself is performing a symbolic act of castration. The power of petrification, however, remains encapsulated in the decapitated head. When Perseus puts the head carefully to rest on the sand, the plants which come into contact with Medusa's head turn into coral. Perseus kills all his enemies by petrifying them to death. One of them understands that the destructive power that Perseus wields is located inside him, not outside and he tries, in vain, to warn his peers:

'You become petrified because of a psychic failure, not because of the Gorgonic forces!' –

"vitio animi, non viribus Gorgoneis torpetis!"

Perseus takes Medusa's head to Minerva-Athene. Since she is the ultimate unapproachable woman, who repels all sexual desire, she uses the head as both a shield and a weapon, displaying the symbolic representation of the terrifying female genitalia.

Here we can see how closely – just as in confused fantasies of little boys and girls – the petrifying terror of castration is linked to the horror of penetration.

---

[23] Ovid P. [1983] IV 792 ff; 770 ff, V 195

The small boy's castration anxiety is mirrored by the small girl's penetration anxiety, an anxiety which was – as André Green pointed out – "underestimated by Freud but which neuroses give us ample scope to observe". This pair of anxieties can be placed "in perspective with another, which depends on the structure of the ego and its limits: namely, separation anxiety [...] and intrusion anxiety." (Green, 2001c, 154) Sexuality and ego are not in opposed relation but rather a complementary one.

The female genitals can seem horrifying for a small boy or immature man if they represent the threat that he might lose his penis, the centre of his most pleasurable feelings. This part of his body might then become the centre of the most unbearable pain, and even endanger his life. For the small girl or immature woman, confrontation with the male genitals can provoke not only the horror that she may have lost a valuable part of her own body, the very part that the boy or man is so proud of, but also that this leaves her vulnerable to intrusion by him into her wound, a fear which is all the more difficult to fend off because it also causes pleasurable feelings.[24]

Sight of the genitals is seductive because of the memory of pleasure, but horrifying because of fearful fantasies. The confused feelings provoked by viewing genitals are often subsumed by using the word "ugly" to describe them. In Webster's Dictionary "ugly" is defined as something offensive or unpleasing to see, and its etymology shows that it derives from the Icelandic term *"ugglier"*, which means "frightening". "Experiencing something or someone as ugly is a powerful aesthetic response accompanied by intense negative affect (fear, horror, disgust and/or loathing), moral condemnation (reprehensibility), and behavioural reactions (being repelled, looking away, fleeing)" [Hagmann 2003, 960 ff]. When beauty is expected, the sudden experience of ugliness disrupts notions of unity and wholeness. "Ugliness" implies the return of

---

[24] I want to remark here concerning the terms which address the most primitive affects *pleasure and pain* that there is sometimes a dissatisfaction in regard to their comparable intensity. For André Green (1999, 4) only the French term *jouissance* (unsatisfyingly translated with enjoyment) would express a similar strong opposite of pain, and he suggests the chain

jouissance-pleasure-unpleasure-pain.

I understand that the word *'pleasure'* might seem to suggest a more superficial, conventional experience, (as in the Latin roots *"placet* = it is convenient for me, I like it") and that it might not convey the sense of a link to deep feeling rooted in the body, powerful enough even to lead to ecstatic states. In German, however, it looks a bit different. In spite of some devaluation of the term in every day language (for instance: "Ich habe Lust/keine Lust schwimmen zu gehen" = "I like/don't like to go for a swim"), our word for pleasure, **Lust,** has preserved the meaning of strong affect, felt with body and soul, and is the word often used by great poets of passion, like J.W. Goethe. For a milder version of a positive affect we often use *Behagen*, and, for its opposite, *Unbehagen*. Both have a touch of uncertainty about the causes of these feelings. So, for German I would like to suggest the chain:

Lust – Behagen – Unbehagen – Schmerz (more common than *Unlust).*

repressed fantasies related to oedipal desire, sexual violence and raging internal conflicts. It is particularly interesting that the original Icelandic term, *ugglier*, signifies the originating state of mind – fearfulness – while modern usage of the English word "ugly" shifted this meaning from subject to the object. Instead of "I am full of fear", we have, "the genitals are ugly". The internal conflict has been externalized by means of projection. *It seems likely that shifts in the meaning of words reflect psychic processes common to many people*, and that words can then function like the *"building blocks of cultural repression"*, in German *"Bausteine allgemeiner Verdrängung"* (Zwettler-Otte, 2005, 229 and 2011, 133). In common language words are lying around ready to be used, easily available for the job of simultaneously preserving and concealing the personal work of repression.

Niobe

In the myth of Niobe petrification expresses the acute pain of separation caused by the wrenching loss of all her children. In Niobe, the wife of Amphion, who was king of Thebes, we find a form of object relatedness dominated by envy, jealousy and competition with any other woman who might be superior to her. Her myth provides material for considering
1. female sexual development, and
2. about the way affects in unconscious psychic processes are bound to the experience of time.

Ad 1)
Niobe was the daughter of Tantalus. He was punished for offending the gods by offering them the body of his son Pelops. He was condemned to stand in water but not allowed to drink; to stand under a tree full of apples but not allowed to eat. Niobe too has to undergo the horrible experience that the presence of quantity is no guarantee of satisfaction.
Ovid begins the story of Niobe with the hint that she should have learned from Arachne, her fellow countrywoman, the discretion to avoid rivalry with a goddess. Arachne's name means "spider"[25]. She competed with Pallas Athene in the art of weaving and, being unsuccessful, was transformed into a spider by the superior divinity. But Niobe was full of envy and jealousy, deeply competitive with Latona, the mother of Apollo and Diana, because, while Latona was honoured by the people, no sacrifices were offered to herself. Niobe, who had seven sons and seven daughters, regarded Latona as virtually childless. Niobe was proud of her husband, her noble descent and her empire, but her greatest prides were her children. This pride brings about her fall. As Ovid puts it:

---

[25] Referring to a note from K. Abraham, Freud stresses that the spider in dreams "is a symbol of the mother, but of the phallic mother, of whom we are afraid; so that the fear of spiders expresses dread of mother-incest and horror of the female genitals". And he links it with Medusa's head, representing the same motif of fright at castration. (Freud, 1932, S.E. 22, 24)

"...felicissima matrum dicta foret Niobe, si non sibi visa fuisset." (VI 155 ff.)
'She would have been called the happiest of mothers, if she had not believed herself to be that.'

What she could not bear was that Latona, who had only two children, was honoured like a goddess while she was not. Beautifully dressed in a golden robe, Niobe angrily shakes her pretty hair and halts the sacrifices being offered to Latona, claiming that she herself can be sure of her fortune in comparison to Latona (193 ff.):

"... sum felix (quis enim neget hoc?) felixque manebo
(hoc quoque quis dubitet?) Tutam me copia fecit.
Major sum quam cui possit Fortuna nocere."

'I am happy (who could deny this?) and I shall remain happy
(who could have doubts also about this?) Quantity has rendered me sure.
I am greater than one whom Fortuna might harm.'

But Latona enters this competition and asks her son Apollo for revenge. Apollo interrupts her complaints and is ready to do as she asks (215):

"Desine!" Phoebus ait: "Poenae mora longa querella est."
'Stop it!" Apollo said: 'A long complaint just delays the punishment.'

Then, with his arrows, he slays Niobe's sons, one after the other. Afterward he shoots at her husband and her daughters. Deeply shocked, Niobe throws herself over the bodies of her children but still she proclaims that she is superior to Latona (284 f.):

"...miserae mihi plura supersunt,
quam tibi felici: post tot quoque funera vinco."
'... In my misery even I have more than you
who is happy: even after so many funerals the victory is mine.'

So Apollo continues this revenge and kills her daughters, who were mourning their brothers. Even Niobe's plea to save her youngest daughter cannot stay his hand (268 ff.):

"... ultima restabat. Quam toto corpore mater,
tota veste tegens "unam minimamque relinque!
De multis minimam posco" clamavit "et unam"
dumque rogat, pro qua rogat, occidit. Orba resedit ..."

'The last one was left. The mother protected her with her whole body,
with her whole robe. "Leave me only this smallest one,
I ask only the smallest from many" she shouted,
but while she asked, the one for whom she asked, died. Without children she
sank back.'

In her pain, Niobe grows stiff. No life seems to remain in her. She cannot move.
Nevertheless, she is weeping. A storm takes her to the top of a mountain in her
native place and there she is converted into marble, with tears running down
(212):

"... *lacrimas etiam nunc marmora manant.*"
'... even now tears are dropping from the marble.'

Of course, there are limits for interpreting the limited amount of material I have
presented, but the theme of competition among these women is extremely clear.
So perhaps we might hazard a guess. Niobe is obsessed by rivalry with other
women because she is stuck in her own female development. Her need to show
herself off, not just with her outward style, but mainly through her children,
makes us suspicious in regard to her femininity. Maybe one can assume that for
her "motherhood purports to fill in the absence which femininity covers over"
(Mitchell, 1986, 398). Maybe Niobe represents a woman who is – as Gregorio
Kohon describes it – " 'stuck' in her divalent stage", unable to "define herself as
a man or as a woman". Perhaps, like many female hysterics, she is already
"petrified half-way" long before her final petrification, "half participating, half
excluded"... "The hysteric disguises herself: she will pretend to be a woman,
she will put on the fancy dress of what she thinks will constitute her 'feminine
self'. What must remain hidden under the disguise is her castration, which she
rejects and which paradoxically is what defines her as a woman." (Kohon, 1986,
379; 376)
The loss of her children robs Niobe of her phallic surrogates. All that remains
for her is to convert herself into stone, a phallus moist with tears, but never
totally deflated.
Losing her husband and her children – all these objects being also a part of
herself – would entail great mourning, a task which includes a renunciation of
the lost objects, as Freud showed in 'Mourning and Melancholia'. The
petrification might represent Niobe's incapacity to renounce and to live without
those objects. For her, perhaps, there is no way of existing without them, not
even for a short time even while they might be replaced by other objects.

ad 2)
This leads to the second aspect I want to address, the aspect of time symbolized
by petrification.

As we have already seen in the Medusa myth, petrificiation represents a *moment* of horror: an unexpected catastrophe is happening, or awareness has dawned of a catastrophe which happened earlier. It is a traumatizing experience, immediate and *present*, and *there is only one aim: to stop this horrible experience.*

We have seen that the origin of this horror lies in the *past,* the catastrophe of the present representing the return of unconscious repressed fantasies. When the unconscious material of the past becomes present, "the present becomes timeless" as Peter Hartocollis put it, a process well-recognised in psychoanalysis in the phenomena of transference (Hartocollis, 2003, 955). Thus petrification is characterized by

- the re-emergence of repressed material (of the past, fantasies about castration)
- prompted by a terrible experience in the present (the sight of something horrible enough to symbolize the horror of castration) and
- the need to stop this unbearable experience and to make a halt at a moment that perhaps (later on) might allow for influence or help.

This last aspect seems to be the motor of the whole unconscious process. An end to the catastrophe offers hope for the *future.* A return of the catastrophe of the past contains not only pain but also the *power of actualisation.* The original trauma is recalled, in disguise, in order to repair it, to undo it.

As in the Medusa myth, so too in the story of Niobe, petrification conceals the fulfilment of a wish: to undo female castration, to transform her into a permanent erection on the mountain top, and so, in fantasy, replacing the lost objects who were her surrogates for a phallus. In stopping, even reversing, time, wishful thinking tries to take over and to find a way of becoming 'real'.

The idea of time blocked by a fixation is an old concept. In 1895, in his 'Studies on Hysteria', Freud already had conceived of strangulated affects and "of the clock which has stopped." (Green, 2002, 9)

But while there the stopping of time belongs to psychopathology, the freezing of processes can have a healthy connotation, as Winnicott showed (see later on). There is no guarantee though that a healthy development will take place. If this hope fails, stagnation may remain connected with "the unbinding processes of the death drive." (Green, 2002, 44) Stopping time and stagnation – represented by petrification – can have the meaning of rejecting processes of growth, development and binding. But it can also symbolize a hidden fulfilment of a wish.

It seems very interesting that – as ever in the antithetical meaning of the primal words[26] – *petrification* can stand for *preservation* as well as for *deadening.*

---

[26] Freud wrote in his short paper about 'The antithetical meaning of primal words': 'I did not succeed in understanding the dream-work's singular tendency to disregard negation and to employ the same means of representation for expressing contraries until I happened by chance

7.2.2 Animated to life

Pygmalion

Animation is a process that can be described as the opposite of petrification, the other side of the coin. While *petrification* leads to immobility, to diminished feeling, curtailed vitality and aliveness, *animation* is a movement in the contrary direction. It brings life into being. While *petrification* is an unconscious process that occurs suddenly and without conscious intention, as if the subject was passively taken over by it, *animation* is based on a desire which is at least preconscious, if not conscious. A great deal of hard work goes into the task of creating an object. Let us listen to Ovid once again (X 243 – 295).

In this story too, the introduction to the main events is important. Pygmalion is an artist from Cyprus. He has seen women turned to stone by Venus for prostituting themselves.

"... in rigidum parvo silecem discrimine versae ..."
'... converted into rigid stone by a small change ...'

Pygmalion felt
"... offensus vitiis, quae plurima menti
femineae natura dedit, sine coniuge caelebs vivebat."
'... offended by the plethora of vices which nature has given to the female mind, and he lived alone, without a wife.'

But he carved white ivory and created a female figure with which he fell in love: she resembled a real girl so closely:
"quam vivere credas ... ars adeo latet arte sua ..."
'one could have believed she lived ... his skill concealed the artifice so cleverly'.

---

to read a work by the philologist Karl Abel, which was published in 1884.'(Freud, 1910, S.E. 11, 153-161). There Abel described the peculiarity in the oldest languages that a fair number of words have two meanings, one of which is the exact opposite of the other. The solution of this riddle is that *our concepts owe their existence to comparisons;* for instance we should not be able to distinguish light from dark, if it were always light; only later on the two sides of an antithesis were separated and hence it could be thought of one without conscious comparison with the other. Now I just used a word which shows this old antithesis: "with-out"; "with" originally had the meaning of both: "with" and "without"; the latter still can be recognized in "withdraw" and "withhold"; "to lock" corresponds to the German word "Loch" (hole); other examples we find galore in Latin: "altus" means high and deep as well; "clam" means secretly - "clamare" means to cry loudly; "siccus" means dry, and "succus" juice (Zwettler-Otte, 2006).

Pygmalion himself was uncertain
"an sit corpus illud an ebur"
'whether it was a real body or ivory'

«oscula dat reddique putat loquiturque tenetque
...ornat quoque vestibus artus
dat digitis gemmas...
cuncta decent,.nec nuda minus formosa videtur....
appellatque tori sociam..."
'He kisses her and believes that she kisses him back, he speaks to her and hugs
her ... he dresses her and puts jewels on her fingers...
Everything fits, and she is no less beautiful when she is naked
...and he calls her the companion of his bed.'

During the celebration of Venus Pygmalion prays:
..."si di dare cuncta potestis
sit coniunx, opto" (non ausus: eburnea virgo
dicere) Pygmalion, "similis mea" dixit "eburnae"
"If you gods can give anything,
I would like my wife to be" (he did not dare to say: the virgin of ivory),
Pygmalion said: " just like the virgin of ivory".

Venus understood what this plea meant: *"sensit ...vota quid illa velint."*
When Pygmalion came home, he touched and kissed the statue and where he
had touched it, the stone became soft flesh:

"... dataque oscula virgo
Sensit et erubuit timidumque ad lumina lumen
Attollens pariter cum caelo vidit amantem."
'... and the virgin felt his kisses
and she blushed, and opening shy eyes
she saw the sky and the eyes of the man who loved her.'

The myth of Pygmalion deals with the horror connected with the frightening
unconscious fantasies about the vulnerable body, which can be wounded and
destroyed. These fears belong to past experience and are repressed, but always
seek to return. Struggling for release they re-emerge at an opportune moment.
With a single word Ovid reminds us of this: that Pygmalion was violated –
"offensus" – by bad women. We are given no clue as to what exactly this earlier,
causative event might have been. We don't know what "l'avant-coup" (Green,
2002, 21) was, but we witness what Pygmalion must deal with afterwards
(l'aprés-coup) and see how he relates to his object. We can surmise that there
may be an unconscious fantasy about the "ugliness" of women, which now

becomes a longing for "beauty". We do not know whether his fear of women was provoked by one of the two familiar and important visual traumas – the primal scene and the female genitals – but we can assume that he had to deal with disturbing fantasies connected to incestuous wishes. This we can deduce from Pygmalion's urgent desire to possess the ivory maiden he has created. "Desire, in human sexuality, is always transgression," Gregorio Kohon points out, "what makes sexuality in human beings specifically human is repression" (Kohon, 1986, 371). Pygmalion recognizes this transgression. He does not dare to ask for the statue to become alive. Aware that he wants something forbidden he disguises his request and only permits himself to ask for a maiden *like* her.

There are hints as to the precipitating cause of Pygmalion's difficulty which are worth considering. There is no memory of the traumatic event. There seems to be no father or any other male figures. Ignoring other men includes ignoring any competition with the "heroic self" (Steiner, 1999, 685 ff.), with other heroes of his own cultural tradition.
It must have been Ovid's intuition to attenuate, in the telling of the myth, just what Pygmalion himself repressed. *Here form represents content by omission.* There is no trace of any male figure with whom Pygmalion might have identified. Such identification is important for the development of sexual identity and can be found to be missing in people with perverse personality structures. The development of a close and exclusive relationship to a non-living object certainly can be considered a perverse trait, with its associative link to necrophilia.

Be this conjecture as it may, Pygmalion certainly has not developed as male adolescents usually do, becoming able to find a female object whom they can love. Rather, he behaves like a girl playing with a doll, identifying with the female figure he creates. The wish to create life can be thought of as an omnipotent wish – a transgression and exaggeration of the natural wish to create life with somebody else, as parents. Feelings of omnipotence, often lurking behind childlike behaviour, are typical of delayed emotional development. Thus in some respects Pygmalion himself has been petrified by his fixations, but he finds a way out of this petrification through creativity. To create a woman out of inert material seems the best way of resolving the unconscious horror provoked by the discovery that women lack a penis. It seems an even better solution than looking for a phallic woman because – as Glen Gabbard noted: "Yet the fantasy of the phallic woman (or mother) is not simply reassuring to the boy child – it also resonates with a darker concern that an omnipotent, penetrating mother may take advantage of his vulnerability." (Gabbard, 1997, 826)
It is not only the statue that comes alive through Pygmalion's love. Pygmalion does too. The change he watches with such excitement is his own, and represents reversal of his petrification. By sculpting an ivory maiden Pygmalion enlarges his repertoire of representations of women. There no longer only is the

horrible unconscious fantasy of licentious women at work. He becomes able to re-create a time of harmonious relationship to a woman, a time, before conflict, danger and destruction turned it into "ugliness". As Hanna Segal put it: "The act of creation at depth has to do with an unconscious memory of a harmonious internal world and the experience of its destructions; that is the depressive position. The impulse is to recover and recreate this lost world" (Segal, 1991, 94).

In this sense, Pygmalion's emotional immaturity is not simply a failure but also denotes a capacity to delay development that could not have proceeded in a healthy way at the time. He had, so to speak, to wait until he was strong enough to move from the paranoid-schizoid position into the depressive position. D.W. Winnicott was correct to call it "normal and healthy for the individual to be able to defend the self against specific environmental failure by a *freezing of the failure situation*. Along with this goes an unconscious assumption (which can become a conscious hope) that opportunity will occur at a later date for a renewed experience [...]." (Winnicott, 1987, 281)

I want to emphasize that *this is true not only for those failure situations where regression is obviously due to environmental failure, but also when an internal failure of development occurred.* By becoming a master sculptor[27], Pygmalion (re-)gained a state of safety. Joseph Sandler, in his "concept of safety" (Sandler, 1987, 1), described the importance of a basic feeling of well-being to the regulation of mental functioning. When Pygmalion achieved mastery in his art, he felt safe enough to confront what had hitherto been repressed in him. His obsession with a work of art was unconsciously aimed at "the conversion of ugliness into artistic knowledge and beautiful form" (Hagmann, 2003, 960 ff.). "Every creative artist produces a world of his own" (Segal, 1986, 188). The world that Pygmalion created was one where women no longer were licentious and dangerous but (again) lovable, tender and beautiful. Auguste Rodin, the famous sculptor, argued that the transformation of ugliness into beauty is the unique domain of the artist, and stated : "[...] let a great artist get hold of this ugliness [...] he makes it into beauty." (Segal, 1986, 200)

Thus Pygmalion's art work implies reparation as well. Doing it involved not only the preparatory work of learning the art of sculpting but also creation of a *"time vacuum"* (Hartocollis, 2003, 940). I borrow this apt phrase from Peter Hartcollis, who used it for the analytic situation that can "throw the patient into a time vacuum, into a limitless time perspective". During his labours the artist too feels nestled in the timelessness of the unconscious. In this atmosphere of safety and creativity the artist unconsciously provides a *space*, a *transitional space* (Winnicott) which can be compared to a *facilitating environment*, enabling further development.

---

[27] It would be another interesting topic to think about anal and aggressive drive-derivates engaged in this work of art.

Concluding, we can see that although petrification and animation are opposing unconscious psychic processes, both have a *common root. This root lies in an overwhelmingly frightening experience, felt at a conscious level - at least for a moment - in petrification, an experience which is repressed in animation,* because animation begins *after* the deadening destruction has happened. In animation, it is dead matter becoming animated. Why it is a dead object in the first place is blurred. In petrification overwhelming affect results in a standstill. In animation, repression erases memory of the events that caused the affect, leaving behind only faint traces. The repressed returns, however, as the expression of an unconscious desire to repair what was destroyed. In this sense, animation of a dead object seems to be, in fantasy, the *re-animation* of a good internal object which became disturbing, and hence bad, and had to be, in fantasy, repelled or destroyed. If the return of the original, desirable object succeeds, the separation can be undone and the bond of love can be re-established.

This sort of standstill, reminiscent of the catatonic state in psychiatry, in an extreme form represents petrification, which contains several different continuums.

- A continuum of time: from a brief cessation to a permanent paralysis;
- a continuum of awareness: from a conscious experience of an overwhelming affect, which is usually a frightening one[28], to a sudden plunge into repression;
- a continuum of control: from averting a catastrophe by freezing the awareness of threat, to loss of control; from preserving to deadening, and lastly
- a continuum of salvation: from banishing the threat of destruction, to finding ways to mitigate and repair the horror, which offers hope for compensation and substitution.

We have seen that in petrification the role of time is of great importance. Repressed material from the past becomes re-activated in the present to seek a better solution in the future.

In animation feelings of horror do not become conscious, but on a preconscious level they get a chance to be elaborated and worked through, guided by wishful ideas. *In animation the horror is eliminated and petrification is displaced from the subject to the object, which then has to be (re-)animated.* There are efforts at repair, supported by strong desires, but it is an invisible repair of

---

[28] Of course there are also moments of overwhelming pleasure which can lead to a full halt because of their surprising effect and the wish to prevent transitoriness. But these moments only become repressed when they are conflictual. As soon as there are conflicts, dangers arise.

unacknowledged damage. The passivity of petrification is converted into the activity of creativity aiming at restoring what was lost.[29]

Thus, on the surface, animation seems the opposite of petrification, because sublimation and the task of enlivening the self conceal the preceding horror and destruction, which belong to petrification. Looking more closely, however, petrification, too, contains not only the aspect of it that deadens and eliminates life, but also a stubborn capacity to endure in the hope of preserving life and pleasure.

7.3 Reparation in mosaics

"Reparation" means "acquiring again", "restitution" and expresses an urgent need to make something that was destroyed intact and whole again. Etymologically the Latin verb 'parare' – to prepare, to create is connected with pario, parere - produce, give birth. "Reparation is the strongest element of the constructive and creative urges." (Hinshelwood, 1991, 412 ff.) Feelings of guilt and love, concern, obsessive defence of aggression and sublimation all play a major role. Reparation is a strong effort to repair and restore in the external world objects that have been damaged in the internal world by destructive fantasies. In the child the urge for reparation arises, if he no longer fixes only on parts of an object, but the whole person, who is good and bad as well, thus again being in danger of being destroyed. This phase Melanie Klein named the "depressive position" because the loss of the object is feared. The child believes that he caused this loss by his own greed and hate. "In fantasy his loved object is continually attacked in greed and hatred, is destroyed, torn into pieces and fragments." (Segal, 1986, 187) The intense experience of loss and guilt generates the wish to recreate the lost object. This process is repeated in the artist, who withdraws into his inner world of fantasies to form it anew. At the same time he returns to external reality by sharing his fantasies with others and communicating with them.

---

[29] There are a plenty of examples of petrification and animation in different cultures worth studying, for instance Lot's wife, the Golem, Prometheus and so on; the most famous modern example of an „animation" is probably „My fair lady", based on Pygmalion by Bernhard Shaw: here Prof. Higgins tries to model Eliza from a - in his eyes - worthless being to a glorious creature. The preceding destruction (denying the object's own life) does not quite function and provokes pleasing tensions in the musical. (Cf. Zwettler-Otte, 2011)

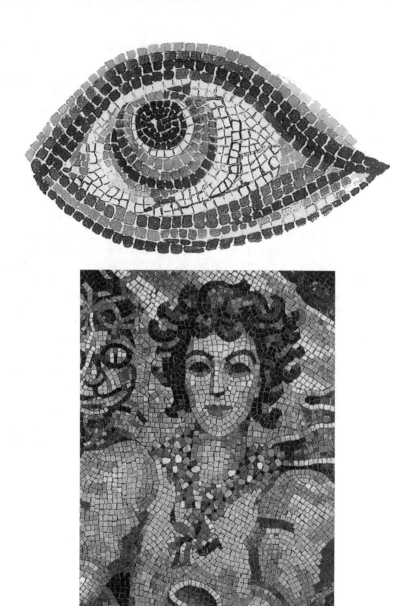

Figures 7 and 8
'The eye of the tiger' and 'The pleasures of life' by Boris Anrep
Mosaics, more than any other form of art, point simultaneously to the
destructive aspects as well as to the reparative forces of creativity.

I have some personal experiences with the art of mosaics, which I first acquired as a self-taught practitioner and later on through instruction in Ravenna. My interest focuses on a special phenomenon. When one is testing the little stones and rearranging them, there is a moment when a *'gestalt'* suddenly is recognized, independent of whether the subject is a figure or an ornament. This moment produces a satisfying feeling that is closely linked with the aim to (re-) make a whole object out of fragmented quarry stones. Both aspects are important. The use of fragments or broken pieces *and* the formation of an image. There is perhaps no other art form that exhibits *simultaneously the aggressive-destructive components and the constructive-synthetic ones so evidently.* Both components remain active. In the process of making a mosaic there is always the danger that a minimal movement of the stones might ruin the image.

In Pygmalion's example we have witnessed the recreation of an object that has been destroyed in a destructive fantasy that was repressed. What we come to see is not just the creation of a beloved girl. The destruction of the dangerous bad women was implied by Pygmalion feeling "offended by their vices". In the mosaic the recreation is constituted by *play with fragmentations* that are an unmistakable proof of a previous destruction. They represent the polarities of creativity. One might say: *The mosaic presents the theme of separation by making it permanently visible maintaining and elaborating it in innumerable variation.*

The mosaic not only makes love an issue but also hate – not only the forming and creation of an object but its dissolution and destruction too. Evidently the technique itself presents form as content for consideration. This is quite concrete, and we can assume that this tendency represents the essence: the delicate balance between creativity and destructivity that must be represented and perceived in actuality in order to assure formation and maintenance in the art work.

Among innumerable books about the art of tessellated work I found only one that considered in detail this peculiarity of mosaics. The author is mosaic-artist Giovanna Galli, who wrote: "The art of mosaic consists of a process of separation and new organisation of material (*un processo di separazione e di riorganizzazione della materia*); it animates a visual system of expression by the processes of fragmentation and composition, characterized by a certain discontinuity" (Galli, 1996, 15 f.). She calls the cut or the fracture of stones an act of fragmentation (*il gesto* della *frammentazione*). The positioning of the tessere is called an act of composition (*il gesto della compositione*), when the little pieces are pressed into the binding agent, which partly fills and animates the interspaces. Fragmentation, the technical essence of the mosaic, is the core of its aesthetic originality and its specific power of expression. The artist plays with the interfaces, with the various structures of the material, with the colours, the irregularities and the refraction of the light on the innumerable small surfaces, like a piano virtuoso plays with the keys of the piano. This fragmentation, caused by multiple explosions, and the return to a unity, are the essence of the art of mosaics. The simultaneous presence of two opposed points of view symbolizes in the mosaic downfall and resurrection. With great economy of material and technical-aesthetical intuition of a high order, an "inextricable play of presence and absence" (un gioco inestricabile di presenze e di assenze) is enacted. This is very far indeed from regarding a mosaic as a mere copy or imitation of paintings, or as an immortalization of one in stone. This art is more an *imploring* than a paraphrase of *palpable reality* .The word "intuition" points to the link to the preconscious and unconscious realm of creativity. Similarly, "implore" contains the idea of an intense, urging desire.

The tessellated work reminds one of the "patched breast" that Andrè Green described in his concept of the "dead mother" (Green, 1993, 152). If a child feels – without understanding – that the mother turned away (to somebody else, to a concern or to whatever distraction), he tries to find this lost feeling in his world of representations. Performance and self-reparation aim at surviving distress about the lost object. This can be accomplished by "the creation of a patched breast": a cognitive fabric that covers the gap, which was made by the mother's decathexis. But the edge of the abyss of emptiness swarms with hate and excitement, the consequences of any incomprehensible loss. Perhaps we could say that the difference between the patched breast and one that is repaired in a mosaic lies in the extent of the repression. In the patched breast the cracks and holes are covered with textile, thus maintaining repression of the agonizing perception, though repression is not a very flexible fabric. The mosaic, however, does not cover but rather integrates the preceding destruction. The cracks remain visible as tolerable separations. The acknowledgement of the destructive elements provide a stronger web than repression alone, and the precipices move closer, becoming interfaces filled with a more elastic binding agent. The art of mosaics provides to a very high degree the condition, which Hanna Segal recognized as a characteristic of all great art: "the degree of denial of the death-instinct is less than in any other human activity" And she observes: "[...] ugliness – destruction is the expression of the death instinct; beauty, the desire to unite into rhythms and wholes – is that of the life instinct. The achievement of the artist is in giving the fullest expression to the conflict and the union between these two." (Segal, 1986, 203 f.)

In the previous chapter we studied a successful reunion after a separation by means of the example of sculpture. If a sculptor creates and animates an object, he can work through a trauma of the past and correct and enlarge his experiences. This chapter dealt with a similar restitution: the artist of a mosaic repairs "exploded" objects and thereby can resume progress in his development.

Artists have the opportunity to create their own world where they might cope better with love and hate than in their everyday life. Often it remains a closed world of their own, and not all virtues and achievements there can be transferred to normal life. Otherwise it could not be explained why some artists "are genuinely creative but totally incapable of love" (Kohon, 1999b, 52 f.). Evidently they remain locked up in the prison of their narcissism, where they have made themselves quite comfortable.

7.4 Venice – flooded by the melody of separation

The previous two chapters examined the creative process in the artist and showed how closely creativity is linked to acknowledgement of loss and destruction. This chapter now deals with the perspective of the lover of art, who does not create art but may be able to identify with the process of mourning and (re-)creating. That I chose Venice for this topic not only has to do with the fact that it is a metropolis of art. It is also a city connected with the threat of sinking, thus being flooded by a melody of separation.

Goethe wrote in 1786: 'Regarding Venice there is already everything said and printed what one can say' (quoted in Grun, 1967, 30). However, the flood of pictures and descriptions never stopped, and thus this prescript enthusiasm permeates authentic personal experience, of course without eliminating it totally. Flirtation with the downfall that is forewarned, but goes unheeded, became a cliché in the literature about Venice. Gaston Salvatore concludes his "Invitation to the downfall" with soft pressure: "Who knows how long the downfall of Venice will still be a pleasant threat?" (Salvatore 2003, 130) And Herbert Rosendorfer urges in his invitation to Venice "to visit this wonder of petrified life as soon as possible, before it will die." (Rosendorfer 2003, Cover)

The pervasive "Memento mori", the ongoing sense of transience enhances the appreciation of the city for many people. Venice contains polarities galore; an essential one is that of future and past: the future is warning of a catastrophic separation; a peculiar, slowed-down tempo which is characterized by softly gliding vaporetti, seduces us into the past. Mark Twain called Venice a funny old city and an elegant black gondola that brought him to the Grand Hotel de l'Europe, was for him a water-borne hearse (Grun, 1967, 185). Dilapidated palazzi, surrounded by gardens running wild, reflect the contradiction of past splendour and present decline.

The dominating presence of the past can be experienced as threat, as when Charles Dickens described his stroll through the palace of the dodge. He saw it as a grandiose dreamlike gigantic edifice, full of golden old mosaics, with the smell of perfume, darkened by incense, bursting with treasures and precious stones, holy as a last resting place of saints, with the colours of a rainbow in the windows of coloured glass, dark with all the woodcarvings, light with the many-coloured marble […] unreal, fantastic, solemn-serious – incomprehensible […]. And walking through the halls and empty chambers he realized he was seeing the former pride and power – dead! Everything here was past – everything past! (Grun, 1967, 194 f.)

Becoming lost, alienation and danger are central themes in Venice's melody of separation.

Herzmanovsky-Orlando explained the crowded narrow lanes by the fact that everyone gets lost there. Nobody, born Venetians included, has ever known his way (Grun, 1967, 152).

For the great conductor Giuseppe Sinopoli, who went astray in Venice one night, it was an inextricable labyrinth whose secret intent was to overcome death (Sinopoli, 2003, 34). The lagoon made Sinopoli aware of the omnipresent contradiction of unity and fragmentation, of clarity and confusion, of life and destruction, similar to the water itself with its antithetic capacity to cause life and death, deadly for the human beings, healthy for fish.

Those who get lost become again the victims of their optical delusions. What at first sight is familiar suddenly appears strange. But Venice is also – especially at carnival – full of wilful deceptions, when masks and costumes hide the real figures.

All these fantasies, conscious and unconscious, are projected into the past or into the future as fears or desires. What kinds of danger become threats of separation? The fear of the city's sinking has its counterpart in fantasies of fusion. For Hippolyte Taine Venice dissolves itself in its own existence: one forgets everything: profession, plans, oneself. One sees oneself lonely, one gathers – one enjoys. And one suddenly feels liberated from everything on earth, high up in the sky, floating over everything – into the light, into the blue (Grun, 1967, 195 f.). And Hermann Hesse dreamed in his poem "Gondelgespräch" (gondola-talk) that they both died yesterday, sliding in their white clothes, with flowers in their hair, in a black gondola towards the sea, listening to sounds, songs and names from far away, words falling in oblivion and dream-death, before they are babbled (Grun, 1967, 117 f.). But even this death-fantasy betrays an unspoken anticipation of a life after death. It allows us to continue to speak of death – yesterday – and to look at the big ships and the summer-sky.

Historic documents of past catastrophes, the decline in the present and the real dangers of the city combine to confront us with the issue of destruction. The beauty and the richness of art in the city suggest the triumph of life and creativity over annihilation. Thus Venice keeps destructiveness – a derivate of the death-drive – and its opposite, creativity, alive in our world of representations. From this vantage-point both pathways are open: a defence against awareness of painful loss endangering our inner and external world, or a confrontation with our own destructive impulses and the human condition of transience. Venice is scenery that provokes such feelings. They might recede again quickly and vanish in the anonymous crowd of tourists and in kitsch. Otherwise, Venice becomes a containing frame for our own anxieties and wishes regarding annihilation. These feelings might be worked through in a new, genuine, creative process that encompasses pain, mourning, guilt, desire and hate. Not only creating art but re-experiencing and identifying with creative action can transform one's own inner beloved and endangered world. In creativity the life-drive regains the upper hand and its downfall is postponed – until further notice.

In Venice one hardly can fail to hear the melody of separation. This can aid us because "it is only when the loss has been acknowledged and the mourning experienced that the re-creation can take place" (Segal, 1986, 190).

7.5 Alberto Giacometti's shrivelling figures

There is hardly a more attractive task than to write a comprehensive psychoanalytic study about Alberto Giacometti, and maybe there will be an occasion for an attempt in the future. Here I want to concentrate on a precious find that one may understand as a hint as to why Giacometti's figures seemed to him to be vanishing over and over again – a recurring phenomenon of separation-anxiety.

Alberto Giacometti was born in 1901 in a mountainous Swiss region. He was the first son of the painter Giovanni Giacometti. One year later his brother Diego was born (who became a sculptor and decorative artist). When Alberto was three, a sister was born, and three years later another brother who later became architect (Breicha, 1985, 186). It was a childhood full of events. Alberto spent a lot of time in his father's studio, which had been a barn before its alteration. Alberto recalled that his first drawing was "Snow White" in her small coffin. He said he had felt very happy when he learned to draw true to nature: 'I had the impression of a perfect command in my task, so that I did exactly what I wanted. How arrogant I was aged ten […]. I controlled my perception, it was paradise, and it lasted until I was eighteen, nineteen: then I got the impression that I was incapable of doing anything! [...] Reality was withdrawing from me' (Matthes, 1987, 154).

From a psychoanalytic point of view one might suppose that his wonderful feeling of being able to control everything was already a reaction-formation following the disappointment that he had no control whatsoever: his close relationship to his mother was disrupted by the arrival of his siblings – and he realized who had caused this rupture. The appearance of rivals provoked feelings of impotence and rage, ready to be expressed in aggression and destruction. Thanks to his outstanding talent and the support of his father Alberto could find an outlet in drawing and painting. His first drawing did not tell the fairy tale of Snow White among cheerful dear dwarfs, rather she was lying in the coffin. Thus he selects the scene where she is the victim of hate and jealousy. Maybe his death wishes did not primarily aim at his 'unfaithful' mother, but at his little sister who already was an irritating rival. Alberto had mentioned that he had sketched a *small* coffin with the dwarfs standing around it. In relation to the dwarfs the coffin should have appeared huge. However, Alberto saw a small coffin in which perhaps in his unconscious fantasy the victim of *his* death wishes rested. Of course, these are all conjectures, but they are supported by facts of Giacometti's biography, and *they contain the nucleus of repressed destructivity that later on – as I believe – became the psychodynamic cause for his fear that his figures might disappear.*

In 1993 in a French surrealistic journal a short autobiography of Alberto Giacometti was published: "Hier, sables mouvants" – 'Yesterday, drift sand' (Breicha, 1987, 111). The volatility of sand that is easily blown to and fro seems to be a telling title. And the dating 'yesterday' points at a past still close and in effect. The text deals with Alberto's childhood and begins with the sentence: 'As a child (between four and seven), I saw of the external world only things that were suitable to give me pleasure. These were primarily stones and trees, and seldom was it more than one object at the same time'. It is remarkable that he was aware of his perception being dictated by the pleasure-principle, and of his capacity to take objects as representations (symbolization) and to concentrate on a single object. This reminds us of the fact that he later chose only few objects, sculpting them again and again. The dense symbolism of the following lines is striking: Giacometti describes a great boulder some 800 metres from the village, 'a monolith of golden colour, opening below to a great cave'. The father had shown the children this rock, which Alberto immediately fastened upon. From now on this cave was the centre of the children's games. It was Alberto's chief pleasure to curl up in the narrowest embayment in the back of the cave. There he was content.

These events during the early years of this highly intelligent child must have drawn his attention to the riddle: out of which cave do little children come? Thus, we might conjecture that it was a regressive pleasure that Alberto enjoyed: returning to the uterus where there was no space for anyone else, just him. We also might assume – following innumerable typical drawings of children – that the tall rock in this phallic form confirmed the hope that cowering in a cave does not mean that a penis is missing. In other words: women also have a penis, and there are no human beings without it. Therefore, one can forget about the danger of castration. The father had shown him the monolith, thus it was presented by the father and also represented him. But the cave within the monolith represented the mother, too. In this retreat everything was fine, there were no rivalry, no conflict and no fear of revenge or punishment; why shouldn't he be in a good mood?

But this peacefulness cannot last. Alberto discovers another gigantic black boulder, which appears extremely menacing. This stone seemed to him a breathing being, hostile and threatening. There was no cave. This was both unbearable and calming too. Maybe he managed to bring some order into his world, giving up denial of his perceptions and acknowledging that there are objects with caves and objects without caves – objects without a penis and objects with it. The unconscious fantasy of a phallic mother was overcome but hostile impulses had to be projected onto the oedipal, phallic object. Alberto kept the discovery of this black menacing rock a secret.

However, the golden monolith apparently soon lost its fascination. Alberto is yearning for the first snow in order to construct his own cave, independent of all stones. He dug a minute and hidden hole in the snow, just large enough for him to slide into, and being in it was utmost pleasure. He did not even want to leave his new cave to go home for dinner and sleep.

When Alberto entered school these fantasies became connected with Siberia. He described exactly what he would see there if he looked out of his warm, small hut which he would call "Isba" in the Russian language. Thus the cave had developed further and was now a hut.

There is, I believe, a decisive passage, which Alberto Giacometti wanted to be the end in the text 25 years later. He added in 1958 a postscript: 'Rereading the final paragraph I recognized that in my imagining of Siberia I described exactly the environment, in which I was and lived at that time.' Thus he became conscious that he had transferred his immediate surroundings far away. The snow-cave and the hut in Siberia have the same source of ice and snow, elements in sharp contrast to passionate heat. Even more important, *Giacometti deleted in 1958 the next paragraph of the original – and with this the whole destructiveness that dominated here.* He reported recurrent obsessive thoughts circling in a daydream. In it he murdered two men in front of a hidden castle and raped two women, whom he afterwards killed too. Then he burned the castle down. Without further speculations about the doubles (two brothers; two women – mother and sister?) we might consider the hypothesis: *it is exactly about this elimination and repression of aggressive and destructive wishes that came out elsewhere and became effective – in the destructive urge, which in Giacometti's inner world threatened that his figures should vanish.* His daydream was full of oedipal material. He first has to kill the men before he can go to the women and penetrate them. This he can do only violently. It is certainly not by chance that in this phase he suddenly could not recall his father's appearance. Not even his numerable portraits and pictures refreshed this visual memory. Alberto's unconscious hostility against his father erased his image. He was dismayed about this incomprehensible amnesia and burst into tears: 'I can no longer remember the face of my father!' (Lord, 1986, 15) What a terrible conflict that in his fantasy he had to kill his father, to whom he owed not only his life but also access to his art! It was a conflict that later was repeated in his creation of figures and the attendant pressure to make them vanish. Claudia Frank elaborated in a careful psychoanalytic study this unconscious struggle between creating and destroying and called this manifestation of the death-drive a reined one (Frank, 2002, 76 ff.).

In 1940 Giacometto complained that to his horror his figures unaccountably were shrinking and shrinking, until they were just one centimetre in size. 'One more pressure with the thumb and jump – the figure is gone!' He conjured rationalisations he needed to make them so small that he could overlook them and that he himself had to remove in order to give an impression of the whole appearance. Nevertheless, this shrinking occurred outside his conscious control and against his will. In 1945 he said that he vowed to himself that he would no longer allow his figures to become any smaller. What happened then, was that he managed to retain to their size, but they became ever slimmer (Hohl, 1998, 100 ff.).

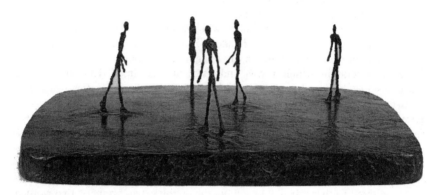

Figure 9
Giacometti's shrivelling figures symbolize the permanent struggle between constructive and destructive forces.

Giacometti's friends called his "micromania" a fixed idea and they could see what he could not: his destructive urge that came out in his art. Michael Leiris, for instance, said that he felt Alberto was a sculptor mainly because it allowed him to destroy immediately what he had created. Giacometti said that he had to reject about twenty figures in order to get the right one, but he was not aware that the act of destruction itself was a personal issue. In an obsessive search for the "right" figure he considered these destructions to be necessary prerequisites. His associates watched this process with concern because he often smashed during the night everything he had worked on the whole day. Once he brought all his sculptures from his studio in a wheelbarrow to the Seine and tipped them into the river. He did not know that what made his figures shrink and vanish was his own destructive impulsion. It was due to his unconscious conflict between perception and denial, and to his perverse obsessive need to oppose to every 'Yes' a 'No'. Nevertheless, he could describe what he aimed at: the figure should be there but simultaneously not be there. They should have volume, but at the same time should not have volume. They should appear to be in motion, but also be immobile. We have discussed this mechanism of simultaneously knowing and not knowing (chapter 2.2). Freud called it a split in the ego. In the chapter about the "dead mother", we noted the strong ambivalence that a child develops toward the mother, who is actually there but simultaneously absent because of some other concern or interest. She makes mourning impossible because she is there. She makes pleasure impossible because she is not really there. The conscious fear that the object will vanish does not know its own unconscious root: the wish to destroy the bad object. Nevertheless, it is always connected with the fear of revenge that culminates in one's own annihilation. Due to the "work of the negative" (Green, 2005a, 223 ff.) the desire and the creative wish come in the wake of the destructive wish, resulting in the unconscious decision to disappear. It is a permanent to and fro of struggling forces. The compulsion to repeat is expressed by perseverations in form and subject. Giacometti could not part with both. He became "the existentialistic Sisyphus" (Matthes, 1987, 99). The impact of his obsession seems to have been stronger than that of his despair about what he could not achieve. Rüdiger von Naso thought: 'Maybe Alberto Giacometti was the 20th century's artist who felt the greatest despair regarding his art – and who was the most content one with his failure.' (Naso, 2001, 58)

Those, who contemplated his sculpture were content, too. His work had a tremendous radiant energy (Matthes, 1987, 347). The concentration on the contradictory tendencies within us, on our ambivalence and on the unconscious conflicts between bond and separation provokes a strong echo. This we have seen in the willing reception of Andrè Green's concept of the "dead mother". Already the first laudatory review that Giacometti received at age 28 from Michael Leiris emphasized ambivalence as a raw characteristic feature of his work: "There are moments that we can call crises, and they are the only one's that count in life. That are moments, when what is outside suddenly seems to respond to the appeal which we are sending out from within. Then the external world somehow opens up in order to communicate suddenly with our hearts. I like the sculpture of Alberto Giacometti, because everything he does is like a perfection of one of that crises." (Lord, 1985, 117)

Final chord

It is a huge bow which bends from bonding and separating as basic principles of life to the coping strategies of separation-anxiety in artistic works and in the experience of artistic processes. In the title of the book, "The Melody of Separation" the inclination was, without conscious intent, expressed to contrast the bonding unity of a melody to separation.

In examples of separation anxiety, whether in everyday life or in tragic mythic fates, harmonic tones (longing, desire, love, pleasure etc.) and disharmonic tones (anxiety, hate, envy, jealousy, rage etc.) can be detected. We have seen several ways to cope with separation anxiety. To be confronted with separation cannot be avoided. It seems a better solution to face it, as it helps usher along a process of mourning that is similar to the process of creativity and sometimes parallels it. The connections between ourselves as subjects and the others who are the objects are so narrow that separation anxiety contains both the fear of losing the other one and of losing oneself. Thus, separation-anxiety is a psychic phenomenon that – if it grows too big – can only be overcome by a new experience of bonding. This can be a happy encounter but there is the risk that one is too frightened or rejecting, even when by chance a lucky occasion is offered. This also can be the intensive effort of reparation that psychoanalytic treatment offers with its specific chance of establishing a new, though limited bond.

An epilogue too has to do with separation, at least with a short delay of separation. I have often heard that readers, who do not only leaf through a book, but read it intently, become sad when the book is ending. It is like a farewell in a relationship. If I confess that it is the same for the author, when he finishes a book, it results again in a comforting connection, to which – perhaps – later on we again might refer.

References

Abraham K. (1909): Traum und Mythos. Frankfurt a. M.: S. Fischer
Aragon L. e.al. (1987): Wege zu Giacometti. München: Matthes & Seitz
Argelander H.(1970): Das Erstinterview in der Psychotherapie.
   Wissenschaftliche Buchgesellschaft Darmstadt
Bahr H. (without year): Das Konzert. Stuttgart: Reclam Jun. (8646/47)
Balint, M. (1959): Thrills and Regression. London: The Hogarth Press
Bion W.R. (2005): The Italian Seminars. London: Karnac
Bollas Ch. (1987): The shadow of the object. Free Association Books, London
Bowlby J. (1998): Separation – Anxiety and Anger. London: Pinlico
Breicha O., Hohl R. (1985): Alberto Giacometti – Paris sans fin.
   Salzburg: Rupertinum
Catull G.V. (1974): Sämtliche Gedichte. München: dtv
Darwin Ch. (1986): Ausdruck der Gemütsbewegungen.
   Nördlingen: Franz Greno
Eckstaedt A. (1991). Die Kunst des Anfangs. Frankfurt/Main: Suhrkamp
Eissler K. (1987): Der sterbende Patient. Zur Psychologie des Todes.
   Stuttgart: frommann-holzboog
Eith T., Wellendorf F. (Hg.) (2003): Fort – Da. Heidelberg: Ansanger
Ermann M. (2004, 4. Aufl.): Psychosomatische Medizin und Psychotherapie.
   Stuttgart: Kohlhammer
Frank Claudia (2002): Mains tenant le vide – Maintenant le vide: Überlegungen
   zu Giacomettis Figuren (von ca. 1947 bis 1952) und zum analytischen
   Prozess.
   In: Jahrbuch der Psychoanalyse, Bd. 44 Ed. F.-W. Eickhoff e.a.
   Stuttgart: Holzboog
Ferenczi S. (1923): On the symbolism of the head of Medusa.
   In: The International Psycho-Analytic Library, Nr. 11, 366
Freud S. (1900): The Interpretation of Dreams. (The Standard Edition of the
   Complete Psychological Works of Sigmund Freud, Vintage: The Hogarth
   Press =S.E.) 4
Freud S. (1905): Three Essays on the Theory of Sexuality. S.E. 7
Freud S. (1910). „Wild" Psycho-Analysis. S.E. 11
Freud S. (1910): The Antithetical Meaning of Primal Words. S.E. 11
Freud S. (1911): Formulations on the two Principles of Mental Functioning
Freud S. (1914): On Narcissism: An Introduction. S.E. 14
Freud S. (1915). Thoughts for the Times on War and Death. S.E. 14
Freud S. (1915): Observations on Transference Love. S.E. 12
Freud S. (1916): On Transience. S.E. 14
Freud S (1917): Introductory Lectures on Psycho-Analysis, rev. S.E. 15-16
Freud, S. (1917): Mourning and Melancholia. S.E. 14
Freud, S. (1920): Beyond the Pleasure principle. S.E. 18
Freud S. (1922): Medusa's Head. S.E. 18

Freud S. (1923): The Ego and the Id. S.E. 14
Freud S. (1924): The Economic Problem of Masochism. S.E. 19
Freud S. (1926): Inhibitions, Symptoms and Anxiety. S.E. 20
Freud S. (1926): The Question of lay Analysis. S.E. 20
Freud S. (1927): Fetishism. S.E. 21
Freud S. (1930): Civilization and its Discontents. S.E. 21
Freud S. (1937): Analysis Terminable and Interminable. S.E. 23
Freud S. (1937): Moses and Monotheism. S.E. 23
Freud S. (1937): Constructions in Analysis, S.E. 23
Freud S. (1938): Splitting of the Ego in the Process of Defence. S.E. 23
Freud S. (1938): An Outline of Psycho-Analysis. S.E. 23
Freud S. (Ed. 1986): Briefe an Wilhelm Fließ 1887-1904.
    Frankfurt a. M.: Fischer
Gabbard G. O. (1997): The Crying Game, In: Int. Journal of Psychoanalysis,
    Vo. 78: 825–827
Galli G. (1996): Technice decorative in Mosaico. Milano: technice nuove
Gavoty B. (1977): Chopin. Tübingen: Wunderlich
Giacometti A. (1999): Gestern, Flugsand. Zürich: Scheidegger & Spiess
Giannakoulas A. (2001): Squiggles and Spaces.
    In: Bertolini M., Giannakoulas A., Hernandez M.:, Vol. 1, London and
    Philadelphia
Goethe J. W. (without year.): Iphigenie. In: Goethes Werke, ed. Theodor
    Friedrich. Leipzig: Reclam
Green A. (1993, 2nd Ed.): On private madness. Madison, Connecticut: Int.
    Universities Press
Green A. (1999): The Fabric of Affect in the Psychoanalytic Discourse.
    Routledge, London
Green A. (2001): The Chains of Eros. London
Green A. (2001): Todestrieb, negativer Narzissmus, Desobjektalisierungs-
    funktion. In: Psyche, 9/10, 55. Jg., Sept./Okt.
Green A. (2001): Life Narcissism, Death Narcissism. London: Free Association
    Books
Green A. (2002): Time in psychoanalysis. London: Free Association Books
Green A. (2003): Geheime Verrücktheit. Gießen: Psychosozial-Verlag
Green A. (2005): Key ideas for a contemporary Psychoanalysis. East Sussex:
    Routledge
Green A. (2005): The illusion of common ground and mythical pluralism.
    In: The International Journal of Psychoanalysis, Vol. 86, June 2005, Part 3,
    627 ff.
Green A., Kohon G. (2005): Love and its Vicissitudes. East Sussex: Routledge
Grun B. (1967): Einladung nach Venedig. München-Wien: Langen-Müller
Hagmann G. (2003): On ugliness. In: Psychoanalytic Quarterly, LXXII, Nr. 4;
    Other Press

Hartocollis P. (2003): Time and the Psychoanalytic Situation. In: Pschoanalytic Quaterly, 72, 2. Other Press

Hinshelwood H.D. (1991): A dictionary of Kleinian thought. London: Free Association Books

Hohl R. (1998): Giacometti – Eine Bildbiographie. Bonn: Hatje

Horaz G. (1982): Sämtliche Werke. Darmstadt: Wissenschaftliche Buchgesellschaft

Jones, E. (1957). Sigmund Freud Life and Work, Vol. 3. Bern-Stuttgart: Hans Huber Schattauer

Kafka F. (1919 <1991>): Brief an den Vater. Frankfurt a. M.: Fischer Tb

Kennedy R. (2002): Psychoanalysis, history and subjectivity – now of the past. N.Y.: Brunner-Routledge

Kellaway N. (1996): The Virago Book of Women Gardeners. London: Virago Press

Kohon G. (1986): The British School of Psychoanalysis. London: Free Association Books

Kohon G. (1999): No lost certainties to be recovered. London: Karnac

Kohon G. (1999): The dead mother. The work of André Green. London: Routledge

Kohon G. (2005): Love in a time of madness. In: Green A., Kohon G. (2005): Love and its Vicissitudes. East Sussex: Routledge

Kristeva J. (1987): In the Beginnings was Love. N.Y.: Columbia University Press

Kristeva J. (1989): Black Sun. Depression and Melancholia. N.Y.: Columbia University Press

Kutter P. (1997): Altern in selbstpsychologischer Sicht. In: Radebold H. (1997): Altern und Psychoanalyse. Göttingen: Vandenhoeck & Ruprecht

Lang H. (2003): Fort – Da. „Ich kann nicht mit ihr leben, und ich kann ohne sie nicht leben" (Franz Kafka). In: Eith T., Wellendorf F.: Fort – Da. Heidelberg: Ansanger.

Lamartine A. d. (1963): Œuvres; hg. M.-F. Guyard, Paris: Plèiade

Laplanche J. (1985): Leben und Tod in der Psychoanalyse. Frankfurt a. M.: Nexus

Leupold-Löwenthal H. (1986): Handbuch der Psychoanalyse. Wien: Orac

Leupold-Löwenthal H. (1985): Zur Frage der psychoanalytischen Nosologie und Diagnostik; Zeitschrift für psychoanalytische Theorie und Praxis, O-Nr., 33-46

Loewald H. (1960): On the therapeutic action of psychoanalysis. In: International Journal of Psycho-Analysis, 41, 16ff

Loewald H.W. (1980): Psychoanalyse. Aufsätze aus den Jahren 1951-1979. Stuttgart: Klett-Kotta

Lord J. (1986): Giacometti – A Biography. London: Phoenix

Matthes A. (1987): Louis Aragon et al.: Wege zu Giacometti. München: Matthes & Seitz Verlag

Merkel I. (1994): Eine ganz gewöhnliche Ehe. Frankfurt a. M.: Fischer Tb
Meltzer W. (1988): The Apprehension of Beauty. Worcester: The Clunie Press
Moore H. (1983): Henry Moore in Wien. Exhibition Catalogue. Wien: Habarta
    Kunsthandel & Verlag.
M'Uzan M. de (1977): De l'art à la mort. Paris: Gallimard
Mitchell J. (1986): The question of femininity and the theory of psychoanalysis:
    in: Kohon G.: The British school of psychoanalysis
Naso R. von (2001): Nichts als die Wahrheit. In: Madame, 7/2001
Ovidius P. N. (1983): Metamorphosen. München: Artemis
Parsons M. (1999): Psychic reality, negation, and the analytic setting. In:
Parsons M. (2000): The Dove that Returns, the Dove that Vanishes. London:
    Routledge
Philipe A. (1975): Nur einen Seufzer lang. Reinbek bei Hamburg: rowohlt Tb
Phillips A. (1999): Darwin's Worms. London: Faber & Faber
Poutalès, G. de (1964) : Der blaue Klang. Fréderic Chopins Leben. Frankfurt
    a. M.: Fischer
Quinodoz J.-M. (2004): Die gezähmte Einsamkeit. Tübingen: edition-discord
Radebold H. (1997): Altern und Psychoanalyse. Göttingen: Vandenhoeck &
    Ruprecht
Ranefeld J. (2003): Im Blick. Der Augenschein. In: Texte, 3. Wien, 28 ff.
Rank O., Ferenczi S. (1924): Entwicklungsziele der Psychoanalyse.Wien: Turia
    und Kant
Rilke R. M. (1987): Werke I, Gedichte. Frankfurt a.M.: Insel Tb
Rosendorfer H. (2003): Venedig – Eine Einladung. Köln: Kiwi
Salvatore G. (2003): Einladung zum Untergang. Wien: Picus
Sandler J., Sandler A.-M. (1983): The "second censorship", the "three box
    model" and some technical implications. In: International Journal of
    Psycho-Analysis 64, p. 413-425
Sandler J., Sandler A.-M. (1996): Das vergangene Unbewusste und das
    gegenwärtige Unbewusste. In: Zwettler-Otte S., Komarek A.: Der
    psychoanalytische Prozess.
Sandler J., Sandler A.-M. (1998): Internal objects revisited. London. Karnac
Saussure J. (1996): Dilemmas und Herausforderung für den Psychoanalytiker
    von heute. In: Zwettler-Otte S., Komarek A.: Der psychoanalytische
    Prozess.
Schmidt-Hellerau C. (1995): Lebenstrieb & Todestrieb, Libido & Lethe.
Stuttgart: Internationale Psychoanalyse
Schnitzler A. (<1892> 1972): Komödie der Worte. In: Dramatische Werke.
    Bd. 2. Frankfurt a. M.: Fischer
Schnitzler A. (<1915> 1970): Sterben. Die erzählenden Schriften. Bd. 2.
    Frankfurt a. M.: Fischer
Segal Hanna (1986): The work of Hanna Segal. London: Free Association
    Books
Segal H. (1991): Dream, Fantasy and Art. London: Routledge

Shakespeare W. (Ed. 1958): Complete Works. London: Hamlyn

Steiner R. (1999): Some Notes on the „Heroic Self". In: International Journal of Psychoanalysis, Vol. 80, 4, 685 ff.

Sterba R. (1932): Das Schicksal des Ichs im therapeutischen Verfahren, Darmstadt

Tichy M., Zwettler-Otte S. (1999). Freud in der Presse, Wien

Tuckett D., 2001: Reflection on M. Hernandez and A. Giannakoulas' On the Construction of Potential Space. In: Bertolini M., Giannakoulas A. e.a.: Squiggles and Spaces Vol. 1. London and Philadelphia

Widlöcher D. (1996): Die Abstinenzregel heute. In: Zwettler-Otte S., Komarek A.: Der psychoanalytische Prozess.

Winnicott D. W. (1983): Von der Kinderheilkunde zur Psychoanalyse. Frankfurt a. M.: Fischer Tb.

Winnicott D.W. (1985, 5. Ed.): Playing and Reality. England: Pinguin Books

Winnicott D.W. (1986): Fear of Breakdown. In: Kohon G.: The British school of psychoanalysis.

Winnicott D.W. (1986): Home is where we start from. London

Winnicott D.W. (1987): Through paediatrics to psycho-analysis. London: The Hogarth Press

Winnicott D.W. (1990): The maturational process and the facilitating environment. London

Winnicott D.W 1991: Human Nature. London: Free Association Books

Yourcenar M. (1967): Feuer. Frankfurt a. M.: Fischer Tb

Zwettler-Otte S. (1991, 3. ed.): Die Repetenten – Warum Lehrer Lehrer wurden. Wien: Perlenreihe

Zwettler-Otte S. (1995): KIP als tiefenpsychologisches Verfahren oder Die rote Mütze des Bahnhofsvorstands. In: Imagination, Zeitschrift der Österr. Ges. für Autogenes Training und Allgem. Psychotherapie.

Zwettler-Otte S., Komarek A. (Ed. 1996): Der psychoanalytische Prozeß. Wien: Turia&Kant

Zwettler-Otte S. (Ed. 2002, 2nd edition): Von Robinson bis Harry Potter. Kinderbuchklassiker Psychoanalytisch. München: dtv

Zwettler-Otte S. (2004): Über die heimliche Attraktivität des Unbewussten. In: Bulletin der Europ. Psychoanal. Föderation, 58

Zwettler-Otte S. (2005): Das vorbewußte dynamische Kräftespiel in der Sprache des Analysanden. In: Zeitschrift für psychoanalytische Theorie und Praxis

Zwettler-Otte S. (2006): The body and the sense of reality – Discussion of Simo Salonens paper. In: Beyond the Mind-Body-Dualism: Psychoanalysis and the Human Body. Ed.: Evy Zacharacopoulou.Athens. Elsevier.

Zwettler-Otte S. (Ed. 2009): „...durch 1000 Kanäle und Poren. Frankfurt-Berlin-Wien: Peter Lang Internationaler Verlag der Wissenschaften

Zwettler-Otte S. 2011: Ebbe und Flut – Gezeiten des Eros. Psychoanalytische Gedanken und Fallstudien über die Liebe. Stuttgart: Kohlhammer

Index

Endless in Love

~ The Maverick Billionaires ~

Book 8

Bella Andre &
Jennifer Skully

ENDLESS IN LOVE

~ The Maverick Billionaires, Book 8 ~

A sexy billionaire and the one woman he can't have...

Dane Harrington is the epitome of power, wealth, and success. The self-made billionaire is used to getting what he wants, when he wants it. And he's well aware he wouldn't be able to get it all done without his brilliant personal assistant, Cammie Chandler.

Cammie is smart, beautiful, and fiercely independent. And before she ever thought she'd work for Dane, the two of them had a steamy night full of sensual touches and passionate kisses. But once he offered her the fantastic position as his personal assistant, they both agreed the only possible way to make it work was if they remained perfectly professional. But no matter how hard they've both tried, neither of them has been able to completely forget their one incredible, sexy night together.

When Dane finally admits the only woman he's ever truly wanted is Cammie, their burning desire becomes too powerful to resist. Can they throw out the rule book that has kept them safe for so long? Or will a love that seems endless be forever doomed?

A note from Bella & Jennifer

Thank you so much for joining us in our journey through the love lives of the Maverick Billionaires! We have been beyond thrilled by how you have taken each Maverick hero and heroine into your heart for the past seven books. Now, we couldn't be more pleased for you to get to know the newest Mavericks – the Harrington family. Like the previous books in this series, regardless of how much money they have in their bank accounts, at the end of the day, each hero and heroine is just like us. They all long for true love, whether they're willing to admit it to themselves, or not.

We hope you fall head over heels in love with the Harringtons! And of course, all of your favorite Mavericks will be in all of the upcoming books, as well.

With love,
Bella Andre and Jennifer Skully

P.S. Please sign up for our New Release newsletters for more information on new books. www.BellaAndre. com/Newsletter and http://bit.ly/SkullyNews.

Chapter One

"Now, that's a lot of pregnant ladies." Eyes on the women on the sidelines, Dane Harrington's sister Ava pulled her glossy, dark red hair into an elastic band.

Dane couldn't tell if that was envy in her eyes. Or terror. Knowing his sister, who was thirty-six and a couple of years younger than him, it had to be terror. She didn't flinch in boardrooms, and a ferocious game of soccer never alarmed her. But babies struck fear into the hearts of all the Harrington siblings—his two sisters and two brothers.

Golden Gate Park on a Sunday afternoon provided the backdrop for one such ferocious soccer game. The Mavericks set up the collapsible goal nets his sister Gabby had brought, and his brothers, Troy and Clay, finished the chalk lines. Since the lawn wasn't an official soccer field, they shared it with kids flying kites, dog owners throwing Frisbees, families enjoying a picnic, and sunbathers catching rays on the first sunny Sunday anyone had seen in six weeks.

January had been wet in the San Francisco Bay Area, with storms hitting hard along the entire West Coast. The rain, thankfully, had let up a week ago, and now, at the tail end of January, the turf had dried out, making an impromptu game possible without it turning into a mud bath. Not that Dane was averse to getting dirty for something important.

And today was important to him.

The Maverick ladies sat in deck chairs on the grassy sidelines, ready to cheer on their husbands and significant others. And yeah, that was a lot of pregnant women. Paige Collins was the furthest along, her due date somewhere around the end of March.

Fernsby, Dane's butler, who insisted on going everywhere with Dane, rolled his ubiquitous tea trolley through the gathering, offering his baked treats and cups of tea.

Dane caught Cammie's eye, and she gave him a thumbs-up. While her hair shimmered red-gold in the sunshine, Cammie's green eyes seemed to sparkle, something he swore he could see even from this distance. Among the women on the sidelines, she formed the Harrington cheering section—along with T. Rex, the long-haired mini dachshund they shared, who'd run to her the moment Dane unleashed him.

His personal assistant for the last twelve years, Cammie Chandler was one of the most caring, loyal people he knew. He felt exceptionally grateful she'd taken time away from her uncle's bedside in the San

Juan Bautista care home to make the two-hour drive north to Golden Gate Park. Her uncle suffered with late-stage Alzheimer's, and Cammie had been on family leave for the past five months to be with him.

But Dane needed her input on the Mavericks before he moved forward with his plans. Cammie's impressions were always spot-on. He thanked his lucky stars for the day Clyde Westerbourne sent her to him for that job interview twelve years ago. His work life had been a shambles, with one assistant after another only making his problems worse. All of twenty-two at the time, Cammie had saved his work life from catastrophe.

Ava kicked his shin. Thinking about Cammie, he'd missed Will Franconi kicking the ball and starting the game. Though soccer normally required at least seven players, there were only five Harringtons. Playing in teams of five, the Mavericks probably thought they had the advantage since they could bring in Cal Danniger or Gideon Jones to spell the others—not that Dane had ever seen an exhausted Maverick.

But they didn't know Gabby and Ava were the Harringtons' secret weapons.

Gabby was right there, taking control of the ball, dribbling it down the field, even though she could have kicked it to one of her brothers. But that was Gabby, totally focused on the goal. Youngest of them all at only thirty, she was blond like their mother, while all the males of the family were dark-haired. Ava, with her red locks, was a throwback to their grandfather.

Both his sisters were holy terrors on the soccer field. And super competitive. Even he found their ruthlessness shocking. They could steal the ball out from under you in a split second. Of all the Harringtons, they were the fastest and wiliest. Soccer wasn't about brute strength. It was about agility and strategy. And they were both excellent tacticians.

Gabby swiftly passed the ball to Ava, just as Matt Tremont made his move, going in for the steal. But he pulled up short, mystified to find the ball no longer there.

Dane and his siblings had played soccer with Gabby since she'd joined her middle school soccer team in the Bay Area, then had gone on to play all through high school. The family had used the game as a way to deal with their parents' deaths in an avalanche while skiing in the French Alps. The blows had continued when they'd learned their parents had squandered their fortune, racking up huge debts. Soccer practice helped them blow off steam and kept the family from imploding. Dane had spent his entire adult life keeping his brothers and sisters together. They were all his best friends, the ones he turned to and counted on, be it critical middle-of-the-night calls or just goofing around.

But now they'd all found their own paths and were doing damn well. Even if each of them had yet to find a partner—or, hell, even a serious relationship. At thirty-eight years old, Dane's life had become about business, his resorts, and expansion.

His team—his family—moved the soccer ball rapidly down the field toward the Mavericks' goal net. While Clay played goalie, Troy and Ava kicked the ball back and forth, but soon Gabby would move in for the kill. Cal and Gideon yelled instructions from the sidelines while Matt, along with Evan Collins, tried vainly to steal the ball. They hadn't a clue it was no use.

Gabby went for the goal. Sebastian Montgomery dove for the ball before it made it into the net, his fingers falling an inch short.

Of course one of his sisters scored first. Dane high-fived his teammates, while the Mavericks stomped the grass like angry stallions.

They were an equally competitive bunch, one of the many reasons they interested him. Since that New Year's Eve gala at Dane's Napa resort, the Mavericks and Harringtons had been feeling each other out over one-on-one lunches, drinks, or dinners. All the proceeds from the fundraiser had gone to benefit Lean on Us, Gideon's foundation for veterans and foster kids. Dane had worked with Cal Danniger and Lyssa Spencer extensively on the holiday gala, getting to know them well. As he learned more about the Mavericks, he discovered a synergy between them he couldn't quite explain. And he envied it.

A couple of days ago, Will Franconi had called him, saying they should all talk.

Dane had suggested the soccer game.

"Sounds perfect," Will said. "Afterward, we'll grab a pint in the city and talk." After a beat, he added, "We feel there's great potential in pursuing some business ventures with all of you."

Dane thought the same thing. His family agreed. The Mavericks would complement everything his sisters and brothers brought to the table.

They got in position for the Mavericks' turn at the ball. Now they'd had a taste of the Harringtons, the Mavericks would be on guard and not as easy to beat.

Dane went for the steal right under Evan's nose. But the man saw him coming, and the ball whirled out of his reach to Matt, who dribbled it down the field. Yeah, the Mavericks were now playing tough.

He'd first met the Mavericks when he anonymously purchased a Miguel Fernando Correa painting from Gideon. The famous artist's work had come into Gideon's hands through an army comrade. After remaining unknown for generations, the painting was now worth millions. Instead of exploiting the windfall, Gideon had used the proceeds to start his nonprofit foundation.

Of course, Dane had heard of the Mavericks long before that. Who hadn't? When Lyssa and Cal came to

London with the intention of hitting him up for a donation, he'd revealed the Correa painting upstairs in his study. And told them of his desire to help the foundation in any way he could. He'd brought in more donations and offered his resort for the gala fundraiser Lyssa had planned.

But it was Cammie who'd first seen the magic in the painting, encouraging him to bid on it. He'd upped the bid until there was no doubt the amazing work of art would be his. After he'd enjoyed the painting in his London townhome for a few months, it was now making the rounds of galleries and museums worldwide. Cammie had set up the tour from her uncle's bedside.

His gaze drifted once more to her on the sidelines. She watched the game as avidly as the Maverick ladies, all of them shouting encouragement as their men kicked the ball between them, moving it swiftly down the field, neither Gabby nor Ava able to check their momentum.

If Cammie hadn't pointed out the Correa painting to him, Dane would never have connected with the Mavericks.

She amazed him with her dedication. She'd taken care of her uncle for years after he was diagnosed with early-onset Alzheimer's. Seven years ago, the disease progressed to the point that she'd had to put him in a memory care facility. He'd lived far longer than most

Alzheimer's patients. A few months ago, however, it became clear he was close to the end of his journey. Dane had insisted Cammie take family leave when he found her sleeping at her desk. The only person who could calm her uncle, she'd been traveling back and forth to the care home several times a week. But caring for him and managing her job at the same time was affecting her health.

After these last few months without Cammie, Dane's life was again in a shambles. Which was why he was so glad to have her here today, though he knew how hard it was for her to leave her uncle. She was more than Dane's personal assistant. She was as important to him as his family. She kept him on track. She was right on about ventures he should go for and schemes he should avoid, seconding his gut feelings. She was smart. She was diligent. And so efficient there'd never been a single hiccup in his work life. Until she left. Even with the temps who'd taken her place, he was barely hanging on. Not that he'd tell her. Her place was by her uncle's side right now.

Except today, when Dane needed her.

The ball thwacked him in the head. He hadn't even realized he'd stopped running. Or that Gabby had gone for another steal. But Matt stole it back. On her feet, his wife, Ari, punched her fist in the air, screaming at Matt to go all the way.

The sidelines erupted with cheers when the Mavericks kicked the ball into the corner of the net despite Clay's dive.

Almost lost among the women on the sidelines, Cammie jumped up and down on the grass, waving her hands, throwing out catcalls. Because she was all for the Harringtons. Always had been. Always would be.

That was his girl Friday.

★ ★ ★

The tied game roused all the passions on the sidelines, everyone shouting hurrahs for the Mavericks, who'd just put in Gideon and Cal to replace Evan and Daniel.

Lyssa Spencer, her dark curls shining in the sunlight, turned to Cammie. "Dane's sisters are crazy good." Even her eyes, a chocolate brown like her brother Daniel's, seemed to smile.

Having taken her seat again, Cammie ran her fingers through Rex's fur as he climbed once more into her lap. Ava and Gabby were the Harringtons' surprise advantage. "They're pretty good."

Letting out a big laugh, Lyssa gushed, "They're out of this world. They could go pro. I mean, my brothers are no slouches." She put a hand on her belly. "And look at Cal out there. He's crushing it." The pure love on Lyssa's face made Cammie's heart stutter. Cal Danniger, the Mavericks' business manager, though quite a few years older than Lyssa's twenty-six, was still extremely attractive and fit, with a hint of silver in his dark hair.

At more than three months pregnant, Lyssa wore that special motherhood glow. Dane had mentioned that Cal and Lyssa had postponed their wedding until after the baby came in July.

Kelsey Collins, Evan's younger sister, nudged Lyssa's arm. "And let me tell you, those Harrington men are no slouches either." She winked, adding a swoony note to her tone. "Talk about tall, dark, and handsome."

The Harrington brothers were definitely a handsome lot—all over six feet, with thick, dark hair and blue eyes that seemed to see everything inside you. At least, Dane's gaze did. Once, long ago, Troy had asked her out. Naturally, she'd turned him down. Working for Dane, it would have been awkward, even if she'd been interested. She was fairly certain Dane had read Troy the riot act for trying to poach one of his employees. He'd even apologized for Troy's harassment, though Cammie had scoffed at his use of that word. Troy had asked, she'd said no, they'd both been fine, end of story. Clay, of course, had never even thought about dating her. They might be drop-dead gorgeous like their older brother, but no way did she need that kind of complication.

But she certainly wasn't blind. They were *all* drop-dead gorgeous. Especially Dane. Not that she actually *looked.*

"I really thought you would date him, Lyssa." Kelsey waggled her eyebrows. "He's such a hottie, with all that thick hair a woman would just die to run her fingers through." She kneaded the air with her fingers like a cat. "Especially after that trip you made to his London townhouse."

Lyssa's gaze rested on Cal, adoration in her eyes as she said, "Dane's London house is stunning, filled with furniture and artwork that should be in a museum." She ignored Kelsey's insinuations about Dane and pointed to Fernsby. "And the house came with its very own British butler."

Fernsby, now busily passing out his baked treats, had been with Dane for years, long before Dane bought the townhouse in the fashionable London borough of Chelsea. Cammie always suspected that baking was how Fernsby showed his love, though you certainly couldn't tell from his manner. With the ageless face of a person who neither smiled nor frowned, he could be anywhere from forty to sixty. Wearing his ever-present stern expression, and with his tall frame and cultured voice, he was the epitome of the loyal manservant, always at Dane's side no matter where, be it the London house, the manor in the English countryside, the Pebble Beach estate, the San Francisco flat, or even the small Caribbean island Dane owned.

But Kelsey didn't let the subject go. "Come on, Lyssa, don't tell me you didn't think about a little—" She fluffed her ponytail of tawny blond-streaked hair and grinned instead of saying exactly what. "—for just a moment during that first meeting with Dane in his fabulous London home."

Hands on her baby bump, Lyssa's gaze fastened on Cal as he masterfully controlled the ball. "You know Cal was always the man for me." Her eyes reflected the dreamy note in her voice. And she nudged Kelsey. "You're the one who should date Dane. He's perfect for you."

Kelsey visibly shuddered. "No way. He's too rich, powerful, and handsome. I want someone I don't have to compete with."

Cammie liked the outspoken Kelsey. From Dane, Cammie had learned that Kelsey and her twin brother, Tony—who couldn't make it today—had appeared in their older brother's life only a year ago. Evan had known nothing about the twins, his mother having left when he was only nine years old. But he'd apparently welcomed them all with open arms, his birth mother included. Cammie was sure there had to be a major story there.

On the field, Dane stole the ball from Cal, and the Maverick ladies erupted in catcalls. Of course, Cammie jumped to her feet cheering. Rex, accidentally dumped on the ground, barked his joy, too, then abruptly ran off to beg Fernsby for a treat.

Kelsey had said she didn't want someone too rich, powerful, or handsome. But she'd forgotten one adjective—perfect. The things Kelsey said about Dane didn't bother Cammie. She wasn't proprietary about her boss. She certainly wasn't jealous. She was just a little uncomfortable with Kelsey talking about Dane as if he were a prize piece of beef. Even if he was. Cammie had done her best not to notice that over the years she'd worked for him. She'd had her uncle to think of, who'd relied on her for so long she couldn't remember a time when he hadn't. And she'd always been there for him.

But even if she had absolutely no designs on Dane—their working relationship was too important— she liked the way he'd introduced her today, not *just* as his assistant, but adding, "I can't do anything without her."

With all the jeering from the Maverick ladies, Cammie cheered the Harringtons. Staid Fernsby, incapable of even cracking a smile, certainly couldn't do it.

Cammie punched the air. "You go, Dane. Crush those Mavericks."

Suddenly, she was the target of all the Maverick females, battle light in their eyes, ready to squash the opposition.

Until Kelsey laughed loudly. Then they all doubled

over, laughing in near hysteria.

Lyssa held her baby bump. Ari Tremont and Rosie hugged each other, both women as far along in their pregnancies as Lyssa. Paige Collins, Evan's wife, had to sit back down. There wasn't a more polite way to say it: She was huge, beautifully pregnant with twins, and due in a couple of months.

Wistfulness fell over Cammie, even as she wiped tears of laughter from her eyes. They were all so happy. And their children would be so close in age. The two boys, Matt's son, Noah, and Rosie's son, Jorge, both almost seven, were dying to be big brothers. One huge happy family, they were wonderful to watch.

And the burst of laughter they'd all shared made Cammie long to be one of them.

Chapter Two

Even as the women wiped their eyes, ignoring the game for the moment, Rosie Diaz stepped up to Cammie. "We're so glad you could come today. Dane talks so much about you."

Cammie smiled, feeling the same thrill that had come over her earlier when Dane introduced her as more than his assistant. "I'm sorry I missed your art show. I heard it was a brilliant success."

Rosie blushed. Like Lyssa, she and Gideon had postponed their wedding until after the baby was born. She would marry her handsome, blond ex-marine—Ari Tremont's brother—in the fall.

"Thank you so much." Rosie's smile reached almost ear to ear. "I appreciate that." She was an amazing painter, according to Dane, and Cammie believed him. He was never wrong. As she tucked her beautifully thick, curly black hair behind her ear, Rosie's smile faded. "You don't need to apologize. We all know how hard it's been taking care of your uncle."

"Thank you," Cammie said softly, feeling the ever-present twist in her stomach.

This was the first and only time she'd left her uncle since he'd worsened last September. But she'd felt deeply how important it was to meet the Mavericks and their partners, rather than just be told about them. When Dane was considering business ventures, she couldn't be left out.

Still, it had been a hard decision to leave Uncle Lochlan, even for the day.

He'd first shown signs of something wrong when she was a senior in high school, and it had been terrifying. She'd planned to start college that fall, and yet, she couldn't leave Uncle Lochlan when they didn't even know what was wrong. Instead, she'd taken a job with Clyde Westerbourne, a good friend of her uncle's. That turned out to be the best decision of her life. It eventually led her to Dane—or rather, to her job with Dane.

The Alzheimer's diagnosis had been a terrible blow, but thankfully her uncle's progression had been uncannily slow. The doctors said he was one for the record books. He'd been able to live in his own home, with her help, until seven years ago, when the police found him wandering more than a mile from home. She thanked God every day for Dane's help, and for Ava, who owned retirement communities, elder care homes, and memory care facilities all over the country and internationally. Ava had found Uncle Lochlan a place.

But now his time was finally running out.

Rosie laid a gentle hand on Cammie's arm. "If you ever need even the smallest bit of help, don't hesitate to call one of us. We're always here for people we care about."

The touch, Rosie's smile, and the kindness in her words warmed Cammie's heart. She'd lost her parents in a car accident when she was seven and gone to live with Uncle Lochlan. He was her only family. And now she was losing him.

And yet, here was a slew of Mavericks entering her world.

As the first half of the game ended, the teammates rushed Fernsby, who'd uncapped bottles of water and laid out an array of tea sandwiches for the players' fortification.

Gabby sniffed one of the sandwiches, looked at Fernsby, then smiled ever so sweetly. "I'm sure the sandwiches are totally amazing, dear Fernsby. The only thing that would make them even better is if there were no eggs or butter and the bread was gluten-free."

Fernsby's face morphed into a rigid mask of horror. "Excuse me, dear lady, but it can't be an egg salad sandwich without eggs. Eggs and butter are the mainstays of a life well lived." Then he drawled, "And I won't address gluten-free bread, as it cannot even be called bread."

Gabby shrugged, laughter dancing in her eyes as

she got right up in his face. "I think you and I need to have our own little bake-off one of these days."

Catching Dane's eye, Cammie shared a smile with him. Fernsby and Gabby had a longstanding rivalry. Vegan and gluten-free for years, Gabby had started her own conglomerate, a franchise of bakeries specializing in vegan and gluten-free products. She managed her own franchise in Carmel. But even after her great success, Fernsby loved his butter, eggs, and all manner of dairy products.

Kelsey leaned close. "Is he just Fernsby? Or does he have a first name?"

Cammie smiled, shaking her head. "If he does, I've never heard it. I think he was just born as Fernsby. He's been with Dane for-like-ever, since Dane bought that first resort."

That drew her gaze to Dane again as he mowed down one of Fernsby's tea sandwiches on thinly sliced bread. That was the British way, so of course it was Fernsby's way.

Seeming to sense her eyes on him, Dane turned, a beautiful smile on his lips that sometimes made her heart race—not much, just a bit. Because, of course, they had rules that kept their relationship purely platonic. They worked so well together, amazing colleagues that they were. One might even say they had synergy. At least, that's what Dane called it. To her, it was the perfect relationship. Even if there were times she thought—

But no way would she ruin what they had. Her job and her uncle's care were her priorities. What if she and Dane started something only to have it end badly? The best twelve years of her life would be nothing more than a memory. And if sometimes she found herself nursing a migraine when he began dating a new woman—though she'd never been prone to migraines—that didn't matter.

Leaning around Kelsey, Lyssa asked, "Did I hear you say the amazing Fernsby has worked for Dane since he bought his first resort?"

Glad for the new subject, Cammie nodded. "It's been that long."

"As I understand it," Rosie said, "Dane was, what, only twenty-four at the time?"

Cammie wasn't giving away secrets when she answered, "Yes. He'd worked at that resort for a couple of years after his parents died. But the owners ran into financial troubles, and rather than see it go out of business, Dane pulled together the financing to take over. That was the beginning. Now he owns resorts all over the world."

All three women smiled at her, as if they hadn't already known all that. "That's an amazing story," Rosie said.

But none of them could know the whole story— how hard Dane had worked to keep his family together after his parents died. "He's a self-made man," she told them with pride.

Rosie smiled at Lyssa, then glanced at Gideon. "That's what these Maverick men are all about. Self-made. And they're all pretty darned incredible."

Cammie had to agree. But they were no more incredible than Dane.

In that moment, Dane looked up from an in-depth conversation with Will Franconi, as if divining he was the topic of conversation.

She and Dane were simpatico. Each knew what the other thought. With that look, he thanked her for moving among the ranks of the Maverick ladies, learning all she could. Which was why Cammie had done a lot more listening than talking today. She was gathering intel. And it was obvious to her that the Mavericks' loved ones had given a thumbs-up to a business link.

As the teams went into action on the field, the women shouted their enthusiasm, screaming for their men to score points. Again. Cammie was unashamed to yell her support for the Harringtons.

Rex chose that moment to run to her, careening into her lap. Cammie nuzzled him. "You're such a sweetie. And I've missed you." He'd been running between her and Fernsby for most of the game.

Kelsey leaned in to say, "Is he your dog, then? I thought he was Dane's."

Fingers buried in the mini dachshund's long hair, Cammie quickly said, "He's actually our puppy. Together." She smiled. "Well, not exactly a puppy. He's seven years old."

Kelsey settled an appraising gaze on her. "I didn't realize you and Dane were..." She trailed off.

Cammie blurted, "Oh, we're not like that. No. I work for him, that's all." Then she laughed, hoping it didn't sound uneasy. "It's just that T. Rex thinks he owns both of us." She buried her face in the dog's soft coat, not wanting Kelsey to see the blush that had crept into her cheeks.

What on earth would the Mavericks think if they knew she lived in Dane's house? Or that she had her own suite of rooms in each of Dane's homes, so they could more easily work together when he traveled? After all, she was his personal assistant. Not a lot of people, though, would understand there was nothing going on between them.

And if sometimes late at night, wherever they happened to be, she thought about Dane in his suite just down the hall and imagined things that could never be, well, that was no one's business but her own. They were PA and boss. And good friends. That was all.

In the end, the game was a draw. Cammie wondered if that was Dane's doing. Or maybe Will's. Though Dane was competitive, and his sisters even worse, he saw no advantage in trouncing the Mavericks. Ditto for Will Franconi.

The Mavericks and Harringtons jogged to center field, shaking hands and giving hearty claps on the back.

Then Will called, "How about going for that pint at the Buena Vista Café?"

The Buena Vista Café served a famous Irish coffee, claiming to have brought the drink to the US. The Maverick ladies darn near squealed, even the pregnant ones. Cammie assumed there'd be nonalcoholic offerings.

Dane caught her eye, and she felt that familiar thrill up and down her spine. That was another of the things she'd never tell anyone.

Reading the question in his eyes, she nodded. Naturally, she'd go for Irish coffee—nonalcoholic, of course, since she had a long return drive to San Juan Bautista.

When they video-chatted tonight, she'd tell him everything.

Except the things she'd never tell anyone. *Especially* not him.

★ ★ ★

Fernsby packed up his tea trolley. He'd designed the contraption himself, with a warming tray, a cooling tray, a battery-powered teakettle, and, of course, a big box fitted below to carry necessities such as serviettes, silverware, and good porcelain. Fernsby never skimped on anything.

Dane looked at him. "Are you coming with us, Fernsby?"

He used his sternest voice. "Sir, surely you can't take the dog to a bar." Then he rolled his trolley away, calling to the animal. "Come along, Lord Rexford, we can't have your morals corrupted by these wastrels." Of course, he said it loud enough for only Dane to hear.

His employer's laughter followed him as he trundled away.

The long-haired dachshund trailed after him, casting longing glances back at Camille. But the little dog was well trained—Fernsby had seen to that personally.

He wasn't a dog person. He wasn't a cat person. In fact, he wasn't even a people person. But the dog, with those sad puppy eyes, had grown on him. As had Camille. She was a hard worker, efficient, no-nonsense. And, above all, loyal. Loyalty was something Fernsby prized very highly. And Dane—he never called him Dane to his face, always sir—had also grown on him during their fifteen-year association. Dane was eminently fair, treating everyone equally, even his personal assistant and his butler. Thus, he'd earned Fernsby's respect. And his loyalty.

He didn't look back, but he felt Miss Gabrielle Harrington's stare right between his shoulder blades, no doubt plotting ways to best his culinary skills with gluten-free and vegan offerings.

Since no one could see, Fernsby allowed himself the smallest of smiles. Her efforts were a lost cause.

When he was finally chosen as a contestant on *Britain's Greatest Bakers*—and vanquished his nemesis Digbert, Mr. Westerbourne's butler, who'd also applied, drat the man—she would naturally have to sing a different tune.

He did, however, respect her unconquerable spirit. She excelled at most things. But she couldn't possibly outdo him.

He admired all the Harringtons. Even if he had his favorites.

After all, that was loyalty.

He turned then, ever so slightly, gazing at Camille and Dane, who stood exceptionally close as the Mavericks gathered their belongings.

Then he smiled, looking down at the dachshund. "Little do they know, Lord Rexford, that the right time for the two of them is almost at hand. You can trust Fernsby on that."

Chapter Three

The Buena Vista Café was a San Francisco icon. Bottles crammed the glass shelves behind the bar, and Irish coffee mugs lined the countertop, ready for the favored libation. Located at Hyde and Beach Streets near Ghirardelli Square, on the first sunny Sunday in what seemed like forever, the bar was filled to capacity.

The waitstaff put together several tables in the tented curbside seating area to accommodate their group. Cammie was sandwiched between Dane and Ava, with Dane's thigh resting along hers, his body heat doing funny things to Cammie's stomach. Something like butterflies. Which meant nothing.

Honking horns and clanking cable cars played a rowdy tune outside the tented parklet, along with raucous voices and boisterous laughter inside. That came mostly from the Mavericks, everyone talking over one another.

Cammie loved the bustle of San Francisco, the happy tourists, the scrumptious food, the salt air, the city skyline, the Golden Gate. Dane had a flat on Nob

Hill, but she hadn't been to the city since her uncle worsened. And she missed the hustle. Though Dane's Pebble Beach estate would always be her favorite of his homes.

Gabby bounded in, a pink bakery box balanced on her hands. She'd said she was bringing a few sweets, but the box was big enough to hold a full sheet cake.

When she opened the flap, the Mavericks went ga-ga at the mouthwatering selection of treats. Noah and Jorge wriggled so eagerly on their seats, they might have bobbed away if Ari and Rosie hadn't been holding them down.

"Those might even look better than Fernsby's of-ferings." Tasha Summerfield rubbed her hands together, while Daniel Spencer leaned close to whisper something into her silky black hair, making her laugh, then bat a hand at him. If those two weren't engaged yet, they soon would be.

Dane jumped in. "Don't let Fernsby hear you say that. You'll never get one of his treats again."

Gabby's eyes sparkled. "That's really why Fernsby left right after the game. I told him I was bringing yummy gluten-free vegan goodies, and he fled in horror."

Everyone laughed except the Maverick men, who'd suddenly gone wide-eyed and leery.

"But we're not vegan," Matt Tremont said, tugging on his hair as if he might pull it out were he forced to eat a vegan pastry.

Dane smiled his lady-killer smile, which of course had no effect on Cammie. At least, not that she'd show. "You'll turn vegan and gluten-free," he declared, "after you taste one of these."

He'd always supported everything Gabby did, just as he had all his siblings.

The Maverick ladies nodded enthusiastically. Ari elbowed her husband. "Come on, Matt. Don't be a fraidy-cat." She ruffled her stepson's mop of hair that was as dark as his father's. "You're dying to try one, right, Noah?"

The boy nodded dramatically. "I'm not a fraidy-cat."

Gabby pulled out a box within the box and set it on the table. Flipping her long blond hair over one shoulder, she leaned close, pointing to a muffin. "This one has an herb that's good for the heartburn pregnant women can get. And here I've got some ginger scones that help the digestion." She held up the box for all of the pregnant women to see. "And this pastry here will help keep your feet from swelling. It's savory, with dill and sun-dried tomatoes."

Ari, her hazel eyes alight, said, "I can't decide which one to try. How about we share?" She looked at Gabby. "They won't cause any reaction with each other, will they?"

Gabby smiled. "Everything here is good for you.

And, of course, there's no cheese."

Rosie, Ari, Lyssa, and especially Paige, the most pregnant of them all, smiled gratefully. Gabby cut the treats into pieces to share, arranging them on plates the waitstaff had brought.

With one taste of the savory pastry, Paige groaned. "Oh my. That is sooo delicious."

Murmurs of appreciation sounded all around. "Thank you so much for thinking of this," Lyssa said to Gabby as Cal tried swiping a piece off her plate. She swatted him. "These are only for those of us who are pregnant. You don't get one."

Once again, the group burst into laughter.

But the Mavericks were a harder sell. Pushing the bigger box to the center of the table, Gabby introduced the delicacies. "This is a cheese blintz."

Sebastian snorted. "If it's vegan, how can it have cheese?"

If he thought he could shoot Gabby down, he was wrong. Gabby Harrington had always held her own around strong men. She simply smiled and said with a slight drawl, "It's vegan cheese. You have heard of that, right?"

"Isn't that an oxymoron?" Daniel said in a dry tone.

Gabby wasn't fazed. "You'd be surprised at the vegan and gluten-free products we have these days. And more are arriving all the time. This one is made with nuts. And it's delicious." Her gaze challenged them all.

Even Cammie, who didn't know them well, understood the Mavericks would never back down from a
challenge.

Troy leaned his elbows on the table, clasping his
hands. "I've got dibs on a cruller, so don't any of you
even think about it. Gabby's raspberry crullers tingle
the tastebuds." He broke into a grin. "And the fudge
glaze is to die for."

Beside her, Dane was grinning, while Ava kept silent, though a sneaky smile played on her lips. The
Mavericks were going down.

Dane reached for Cammie's hand under the table,
squeezing her fingers before he pulled away. He
couldn't know what his touch did to her. And she'd
made sure he never guessed.

Having been the first to question Gabby, Sebastian
had to take the cheese blintz.

Gabby had baked muffins, croissants, crullers, cinnamon rolls, pound cake, zucchini bread, Danish
pastries, and more. Each Maverick chose only one,
while most of the ladies decided to share. There were
no duplicates. Gabby was a smart cookie, not wanting
them to think any one treat was a fluke.

Just as Sebastian had been the first to choose, he
was also the first to take a bite, his mouth pinched as
though he might have to spit it out. But he chewed
thoughtfully. And took another bite. Finally, he looked
at Gabby, his coffee-colored eyes gleaming. "Gabby,

where have you and your delicious goodies been all our lives?" He held out the fork for his fiancée, Charlie Ballard, to try. "You're going to love this, sweetheart." Of course, she did.

Daniel cast a sideways glance at him, as if he suspected Sebastian of trying to pull a fast one.

Then his eyes went wide as he tasted the zucchini bread. "Wow!"

The boys were bouncing in their seats. "Can I, can I, can I?" they cried in unison.

Gabby looked from Rosie to Ari, who both nodded, smiles stretching across their pretty faces. Then she held out the box. "Pick whichever one you want."

Noah chose a frosted cupcake. But Jorge wanted to taste his mother's vegan treats. Rosie gladly shared.

"I never thought I'd say it," Evan admitted, a huge bite missing from his cinnamon roll, "but vegan and gluten-free—at least the way you bake, Gabby—are amazing. I second Sebastian. Where have you and your treats been all our lives?"

And every Maverick chimed in with praise.

Dane smiled broadly as he took in his sister's joy. Cammie knew Gabby didn't lack self-confidence. But these were Mavericks—assured, powerful, assertive men who would obviously balk at her specialty. It had been a test, and she'd passed like a gold medalist racing over the finish line and knowing she'd run her best time ever.

"You—" Matt pointed a finger at her. "—are unbeatable."

Gabby's biggest challenge, however, would be Fernsby. And that day was coming.

Two servers arrived, each carrying a massive tray of drinks, hot chocolate for the boys, nonalcoholic Irish coffees for the pregnant ladies and Cammie, and full-bore Irish whiskey and dark roast coffees for the rest.

The Mavericks were soon to learn that Ava and Gabby could outdrink them as well as outplay them.

With her first sip, Cammie groaned. "This is ambrosia." She closed her eyes to relish the coffee concoction, made with an alcohol-free extract rather than whiskey.

Opening her eyes again, she found Dane staring at her, his Irish coffee in midair. She laughed. "Are you waiting to make sure I thought it was good before you tried yours?"

His eyes as blue as the sunny sky, he smiled and drank. And she could breathe again.

A dab of whipped cream remained on his lips after the first sip. Cammie reached out to wipe it away, as if it were an automatic gesture. But touching had never been automatic between them. So she simply pointed. "Whipped cream." Dane licked it off, sending shivers through her that she barely managed to contain.

What was up with these weak moments? Maybe it was the months she'd spent away from Dane, making everything as fresh as the first time she'd seen him.

But she was tough. She had amazing control. Things would go back to normal.

Will Franconi drummed his fingers on the table, breaking the spell. "We've been thinking a lot about your family."

Dane grinned, and Cammie looked away quickly before his smile brought back those butterflies. "We've been thinking about yours a lot too."

The table went silent as a cable car rang its bell on the street. Then, as if by magic, or synchronicity, they all called out in unison, "Merger!"

When Dane once again reached for her hand under the table, she squeezed back lightly, telling him without words that she agreed. They often communicated with gestures, a smile, or just a look. And his smile warmed her, as if it were only for her, even if their rules made anything personal off-limits.

"If we look at the potential numbers," Will began, only to stop when the Harringtons shook their heads as one.

Troy spoke for them all. "We don't need to look at numbers. This is going to work. Big-time."

The Harrington siblings had taken a month to think it through and talk it over, conducting one-on-one meetings with different Mavericks, each side testing the other's mettle.

They all, especially Dane, knew a good thing when

they saw it.

Cammie took that moment to check her phone. Her uncle lived in Ava's stylish San Juan Bautista facility. But during the entire soccer game, Cammie couldn't help looking for updates. She trusted Ava's people implicitly, yet she couldn't dispel a nagging fear that without her at his bedside, things could go sideways, and he'd be gone before she could get back.

Ava patted her hand, her lips close to Cammie's ear. "Don't worry. I've got my people with him all the time." She held up her phone so that Cammie could see a text with a photo of Uncle Lochlan sleeping peacefully.

She should have known Ava would make a special effort. "Thank you."

She would forever be grateful to Dane and Ava for making it possible to keep Uncle Lochlan with such comfort and oversight. Cammie could never have afforded the care home in San Juan Bautista without their support. Their kindness brought tears to her eyes even now. She'd sold Uncle Lochlan's house right after the move seven years ago and put all the proceeds toward his support. When that was exhausted, she paid whatever she could out of her salary. Of course, it wasn't enough. But she would pay them back over time. Every penny.

Dane had stopped by to see Uncle Lochlan last week, and he'd talked with Cammie about this game.

"You don't have to come," he'd said.

Cammie had immediately shot back, "You think I'd be on board with making such a massive decision without meeting the Mavericks too?"

When he raised his arms, she'd been sure he was about to envelop her in his comforting embrace. Nothing personal, just gratitude that she would do this for him. It warmed her to know how much he valued her input.

Dane was an amazing boss.

She would never leave him. Especially since it would take years to pay him back for all he'd done for her and her uncle.

★ ★ ★

He and Cammie were on the same wavelength. This merger was the best thing for the family. But Dane was glad for the simple agreement in her squeeze of his hand.

If her touch shot a bolt of lightning through him, that meant nothing. He needed Cammie for her smarts, her diligence, her efficiency, her quick mind, and her intuition. Anything else took second place. Even if sometimes…

But now he needed her impressions. Dane wanted this merger for his family. Badly. And he needed Cammie to agree.

His family had good lives. They'd come a long way

since losing their parents. He and Ava had to quit college back then, but the sacrifice had been worth it, because together they'd helped their younger siblings achieve their goals. Troy pursued his dream of Olympic diving, Gabby had visions of cooking school, and Clay was their computer geek. Ava, too, had finished business school, getting her degree in healthcare management. Now they never had to want for anything again.

Except love.

After meeting Bob and Susan Spencer at Gideon's New Year's Eve gala, Dane had recognized the potent, cohesive, loving element that parents added to the mix. His family had so much to learn from these Mavericks, not just businesswise, but emotionally.

Their parents had never provided the stability that Susan and Bob did. Partying in the world's hotspots, Dane's parents had left their kids with indifferent nannies, while Dane and Ava had given their younger siblings all the care they could. How often had he begged his mom and dad to take all the kids with them? Yet, every time, his parents had returned alone to Europe's playgrounds and the ski slopes of Vail or Chamonix or the Swiss Alps. They'd been risk-takers, and in the end, risk had won.

It was no wonder his brothers and sisters were still single. They'd never known a parent's love or witnessed real love and commitment.

They'd all been stunted. While they'd reached for the stars in their careers, none of them had ever found the kind of loving relationship Dane saw in abundance at this table. He wasn't sure any of them would know what to do if the perfect partner came along.

He looked at this impressive Maverick bunch, with the recent additions of Gideon Jones and Cal Danniger to the fold. Each had found a love that surpassed anything Dane had ever imagined. When a Maverick looked at his lady, it was as if love enveloped her. It shone out of their eyes. It softened their features. They might be ruthless men in business, but with the women they brought into their lives, they were compassionate, caring, loving, and loyal.

It could only be due to Bob and Susan Spencer's upbringing. It was the love the couple had felt for the lost boys they'd brought into their family, equal to that for their biological children, Daniel and Lyssa. They'd raised this family in a poor Chicago neighborhood when times must have been unfathomably tough. Yet they'd forged an extraordinary bond with their love and raised extraordinary men and women.

He didn't see the Spencers ever leaving their boys behind, even if they'd had the money to travel. And now, they'd moved halfway across the country from Chicago to join the family on the West Coast. They were fixtures in their children's lives. To their foster sons, they weren't Susan and Bob, but Mom and Dad.

Dane also had an unbreakable bond with his brothers and sisters. He could call on any of them night or day, and they would be there, just as he would be there for them. They weren't just siblings, they were best friends.

But there was so much more out there for all of them. The Mavericks had it. And Dane wanted it with every fiber of his being. He wanted it for all of them.

And for Cammie too.

Thank God for Cammie. She was as much a best friend as any of his family. He could talk over any idea with her, tell her anything. She couldn't know how much he'd missed calling her at any hour since she'd been on family leave. Neither the nightly video chats nor the weekly visits he made to check on Lochlan were enough. She had to do this for her uncle, and Dane had to be supportive. But working without her by his side, it seemed as if he'd lost not only his right hand, but the whole arm. And sometimes it ached like a phantom limb.

With all his woolgathering, he realized Will Franconi had taken over the meeting.

"We actually have a lot of synergy going on," Will was saying, echoing Dane's thoughts. As if taking roll in class, Will introduced each of the Mavericks. "Sebastian is our media mogul with Montgomery Media International." He pointed to Clay. "You both have totally different contacts, and yet, what you do converges. That new YouTube platform you've got going is an amazing feat."

Clay jumped in immediately, not defensive, but wanting everyone to understand. "In reality, it's completely different from YouTube. It's a space for artists, musicians, writers—all forms of artistic endeavor, in fact—to display their work without fear of a hostile environment."

The new platform was already taking over the web. Clay totally knew his market.

Dane started the next round, looking to Matt. "I see a lot of synergy between Troy's sports empire and Trebotics International. With you being the inventor and robotics guy and the new sports machines Troy has in mind, there's immense possibility in what you two can do together."

"I've got tons of ideas." Troy grinned at Matt. "But I need an expert to make them viable."

Matt was nodding, and Dane could see the interest flashing in his eyes. "We've talked a bit," he said. "But we really need to put our heads together."

Dane went on, jutting his chin at Gideon. "Your foundation, Lean on Us, is all about veterans, many of whom are fresh out of the forces." He pointed at his sister, who sat on Cammie's other side. "And Ava is our expert on retirement facilities. You help them when they're younger. She can offer support when they get older."

"I hadn't thought of that." Gideon leaned forward to look at Cal and Lyssa, who were instrumental in running the foundation for him. "Sometimes the older vets don't even know what benefits they actually have." He smiled broadly at Ava.

Full agreement sparked in Ava's eyes. "We've got a lot to talk about."

Will took over again. "Daniel's Top Notch DIY conglomerate has a place in everything we do. As well as The Collins Group, with Evan being our finance guru."

Dane agreed. "We all complement each other, yet bring something unique to the table."

Evan popped up with, "And Gabby can feed us."

As the Mavericks clapped, Dane turned to catch Cammie's eye. Without a word, they were thinking the same thing. *Don't let Fernsby hear that.*

Will waved a hand between the two of them. "I see lots of crossover between you and me, Dane. With Franconi Imports, we can add products and foodstuffs your guests at DH International Resorts have never even dreamed of."

As he lifted his hand in the air, Dane stood to high-five him.

Oh yeah, the Mavericks and the Harringtons together would be a powerhouse.

This was what Dane wanted—synergy, working together, bonding. He could almost feel the magic he,

Cammie, and his siblings could create with the Mavericks.

He rapped his knuckles once on the table. "Let's do it. A partnership." His family were as gung-ho as he was.

Will punched a fist in the air. "Let's do it," he repeated. "I suggest meeting once a month to go over what deals we're all working on, discuss how they can benefit the group, and what each of us can add to them." He looked to his brothers, all of them nodding agreement.

"Sounds good," Dane said. "I see this growing organically. We don't need to shove ideas down each other's throats. We'll work on things that are mutually beneficial."

"Absolutely," Will agreed. Then he grinned. "Let's draw up a partnership agreement." He directed that at Cal Danniger, who in addition to running Gideon Jones's foundation, managed many of the Mavericks' joint ventures.

"I can get that done within a couple of days," Cal agreed, enthusiasm lighting his eyes.

Will gave him a thumbs-up. So did Dane. Beneath the table, Cammie tweaked Dane's hand, a *pinch me, I can't believe this* gesture, signaling her approval of everything he was doing. It was why he'd needed her here.

The sparkle in her eye heated him as she leaned

close, a subtle citrusy scent that was uniquely her own drifting over him. "I'm going to take off now," she murmured.

He held her hand a moment under the table. "I'll walk you to the car."

She shook her head. "You stay here. Talk more. Then call me tonight. We'll discuss it all." Her smile wrapped around him. "But I already know this is going to be the most astounding alliance ever."

Chapter Four

In the quiet study of his Pebble Beach house, Dane slid down into the buttery-soft leather sofa, T. Rex nestled against his side. The mini dachshund grumbled in his sleep, as if he were dreaming of hunting squirrels, and Dane ruffled his long hair. Being such a tiny thing, the dachshund needed a big-dog name, so Dane had dubbed him T. Rex. To him and Cammie, the little guy was anything from T. Rex to Mr. T to just plain Rex. Fernsby always called him Lord Rexford.

Before quitting college to take over as the family guardian, Dane had been on his way to becoming a veterinarian. He'd always loved animals, forever rescuing wild creatures—caring for an injured bird, nursing a chipmunk back to health. His parents' deaths ended that dream, and now he had the resorts and a dog who traveled with him wherever he went. Cammie, a whiz at everything, had streamlined the procedure, making it easy for him to breeze through Customs in various countries without even a quarantine.

He tapped out a text to his whiz: *OK to chat?* Cammie was the first person he wanted to talk to about this afternoon's events.

Sitting back to wait, he propped his feet on a hassock. The study was his leisure room, with a massive flat-screen TV, state-of-the-art audio system, and built-in oak bookcases filled with first-edition classics, hardback bestsellers, genre fiction, business books, and whatever else took his fancy—or Cammie's. Floor-to-ceiling windows afforded a magnificent view of the ocean, though now the sky was socked in by fog, with not a single star visible.

It still felt odd wandering around the huge house without Cammie here. Or sitting at his office desk without being able to look up and see her typing away on her computer, surrounded by her desk and credenza and the files she was working on.

She got back to him in a matter of minutes, as if she'd been anticipating his text: *I'm at your beck and call, Lord Fuzzybottom.*

Rolling his eyes, he laughed even though she couldn't see him. She'd called him Lord this and Lord that since he'd bought the English manor house a few years ago. Bradford Park happened to come with a title he'd never used. Cammie never used the proper honorific, Lord Bradford, but made up funny names instead. He loved that she always ribbed him about it.

On his laptop, he clicked a button for the video

chat to Cammie. She answered with a wan smile and drawn features. Seated by her uncle's bedside—Dane recognized the landscape painting behind her—she was as beautiful as ever, despite the weariness marking her face. Cammie Chandler was a beautiful woman, her wavy, rose-gold hair falling past her shoulders, her eyes the color of jade. But now she appeared drained by the long day and the drive from San Francisco back to San Juan Bautista.

He didn't point that out. "Hey there, how you doing?"

"Is that my little T. Rex beside you?" As he angled the laptop's camera, she cooed at the dog. "It was so good seeing you today, you little sweetie." If dogs could smile, Rex smiled at his favorite woman in the world. "I've missed hugging and petting you."

Dane wouldn't have minded trading places with Rex and being the recipient of those hugs. Of course, she'd be horrified at the direction of his thoughts—it was against all their rules—so he turned the conversation around. "Thanks for coming today. I really appreciate it. I promise I won't keep you long. I hope the game and that long drive didn't wipe you out."

She denied the evidence on her face and in her tired eyes. "No. But Uncle Lochlan got restless, thrashing about in the bed. It took a bit to calm him down after I got back."

"I'm sorry."

"It's not your fault. You know how he gets." She shrugged as if her steadfast loyalty and compassion were nothing more than what anyone would feel or act on.

He could have jumped into the business discussion right then, but she had bigger things hanging over her, and he needed to offer his support. Their relationship wasn't just that of assistant and boss, where all she did was look out for his needs. He cared for her too.

Though her uncle lived at one of Ava's premier facilities in the Bay Area, he was at his best when Cammie was nearby. Without her, he was often quarrelsome, even combative. She'd been going to San Juan Bautista as often as she could, but Dane had seen the toll it took on her, and last September, he'd finally told her to take family leave.

Now, with Lochlan unable to recognize her, even unable to walk, and sleeping most of the time, Cammie was on the fence, hating to see him suffer but powerless to let him go. It was obvious Lochlan wouldn't last much longer. And Dane needed to be there for her when it happened.

He hadn't told her what a mess his work life had become since she'd been gone or how subpar her temporary replacements had been. Adding that burden to her shoulders might have crushed her. And yet, without his saying a word, a few weeks after she'd left, Cammie had contacted her network of personal assistants, and the next candidates had been far more tolerable. But none of them was Cammie. None of them knew him the way she did, anticipating what he wanted even before he said it.

She sighed. "He's been comatose off and on for the last few days, hardly responding."

Dane detected the tremble in her voice. She'd told him none of this while they were together today. Then again, they hadn't been alone.

And now he gave her the space to get it all out. "The in-house doctor suggested we could stop feeding or hydrating him." She swiped at her eyes and glanced away from the camera, obviously looking at Lochlan in the bed. "But I won't do that. He can't really eat, so I just dribble things in his mouth. And I put ice chips on his tongue. If I give him too much water, it comes back up. But he gets so restless, his legs and arms moving."

He wished he could be there to at least hold her. "I'm sure Ava wouldn't starve someone."

She shook her head, her hair falling across her cheek. "It's not Ava. But I understand where the doctor is coming from. It's like I'm prolonging his agony."

He reached out, as if he could touch her face. "Of course you're not. You're doing everything possible for him. Don't get down on yourself. You've taken care of him for years."

"I know." She sighed, but he was afraid she didn't believe him. "I can never thank you and Ava enough for bringing him here."

"I've told you a million times, you don't have to thank me." He'd gotten to know Lochlan, too, after Cammie came to work for him, and he wanted the best for the old man.

When Cammie realized she could no longer care for Lochlan on her own, Ava had opened up space in her five-star San Juan Bautista facility, the closest one to Dane's Pebble Beach estate. Cammie had balked, knowing she could never pay for it on her own, but he'd convinced her that not taking his offer would reduce Lochlan's quality of life. Maybe that was dirty politics, but he'd needed her to give Lochlan the best, knowing full well she'd regret it for the rest of her life if she didn't.

Cammie had him deduct a portion of her salary every month, even though Dane didn't want the money and Ava had a fund to subsidize the care of those in need. He'd never met a more admirable, caring person in his entire life. Except perhaps Susan and Bob Spencer.

"Ava's people took such good care of him today," Cammie told him. "I'm so grateful for that. I talked to her, but will you tell her that for me?"

"Of course I will." Ava admired Cammie's loyalty as much as he did.

"It's been such a struggle for Uncle Lochlan. First, he had to take care of me after my parents died. And then the Alzheimer's started so early."

When her parents died in a car crash, Lochlan, her father's older brother, had taken her in. Unmarried and childless, he was totally unprepared to care for a seven-year-old. Yet he became her surrogate father and raised Cammie to become the amazing woman she was. Dane had lost his parents when he was twenty-one, and though he hadn't been a child, somehow both of them becoming orphans at a younger age and through tragedy was part of why they'd formed such a strong connection.

The bond had only grown between Lochlan and Cammie when he'd needed more and more care as she grew into an adult.

She'd been lucky to have Clyde Westerbourne, Lochlan's longtime friend, who became like a father figure to her too. It was Clyde who'd sent Cammie to Dane. When Westerbourne decided to retire to his Caribbean island estate, Cammie couldn't accompany him, not with her uncle growing worse.

Lochlan reminded Dane of his grandfather, who'd returned from the Second World War a changed man. Dane now knew he suffered from PTSD, but no one had understood that back then, and it was never treated. He'd heard stories of the fun-loving, laughing guy his grandfather had been before the war, but Dane had known only the quiet, withdrawn man he became. Just as the war had changed his grandfather, Alzheimer's had changed Lochlan. Dane understood how difficult it was for Cammie, but he was also glad she'd had all the good years with Lochlan before the disease took him away.

She tapped her temple, obviously having had enough of that conversation. "Okay, let's get down to the Mavericks."

"We can let business take a backseat right now." Even though he was dying to hear her impressions.

Cammie snorted. "Are you kidding me? I feel like an emotional mess when I'm not working." Which was why Dane gave her projects to work on even though she was supposed to be on leave. Nothing huge, just enough to keep her mind occupied, like setting up the gallery and museum tour for the Correa painting. "So tell me how the temps are doing," she said.

"They're fine," he said, working his mouth into a half smile. "But it takes three of them to do what you do."

She smiled. How he'd missed her dazzling smile in the months she'd been gone. "It's only because we've worked together so long. And I've watched your business grow."

She'd skillfully sidestepped his compliment, but that smile told him how much she liked knowing she was irreplaceable. He'd never had any compunction about telling her—in fact, he enjoyed it. She kept his life on track. Just as Fernsby kept his houses in order.

"Okay, the Mavericks." He hadn't wanted to sign any contracts with the Mavericks until Cammie had met them. But she'd given him that nod and a wink right there in the café. "What do you really think about this merger of our two families?"

He included Cammie in that comment. She wasn't just his assistant. He wanted her opinion as if they were peers, as if he weren't a billionaire talking to the hired help. What she thought was just as important as his siblings' opinions. The fact was, Cammie had been personally responsible for many of his big deals. He could take her to an exhibition or an art show, and she'd find a way to turn something they saw into an idea for a profitable business venture or a new feature at a resort. The Mavericks had been one of the few deals he'd found on his own, but only because of their close association with Gideon Jones and his foundation.

Of course, Cammie had brought Gideon's painting to his attention.

He had to tell her, "Come on, my little idea genie, give me all your words of wisdom."

She blushed. "Would you stop with that?" she groused at him.

He snapped his fingers. "It's true. Great ideas come like you've pulled them right out of your magic lamp." He gave her a quirky grin, miming rubbing a genie's lamp. "Like buying Gideon Jones's painting."

As her blush deepened, she made a joke, taking the

attention off herself. "What would the Mavericks say if they knew you were Lord Muckety-Muck?" She couldn't truly accept compliments.

"It's Lord Bigwig to you."

She laughed then, the hot color fading from her cheeks. Then she got down to business again. "I'm rubber-stamping what you already know, but this is going to be amazing. The Mavericks will bring new blood to all the family ventures, yours included. Will Franconi said it right—what the Harringtons do complements what the Mavericks do."

"You might be rubber-stamping, but I wasn't about to act on it until I talked to you."

She huffed out another laugh. "But you did act on it before we even talked. You brought up a merger right there at the café."

He shrugged. "You pinched me under the table, giving me permission."

She gaped at him. "I didn't pinch you until after you'd already talked about a merger."

He grinned. "But I could read your mind, and I knew you thought it was a great idea."

She shook her head at him, as though he were a recalcitrant child from whom she didn't believe a single word. "Whatever. I liked them. And I liked all the Maverick ladies. They might've married billionaires, but they're all so down to earth. And kind. They didn't talk to me like I was just your assistant."

He jumped in quickly. "That's because you're not *just* my assistant. You're my girl Friday and my idea genie. I'd be nothing without you."

She rolled her eyes at him again. "Oh, will you just stop that?"

He didn't want to stop. With her uncle so gravely ill and close to the end, showering her with compliments was the least he could do for her.

Even if sometimes, especially late at night, he wanted to do far more.

★ ★ ★

The house was so damn quiet after they said goodbye, even with Rex snoring softly beside him on the couch. Dane wished with everything in him that Cammie would come home. Because this *was* her home. The moment she'd decided to sell Lochlan's house where they'd both lived, Dane had set her up with her own suite of rooms in the Pebble Beach house. He'd wanted to make the transition as easy as possible for her. Searching for an apartment with all the other things on her plate at the time would have been a nightmare. There was the added bonus that it saved her rent and utilities, especially when she traveled so much with Dane anyway.

So he'd cleared out the office space on the San Francisco Peninsula and moved his headquarters to his Pebble Beach estate. He'd had the office there only because it was close to Lochlan's home and therefore cut down on Cammie's commute. But Pebble Beach was closer once Lochlan went into the San Juan Bautista memory care facility. And Dane made sure neither Cammie nor her uncle wanted for anything.

He admitted only to himself that Cammie living just down the hall had been seven years of torture. The need to knock on her door sometimes overwhelmed him, and he'd march to her suite with some crappy idea just so he could talk to her, look at her, smile at her. The worst was resisting her lure when the darkness was so complete he could barely see his hand in front of his face. When he'd lain awake for hours thinking of her.

But of course he couldn't go to her then. He wouldn't. There could be no excuse for an after-midnight excursion. But damn, it was hard.

Cammie wasn't just his assistant. She was his best friend, as important to him as any of his brothers or sisters. Cammie had become part of the family unit.

And yet, late at night, the questions plagued him. What if everything about the way they'd met had gone down differently?

What would have happened if Clyde Westerbourne had never sent her to him as a job candidate twelve years ago? What if, when Dane had met the beautiful young woman on the golf course the day before his interview with Clyde's assistant, when he had no clue who she was... what if there'd been no interview at all the next morning? What if, after that sexy golf game they'd shared, after he'd made love to her in his condo all night long... what if he'd never had to let her go?

What if there'd been no impediments to a relationship?

But there'd been so many impediments. He'd seen his own shock mirrored in her eyes the following morning when she'd walked into his office. The morning after one of the most incredible nights of his life. His one and only night with her.

They'd both had to agree their one-night fling could never happen again.

He'd badly needed an assistant who would take his work life in hand and keep him on track. Not one of the umpteen secretaries he'd been through could handle it. Fernsby had been ready to desert him if he didn't do something. Then Clyde Westerbourne had called, swearing that Cammie Chandler could do the job. Dane had never met her, had no idea what she looked like. He'd actually imagined someone matronly, in her forties or fifties. Because how could a person Cammie's age be such a paragon? All he'd cared about was that she'd totally organized Clyde's life. If Clyde could have taken her with him on his permanent move to the Caribbean, he would have. But Cammie badly needed a good job in the Bay Area, where she could take care of her uncle, who'd been going quietly downhill.

The fact that she and Dane had both been on the same golf course at the same time just one day before the interview was a fluke. They could have exchanged names and changed everything. He would have known immediately that she was off-limits. But they hadn't. Was that a fluke too? Or was it the universe granting them that one night?

The next morning, during that strange job interview, they'd both had good reasons to agree never to indulge their fantasies again. So they'd made their rules. No inappropriate touching. No longing looks. No sneaking away for a night of passion. He honestly hadn't known he'd never experience another night like that with any other woman. Not then.

Over the subsequent years, his belief in the rules had grown only more solid. She turned his chaos into order. He relied on her good sense. She was the one who made sure he added heart to his ventures. They couldn't risk screwing up their perfect work relationship. Romance was out of the question.

Besides, if he ever made a move, ever pushed for anything more, he would totally lose her. And he could not bear to ever lose her.

She'd dated. Of course she had. She was gorgeous, funny, smart, and men flocked to her. But he was so damned glad none of those relationships had come to anything. They were all jerks who weren't good enough for her anyway. And that one creep who'd let her down so badly? Dane could have pummeled the guy into the ground. Truth be told, he could even have pummeled his brother Troy for asking her out. For God's sake, she'd been his assistant for four years at that point. What had Troy been thinking? Still, Dane didn't like to remember how he'd completely lost his cool that day, accusing his brother of harassing his employees, and a lot worse. Especially when he learned Cammie had turned Troy down.

Of course, he'd only ever wanted to protect her from jerks who'd screw her over. Sure, he had thoughts. But he never acted on them. He didn't even want to. He liked his life just the way it was. He absolutely wasn't one of those jerks.

But sometimes at night—not every night, mind you, maybe once a month, or once a week—with the darkness surrounding him and her room just down the hall, he remembered the softness of her hair, the scent of her skin, the sweetness of her lips.

And he regretted every damned rule they'd set up between them.

* * *

Cammie sat in the chair next to her uncle's bed, his hand securely tucked in hers.

Sometimes it seemed as though he was in a coma, others that he was only sleeping. She put an ice chip against his lips, and he opened his mouth, taking it in. She wished he would open his eyes. She couldn't remember the last time he'd actually looked at her. She talked to him, and sometimes he would mumble an answer she couldn't understand. She'd tell him a joke, and once in a while, he would make a noise that sounded like a laugh. Or she'd tell him she loved him, and he'd grunt as though he had so much more to say. But he never opened his eyes. Somehow that was the worst. She wanted him to see her. Even in his last few days, or even hours, she wanted to know that he'd seen her, that he knew she was here with him.

But it had been such a long time since he'd even known who she was, though somehow, having her close calmed him.

She'd felt guilty leaving him today. But God, it had been good to get out. To see Dane. And how she'd missed Rex. When he'd bounded to her across the soccer field and barreled into her lap, all she'd wanted to do was hug him close and drink in his doggy scent while he slathered kisses all over her face. She missed her work. She missed her suite of rooms in Pebble Beach. She missed Fernsby's cooking. She even missed Dane knocking on her door in the late evening to share an idea that had suddenly come to him. The feeling was something like homesickness. For Rex, for Fernsby.

And maybe most of all for Dane.

Chapter Five

Dane lounged against Susan Spencer's kitchen counter as Fernsby took over the space, providing both the meal and the dessert. T. Rex lay under the kitchen table in the dog bed Fernsby had brought for him. Because Fernsby and the dog went everywhere with Dane.

Especially with Cammie gone and Rex pining for her.

It had been two weeks since their defining soccer game and the roundtable at the Buena Vista Café in San Francisco. After Cal had drawn up the merger agreement, they'd all participated in the signing meeting a few days ago.

Susan and Bob wanted to host a dinner party at their new home in Portola Valley, completely renovated for them by the Mavericks. "Now that you're all in business with the boys—" The Mavericks would probably always be *boys* to Susan. *Her* boys. "—Let's have a party. Though we met at Gideon's New Year's Eve gala, we should all get to know each other better."

Dane had readily agreed, and here they were—

Troy, Clay, and Ava chatting with the main group in the living room, while Gabby oversaw everything Fernsby did, much to the butler's consternation. Susan joined them, though she'd ceded control of her kitchen to Fernsby for the night.

Swiping an appetizer off an almost empty tray Fernsby had just replaced out in the great room, Dane squatted by Rex's bed to offer the dog a tasty bite.

"He's adorable." Susan leaned down to pet Rex's head.

Dane stood again, taller than Susan, who was a tallish, kind-eyed woman with a cap of silver hair and a lovely smile. "Thank you for allowing us to bring him."

"He's so well trained." She lowered her voice to add, "We have three new puppies in the family, all of them a year old. We're still in training mode."

Fernsby interrupted with a loud gasp rumbling up from his throat. "Sir," he belted out, "the dog is getting fat. He waddles. No treats. How many times must I convey that fact to you?"

Dane looked at the outraged man and chuckled. "But you're making roast beef and Yorkshire pudding. It's driving Rex crazy."

Fernsby eyed him balefully. "Lord Rexford," he intoned, "was sleeping before you disturbed him. He wasn't even aware there was roast beef nearby."

Susan gave Dane a sympathetic smile.

Fernsby bent to open the oven door, the scent of

Yorkshire pudding and roast potatoes wafting into the air. "The Yorkshires are done," he declared, taking them out and setting them on the stovetop. The roast beef rested on the counter under a foil tent. "They're perfect." Fernsby allowed himself a swift nod of congratulations. He'd made the Yorkshires in a muffin pan, turning them into popovers, with a hole in the center for his rich, homemade beef gravy.

Dane's mouth was already watering.

"They look absolutely amazing." Susan gave Fernsby the praise he required.

Then the man looked to Gabby, his mouth stretched into something resembling an evil grin. "I know you want a Yorkshire. With gravy. Lots of it. And butter on your roast potatoes."

Gabby screwed up her face, lips pinched, eyes squinty. "That is just so gross." She turned to Susan. "If you let him in your kitchen, he'll add butter to everything, even if it doesn't need it. He's a butter fiend."

Face devoid of any expression now, nose imperiously in the air, Fernsby said, "Butter and eggs are the staff of life."

But Dane knew Fernsby had prepared a special meal for Gabby—vegan meatloaf, a baked potato, vegan sour cream to top. He just liked to rub Gabby the wrong way. The feeling was mutual.

Susan tied on her apron. "I'll help serve."

His tone immutable, Fernsby said, "Dear lady, you

go be with your guests. Let me handle this. It's what I do." He put a hand to his chest. "I'm Fernsby!"

Then he handed her a glass of champagne and shooed her away like the Grinch patting Cindy-Lou Who on the head after she'd just walked in on him trying to stuff the Christmas tree up the chimney.

Susan Spencer hooked her arm through Dane's and led him out to the living room, where all the Mavericks were gathered. She whispered, "He's really amazing."

"And he's bossy."

They shared a smile.

The dining table had been set with crystal, porcelain, and silver, two leaves added to accommodate them all. The massive great room held the seven Mavericks, their ladies, and all the family that went with them, including Charlie Ballard's mother, Francine, and Evan's birth mother, Theresa, who hadn't made it to the soccer game. Tony Collins, Kelsey's twin, had come tonight too.

They all rather overwhelmed the small group of Harringtons. Dane wished once again that Cammie could have been here for the celebration. If he closed his eyes, he could almost imagine her next to him, her sweet scent seeping into him, her warm hand on his arm as she pointed out this or that.

He had to shake himself back to reality.

Ava had cornered Will Franconi's wife, Harper. He was glad his family was making the rounds. He hoped they felt the same emotional impact he did.

Dane had spoken with Harper earlier and learned she was a recruiter, handling placements for high-powered business executives. What intrigued him most was her love for her brother, Jeremy. The young man had been hit by a car when he was a child. Now, at the age of twenty, he still had the mind of the boy he'd been. And he was delightful. Harper had become his guardian when their parents were killed in a plane crash, and he admired how she'd taken responsibility. Much the same as Cammie took responsibility for Lochlan. He hadn't missed that Harper had been just about his age when his parents died, and he'd taken on the role of head of the family.

Troy was engrossed in a conversation with Matt and Ari Tremont. Clay had just stepped away from Rosie to snag an appetizer off Fernsby's tray, and Dane took his spot. "I have to congratulate you again on your gallery showing back in January." All the Harringtons had complimented her on the great show after the soccer game, but Gideon had given Dane more news. "I hear you sold almost every painting. Your art is truly amazing."

Gideon wrapped an arm around his pregnant fiancée, pride gleaming in his eyes. "It was so successful that she never has to crunch another number again in her life."

Rosie had been an accountant, and Gideon met her

through his sister, Ari. Rosie and Ari had been best friends since they were girls in foster care.

All the Mavericks had come from troubled backgrounds. Gideon joined the Army right out of high school to take care of his mother and little sister. And yet, for all his loyalty, after their mother's death, Ari had been lost to him when she disappeared into the foster care system. He'd spent years trying to find her. It was an amazing story. Now he'd joined the family, along with Rosie and her son. And Jorge was treated like a treasured grandson, the same as Noah, Matt's boy.

With Susan and Bob, Dane knew instinctively, there was always more love to go round.

Dane moved through the crowd—and it *was* a crowd. He'd spoken with Ari earlier, the kindergarten teacher. She'd met Matt when she became Noah's nanny. Dane figured it had been love at first sight for both father and son.

He'd also talked with Paige Collins, who was a family therapist. From things she'd said, Dane had a feeling she'd helped bring Evan back together with his long-lost mother and the twins. Obviously, twins ran in the family.

Tasha, Daniel's girlfriend, was a web designer, executing brilliant ideas for Daniel's DIY empire, creating an amazing 3D application for Daniel's customers to design their own kitchens, bathrooms, bedrooms, and living spaces, both indoors and out.

Dane was good at getting people to talk about themselves. He gleaned information by listening rather than talking. Cammie often told him that was his superpower, getting people to open up. He supposed it was true, but only because he was genuinely interested. Besides, he wasn't one to talk much about himself.

Fernsby entered then, clapping his hands to gain everyone's attention and saying in his sonorous, cultured British voice, "Dinner is served."

Everyone took seats while Gabby helped Fernsby carry in the plates. He did not do buffet-style, instead plating everything himself and giving everyone a portion of each selection.

Dane managed to sit between Charlie and her mother.

"This all looks so scrumptious," Francine enthused before delicately tucking in.

As they ate, he took the opportunity to tell Charlie, "I've seen your magnificent sculpture at Montgomery Media. *The Chariot Race* is one of the most amazing pieces of artwork I've ever seen."

Charlie and Sebastian met when he'd commissioned her to create the stunning sculpture for his new San Francisco headquarters. Next to her, Sebastian beamed with pride, just as Gideon had over Rosie's art.

Francine Ballard covered his hand with hers, her papery skin slightly cold. "You should see her dinosaurs. Charlie makes awesome dinosaurs. She even has a T. Rex. And I know your little dog is named after that ferocious beast. Maybe you need a big Tyrannosaurus Rex in your yard."

Charlie laughed. "That might be a bit much for a little dog."

Dane shook his head. "But that's why he's named T. Rex. He needed a big-dog name since he's a big dog in his own mind. He'd love a big T. Rex."

"He'd probably pee on its tail," Charlie said, pretending indignation.

Francine giggled and flapped her hand. "They're all rusty anyway, so it won't matter."

Dane saw a big T. Rex in his future to go along with his little T. Rex. Cammie would love it.

God, how he wished she were here. The need was a sudden ache in his chest, a hole she'd left behind. But Lochlan needed her now more than ever.

The meal was delicious, everyone complimenting Fernsby. He beamed with pride, though no one else but Dane probably noticed that shine in his silvery gaze. For dessert, he'd made his to-die-for mille-feuille.

Matt took a bite and moaned. "This is the most incredible dessert I've ever tasted."

Gabby took her seat after helping to serve dessert. "Maybe we could try it without butter. What do you think, Fernsby?" She held up her vegan, gluten-free peanut butter brownie.

Fernsby gaped. "No butter? Have you gone mad? One must use as much butter as possible. How else do you get the pastry in your mille-feuille to puff?"

He returned to the kitchen in a huff, exiting to peals of laughter.

After Fernsby's luscious dessert—why did that word make Dane think of Cammie, of her smooth skin and her luscious lips he'd tasted only for one night?—they moved once again to the enormous great room to chat over coffee and after-dinner drinks.

Dane joined Susan and Bob Spencer by the grand fireplace. Since it was mid-February, Bob had lit the fire.

"You have a great family here," Dane told them.

"And it's growing all the time," Bob said with a big belly laugh, his gaze floating over his daughters-in-law and their baby bumps.

Daniel joined them, while Tasha chatted excitedly with the pregnant group. Paige placed Tasha's hand on her round mound, and they all squealed with delight when it seemed the babies kicked.

"Tasha seems a little too interested." Daniel eyed her with what could have been longing.

Susan patted his arm. "Don't worry. Your time will come." And that could have been a twinkle in Daniel's eye.

"I want to thank you all for having us here," Dane said. "My brothers and sisters and I are enjoying ourselves immensely."

Daniel clapped him on the back. "This merger will be good for all of us."

He couldn't know how much his words meant. Now more than ever, Dane wanted to be part of this family, not just for himself, but for his brothers and sisters. He wondered if Bob Spencer, with his comment about a growing family, had included not only the coming babies, but the Harringtons as well.

Susan and Bob were the glue that held this band of brothers—and more—together. They'd married young, had little money, and lived in an apartment barely big enough for them and their two children. Bob had been a baggage handler at O'Hare and Susan a waitress. Yet, when Daniel brought home his friends, all of them in bad places in their young lives, Susan and Bob had taken them in. They'd given each Maverick exactly what he'd needed—love, support, discipline, and life lessons. And these Mavericks had even taken on the responsibility for their little sister, Lyssa, who was just a baby at the time, being ten years younger than Daniel.

And all the while, Dane's parents had been roaming the globe. Dane recalled holidays when they'd been absent because the skiing was too good in the Alps. It was as if the Harrington children were afterthoughts. His parents had never offered the love he and his siblings craved, as much as they'd all wanted and needed it. Maybe Dane had craved it the most.

Their answering refrain when he'd begged? *You always want too much from people, Dane.*

What would his family have been like if they'd been raised as the Mavericks had? Maybe he would have been an uncle by now. Maybe they would have learned how to love instead of fearing and mistrusting it.

He flicked his gaze to his brothers and sisters as they worked the room, talking, laughing. Did they feel what he did—a craving to be part of this family? He wondered, too, about Cammie. After losing her parents so young, after having only her uncle, even as much as she loved Lochlan and was now on the verge of losing him, did she crave something bigger?

As if thoughts of Cammie had conjured her up, his phone rang, her ID on the screen.

Excusing himself, he stepped away to answer, his gut roiling. "Hey, what's up?" he asked even before she could say hello.

Her voice quivered. "It's Uncle Lochlan. His aides are here." She choked back what could only have been a sob. "He's barely breathing, and his pulse is almost nonexistent. They told me that if they turn him, he'll probably go."

"I'm leaving now." He hated that she was so far away, that he couldn't be there with a snap of his fingers. It would take him over an hour.

Her voice whispered across the airwaves. "Thank you."

"You hang in there. Wait for me."

"I will. I better go now."

She was near tears, and her pain tore at him like a fist closing around his heart. He had to go. Now. He couldn't waste a single minute getting to her.

Approaching the Spencers again, he said, "It's Cammie. Her uncle. I'm sorry, I have to leave." On the way out, he squeezed Ava's arm. "It's Lochlan. I have to be with her in his final moments."

She pressed her lips together, her face solemn. "You go. Give her our love. Call me later."

Dane knew she'd check with her own people and was, in fact, already reaching for her phone.

In the kitchen, he found Fernsby with his hands in soapy dishwater, an apron around his waist. "It's Cammie's uncle," Dane said.

Fernsby's eyes turned a misty gray. "You must immediately go to Camille. Don't worry about Lord Rexford and me. Gabby can drop us off in Pebble Beach on her way home to Carmel. It'll be a perfect opportunity for me to give her a few pointers about the health benefits of butter and eggs when she's driving and can't hit me," he said with a straight face.

Dane wanted to hug him. Trust Fernsby to break the tension.

Then he headed out, thinking only of how quickly

he could get to Cammie.

★ ★ ★

Daniel stood with his parents by the fireplace.

"What a caring family you've connected with," his mother said, that look in her eye when she was wondering exactly how she could help someone in need.

Daniel couldn't smile after witnessing the anguish written on Dane Harrington's face. "They were orphaned at a young age. Dane was barely twenty-one and had to drop out of college. Ava did too. The others were still in high school or middle school."

"You know what I think, honey?" His mother's gaze roamed over the remaining Harringtons in the room.

This time, Daniel chuckled softly. "I already know, Mom. You're always wanting to take in strays. Now you want to take in the Harringtons."

"I barely know Dane, but I can see he's a man who's always taken care of other people. Maybe he needs someone to lean on too."

Tonight allowed him to see the Harringtons in a new light. They might be leaders in their fields, but they were also orphans, without the love of inspiring parents. While they seemed exceptionally close, they hadn't had Susan and Bob Spencer in their lives. Daniel and his brothers had achieved what they had only because of his parents. They'd taught him how to love.

He wondered if he'd have recognized his love for Tasha without their inspiration in his life.

Maybe the Mavericks could bring more to the table than just some good business ventures. Maybe they could bring his parents and a share of the love he'd known all his life. Lord knew his parents had so much of it to give.

★ ★ ★

The bed stood in the center of the room, paintings of flowers and landscape scenes on the blue walls. Comfortable chairs sat on either side, and a long bureau held Lochlan's things, though he no longer needed them and hadn't for months. Cammie stood by the quiet form, holding his hand. She was exactly where she'd always been, at her uncle's side.

That's who Cammie Chandler was—steadfast, caring, and loyal.

The pain cracking her features nearly broke Dane.

Though he hadn't made a sound, she turned, the tracks of dried tears on her cheeks. The moment she saw him, they flowed once more, and in the next moment, she was in his arms.

He held her tight as she shook against him.

She put on such a strong front. She *was* strong. That's how the Mavericks had seen her at the soccer game. But inside there was a fragility she hid from the world, growing right along with her uncle's disease.

Dane knew how hard this was for her. It was why he'd rushed to her tonight, why he visited every week, why he video-chatted with her every night, trying to take her mind off the agony of watching her uncle deteriorate.

Holding her now, he whispered words she needed to hear. "You are the best niece in the world. You've done everything possible for Lochlan. And I'm not leaving your side while you go through this."

She pulled back, swept a fresh wave of tears from her cheeks, and gave him a weak smile. "Thank you. I don't want to be alone for this."

He cupped her face in his palms. "You're never alone. I'm always here."

Then together, hand in hand, they turned to her uncle's bed.

★ ★ ★

At dawn, Fernsby stood in the kitchen window of the Pebble Beach house, Lord Rexford in his arms. Dane pulled the Jaguar into the garage, and Fernsby fed Lord Rexford a bit of leftover roast beef. "You need a treat too," he cooed to the dog. "You feel bad for Camille. As we all do."

After Lochlan Chandler's passing a few hours ago, Dane had stayed with Camille until she'd fallen asleep. But when she woke, she'd sent him packing. That was her way, always needing to show people how strong she was. Dane had respected that. So did Fernsby. But he knew it had been a long night for them both.

He shifted Lord Rexford in his arms. Camille would be coming home soon. It had been a terrible time for her, and Fernsby would treat her gently. Tomorrow, when she was rested, he would call her with his condolences and the words of comfort he could offer. "But it's best she comes back where she belongs very soon," he told the dachshund.

As he heard the garage door close, he gave the dog one final command. "Now it's time to show those two they belong together. No matter how hard it is to get them to see that romance is inevitable. She needs him just as much as he needs her." He kissed the tip of the dog's nose. "We're in this together, Lord Rexford. It's going to take all our skills."

Chapter Six

Cammie stayed an extra couple of weeks in San Juan Bautista. Ava had arranged a room for Cammie's use while she'd cared for her uncle and hadn't kicked her out even after Uncle Lochlan passed. She could never thank Dane or Ava enough for how much they'd both done. She'd known she couldn't put her beloved uncle in an inferior home just because she was too proud to accept their assistance. And she would pay back every penny, even if it took the rest of her working life.

She still ached deep in her belly, but she'd lost Uncle Lochlan a long time ago. It had been years since he'd been the loving uncle of her childhood. The knowledge that he was at peace was her only solace. Wherever he was, his mind was once again clear, and he was himself.

This room had been her home for the last five months, decorated soothingly with a wallpaper border around the ceiling, landscape scenes on the wall, and a comfortable bed fitted with the finest linens and a warm duvet. Sitting at the desk, she went through the necessary paperwork.

She'd held no funeral for Uncle Lochlan. His friends were long gone, all except Clyde Westerbourne, who'd called to offer his condolences. "Oh my dear, I am so sorry. I know how hard this must be for you."

The loss had been only a couple of days old when he'd phoned, and she'd felt the tears rising again. But she didn't let them fall. "Thank you, Clyde. I miss him, but this was truly a release for him."

"This may sound harsh right now, but I hope you see it as a release for yourself too, my dear. You've suffered, watching his decline."

She didn't want to admit it, but Clyde had known her so long. And he'd found Dane for her, the man he'd said would be the perfect employer.

Over the twelve years she'd worked for Dane, Clyde's words had proven to be prophetic.

It was only with Dane's comfort that she'd made it through the night of Uncle Lochlan's passing. And every day since, she'd worked diligently on the estate, wanting the paperwork finished before she returned to Pebble Beach. Her uncle didn't have much, since she'd sold the house and everything in it to pay for his care. But there were still government agencies to be informed and details to take care of.

The harder she worked, the more she was dying to get back to Dane. To get back to work. They'd already bounced around projects and ideas that might be good for the new merger.

Needing a break, she typed a quick text: *Dear Lord Barnacle, have you seen Charlie Ballard's work?*

Of course Dane would have. He'd probably learned all about Charlie's talents while chatting at the signing dinner.

He opened a video chat immediately. "Now I'm a barnacle?" he muttered, his face unshaven, as if he'd only just gotten up, though it was past ten.

She shrugged, suppressing a smile. "You can't help it." Then she rushed on to make her point. "I'm just wondering how we can incorporate Charlie's artwork in some way at the resorts." Then she thought of Ari's background in child development. "And what do you think about Ari Tremont checking out the daycare facilities at the resorts and making sure they're up to snuff?"

"As always, you're my brilliant idea genie."

She hoped his words hadn't made her blush. Dane always filled her up. Someday, she hoped to run a project herself. She hadn't been able to think about it while she had her uncle to care for. And she had to be completely honest with herself—being one hundred percent in control of a project was a little daunting. If anything went wrong, the burden would be on her shoulders. But one of these days, she'd do it. She just needed to get her feet under her after Uncle Lochlan's ordeal.

What she really needed was to get back to Dane.

★ ★ ★

Practically the moment Cammie brought up Charlie Ballard's work, Dane set up a meeting with her. And now, only two days later, he sat on a camp chair in Charlie's studio on Sebastian Montgomery's sprawling estate in the Hayward Hills.

Workbenches filled every wall, along with tool chests and stacks of supplies, barrels of nuts and bolts, and great wooden crates holding metal, ceramic, stone, and piping—anything Charlie could use to create her art. Despite the vast quantity of materials, the studio was the picture of orderliness, everything at hand or easily located.

Which was in complete contrast to the beautiful mess of a woman before him. Tendrils of curly red hair fell from a hastily secured knot on the top of her head. She wore stained overalls over a torn sweatshirt. But none of that mattered when her work was so pristine.

She'd removed her goggles and turned off the blowtorch when he arrived, but even as they talked, she assembled bits and pieces of what would become a...

"I'd like to say I know exactly what you're making." Dane leaned closer to the metal pieces covering the floor, as if that would help. "But I can't tell."

Charlie laughed, a musical sound that reminded him of Cammie. He couldn't stop the errant thought that he wished she'd come back soon. But he had to give her these two weeks. After everything she'd been through, she needed the time.

Charlie eyed the metal surrounding her. "Eventually, it'll be a cowboy on a horse roping a steer. It's a commission for a Texas oilman."

Dane snorted. "Of course he's a Texas oilman. And his family were probably ranchers way back when."

Charlie's eyes twinkled. "How did you know?"

He shrugged. "Only an oilman from a ranching family would want a life-size sculpture of a cowboy and a steer."

With that same twinkle, Charlie changed the subject. "Have you come here to talk about a Tyrannosaurus Rex for your yard?"

His thinking cap had definitely been on. "Depends on how big."

"I haven't seen your estate, but from the little I know of you, I don't think you want something as large as the dinosaurs at the Flintstone House in Hillsborough."

He'd passed by the house many times driving up Highway 280 on the way to San Francisco. Some people thought it an eyesore, but he found it charming, with its domed style and all the massive metal creatures populating its yard. "You're right. Rex might be intimidated by something that big." He grinned. "He needs something he can look down on and feel like he can vanquish."

Charlie pursed her lips into a half smile. "I have the perfect thing." She opened a pair of cabinet doors and waved him over. "These should be perfect for T. Rex. He can lord it over them."

Dane couldn't stifle the half laugh, half snort. "What the hell are they?"

She held one of the metal sculptures on the palm of her hand. "It's a Zanti Misfit."

He eyed her. "What the heck is a Zanti Misfit?"

Charlie rolled her eyes. "Haven't you ever watched *The Outer Limits*?"

"Can't say I have."

"It was an old episode with Bruce Dern. Zanti Misfits are aliens who land in the desert with nefarious intentions."

He looked at the creature, shaped like an ant with a huge, garish grin of metal teeth and bulging painted eyes. "That might be a bit too terrifying for Rex."

Charlie snorted. "If Bruce Dern could vanquish the Zanti Misfits, you can be darn sure T. Rex will too."

He laughed outright. "Charlie Ballard, you are one very odd woman."

She smiled, accepting the compliment. "Thank you very much. I've never wanted to be normal."

Then he added, "I need at least five."

She waved her hand toward the cabinet as if she were a magician. "Take all you want."

They still might terrify Rex, but Cammie would love them. "Thanks. That's very generous."

"I just make them when I need to think," Charlie explained. "Making something I can practically create in my sleep frees up my mind to brainstorm other ideas."

"That's an interesting observation. I feel the same way about golf. It frees my mind to think." Especially when he played with Cammie. Then, his mind could wander back to their first golf game, to that one night, her skin so sensitive, her touch on him so exquisite, her taste so sweet.

Damn, he needed to slap himself.

He dragged his thoughts back to why he'd asked for this visit. "Cammie and I are excited to talk to you about a new project we have in mind." He opened his computer on Charlie's workbench. "It was her idea, so I'd like to include her, if that's okay with you."

"Of course."

Dane brought up the video app. Cammie answered, her face lighting up the screen as if she'd been waiting all day for his call. Dane suspected she was glad to step away from her uncle's estate management.

"Hey, Charlie." Cammie waved.

Charlie fluttered her fingers. "I'm so sorry about your uncle."

Cammie blinked, as if she needed to hide the tears that suddenly pricked her eyes. "Thanks so much. I miss him, but I'm glad he's not suffering anymore."

"I understand completely." Charlie would understand more than most, since she took care of her mother, Francine. She'd settled her in a Los Gatos facility, which happened to be one of Ava's. The small bedroom community sat at the base of the Santa Cruz Mountains, and Dane knew Charlie was over there regularly. Of course, Francine could have lived with Charlie and Sebastian, but she claimed she wanted her independence.

Dane started the conversation. "Since it's your idea, Cammie, why don't you tell Charlie what you had in mind?"

Cammie huffed a breath. "It wasn't really my idea. I just posed a question, and you ran with it."

They'd brainstormed, tossing ideas back and forth, but using Charlie's work at the resorts had come from Cammie. She didn't even realize that she truly was his idea genie, no matter how many times he told her. Cammie's touch was pure magic.

She jumped into the proposal. "We'd love to have you create a sculpture for the lobby of each of Dane's resorts. Some of them have courtyards, some are marble entryways, some are open air. But we thought greeting his guests with an accent signifying the location of each particular resort would be amazing. A bald eagle for the Montana resort. A Joshua tree for the desert. But really, it should be whatever you feel is appropriate."

Charlie's mouth dropped open.

Cammie rushed on. "We wouldn't expect this to take precedence over your other commissions. But if you're interested, we'd like you to you work us into your schedule whenever you can."

Something unfurled in Dane's belly when she said *we.* They were a team. They always had been. But now, it felt as if she was finally taking partial ownership of the things they did together.

"Wow." Charlie put her hand to her mouth. "That all sounds incredible."

"The other thing we'd like you to consider," Cammie went on, "is putting together some art classes. Since metalwork is your specialty, we'd create a workshop in some of our resorts where you could teach. The building could be whatever size you need, with room for your materials, as well as other types of art like painting, pottery, and so much more."

The way her mind worked stunned him. They'd talked in general terms, but she'd dreamed up an extraordinary idea with more specifics than he could have imagined.

Cammie's ideas just kept flying. "You could visit a different resort once a month, or whatever fits your schedule, and give a class, showing other people how to do what you do."

Charlie's face flushed, and with a beaming smile, she jumped off her stool, waving her arms. "I'd love to fly out to your resorts once a month. I can even take people shopping for junk. That's what I use for raw materials. I love junkyards and flea markets. Then we can bring back the treasures we find and make art."

She lunged at Dane, as if she wanted to hug him. "This is just amazing. Thank you so much for thinking of me. Sebastian will go wild."

Dane held out his hands. "Don't thank me. This was all Cammie."

Charlie hugged the computer screen. "Thank you, thank you. I will absolutely love doing this."

Cammie beamed. He hadn't seen her eyes sparkle like this in months. His heart wanted to leap right out of his chest, and he, too, could have hugged the computer screen. He could have hugged Charlie as well, for making Cammie so happy.

When Cammie was happy, he was happy.

★ ★ ★

The next day, Cammie and Dane had a three-way video chat with Rosie. Once again, Cammie laid out their idea.

"You two stagger me." Rosie's eyes shone as brightly as Charlie's had. "You really want my artwork in all the rooms of your resorts?"

Dane explained, "If you're willing to take on the task. Nothing has to be completed right away, of course. We can make prints from the originals, so you don't have to paint something for every single room."

Laughing, she put her hand on her stomach. "This little one would be a college graduate by the time I finished an original for each room."

"We wondered if you'd like to teach classes at different resorts too," Cammie said. "Just one a month, or whatever you're comfortable with. We'd like to offer an art program for our guests who want to learn."

Tears shimmered in Rosie's eyes, and her voice wobbled. "You're both just freaking amazing. I'd love to do it. The art *and* the classes."

"As long as it doesn't interfere with your next show," Dane assured her.

"Would you mind if I used some of those paintings?"

Dane nodded heartily. "The originals would all be yours. We'll just use prints. That's what will make this thing unique. They'll be in your show, and we'll promote them as being an eventual feature in the resorts. Two-way marketing."

"Wow," Rosie exclaimed. "I'm totally in. Thanks so much for this opportunity."

When Rosie left the meeting ten minutes later, after talking logistics, Dane smiled at Cammie. "I'd say that went really well."

The brainstorming had brought back her natural glow. Her smiles came more readily. Her enthusiasm shone in her eyes. "Exceptionally well," she said, clasping her hands as if she couldn't contain her excitement. "I'll set up a meeting with Ari. We can tackle her about reviewing the resorts' childcare facilities."

Dane loved that Cammie was completely on board with the projects, doing most of the talking without even realizing how much ownership she was taking.

Cammie was back in the game. And soon, she'd be back physically as well. Back in his office and back in his house. Right where she belonged.

Chapter Seven

The call with Ari Tremont two days later went as well as the others. Cammie felt her strength rebuilding, her confidence coming back after all the months—all the years—of watching her uncle literally fading away. She felt in her element now, trading ideas, watching the projects grow. More than anything, she needed to get back to work.

Ari was all in, even suggesting that Noah could help too. As well as Rosie and Jorge. Seeing how the boys played together in the different resorts would help them evaluate what worked and what needed more attention.

Dane once again stayed in the meeting after Ari signed off. Cammie loved their online chats, which gave her a chance to gaze at him without a qualm.

"She's really on board with this." He leaned back in his chair and stretched, his hands behind his head, his chest broad across the screen.

Excitement welled up inside Cammie. "This will be great." She loved the work they were doing, talking with the Maverick ladies, bringing to life these amazing ideas. With Dane encouraging her to do all the talking, it felt as though she could actually be in charge of these projects. "Do you want me to set up the interview with Tasha?"

He nodded. "You have my schedule. Just let me know the time."

They needed an interactive website for the resort conglomerate that would drill down into categories, then into each individual resort. "I hope Daniel can spare her. I know she does a lot of work for him."

"I'm sure Daniel won't mind," Dane said with a shrug.

"Good. Because I also wanted to talk to you about some ideas I had involving Harper Franconi."

Dane was staring at her, the features of his handsome face softened, his sapphire eyes mellowed to the color of cornflowers.

"What?" Her voice sounded natural, but her heart beat with unexpected trepidation.

"I feel like I'm rushing you into coming back. I've involved you in all of this Maverick stuff, but you're still grieving for your uncle and hip-deep in his estate."

For a moment, she felt as if she'd choke up. But she banished it. "I would tell you if I couldn't handle this. But really, these projects help me keep my sanity."

He eyed her skeptically. "You've been running at a hundred and ten percent. And now you look tired."

Her hands flew to her cheeks. She'd been working with Uncle Lochlan's bank just before the meeting. Time had flown, and she hadn't had a chance to put on makeup. But Dane would accept nothing less than the truth. "It's just that I received his death certificates today. I expedited them." And paid a fee to do it. The certificates made her uncle's passing all the more real.

"I'm so sorry." Dane's voice held so much compassion she wanted to weep. "I know how hard this must be for you. That's why I want you to take more time."

She blinked, staving off her emotions. "The best thing I can do is work. And come home."

Home. With the suite she'd decorated herself, Pebble Beach felt like home.

Being with Dane felt like coming home.

Was it really all that bad if sometimes she lay awake in her king-size bed with Dane just a few steps down the hall and let thoughts of him take over? During the day, she was efficient, dedicated, knowing exactly what he needed right when he needed it. But the nights were hers, and sometimes she simply wanted to close her eyes and remember his hard muscles beneath her fingertips, his silky chest hair against her cheek, his lips on hers, his tongue teasing her. It should have been torture, but she relished those private moments, those private memories.

But she couldn't afford them now. "I'm coming home in just a few days. The first week of March." It wouldn't be long. "Right now, I have too much time to think."

After a long slice of silence, he said, "Even if it's for my own selfish reasons, please come home."

Their work was his reason. It wasn't as if it was about *her*. Despite everything Dane said, she knew he was tired of the temps.

She'd lived with these fantasies about Dane locked deep inside all this time. She'd go on living with just that—fantasies.

Because she knew the rules. Better than anyone. Maybe even better than Dane.

★ ★ ★

Fernsby ticked off the day in early March on his secret calendar hidden deep in the pantry. Thank heaven. Camille had returned. He stepped into the entry hall just as Lord Rexford rushed her, barking, jumping, ecstatic. Smiling at the display of affection, Dane set down Camille's bag.

Only Camille could be away from home for five months and need only one suitcase.

If he were a different man, he might have hugged her. But he wasn't the hugging type.

In his sternest voice, disregarding Dane altogether, he said, "Thank goodness you're back, Camille. Your employer has been absolutely impossible for the last five months. He simply cannot function without you."

Dane scored him with a glance. "Aren't you over-stating things a bit, Fernsby?"

Nose in the air, Fernsby droned, "You know my policy is always to tell the truth." Then he added, "Sir," in his deepest intonation.

His employer made a move for the bag, but Fernsby got there first. "I will escort Camille to her suite of rooms." He grazed a look over Dane. "She needs time to adjust." Then he turned to Camille. "Shall I unpack for you?"

Dog in her arms, Camille laughed that most delightful laugh of hers, a laugh that should have brought a man to his knees in worship. Dane, however, wasn't on his knees. When would the man learn?

"No, Fernsby," she said sweetly, for Camille was always sweet. "I can unpack for myself. Honestly."

He headed up the stairs with her bag, which weighed almost nothing, and left the two alone in the marble entryway.

Only then did he permit himself a smirk. His thoughts pleased him. "Let's get cracking, you two."

They'd dawdled enough. They were meant to be together. And he would make sure it happened.

It was what Lochlan had wanted just as much as he.

★ ★ ★

In the late afternoon, when Cammie finished unpacking, she took a moment to sit on the bed and drink in the sense of home she'd longed for over the past five months. How she'd missed this place. She'd chosen everything in the room—the flowered border around the ceiling, the seafoam walls, one of them a darker teal that complemented the rest. The seafoam bedspread with splashes of teal. A lounge chair in the corner where she could read comfortably or use her laptop to do some paperwork. The only thing she hadn't chosen was the stuffed teal-colored Tyrannosaurus Rex Dane had brought her the day they'd decided on the little dachshund's name. As a puppy, he'd almost fit in her hand.

She treasured that stuffed dinosaur. Sometimes, lying in her bed, knowing Dane was just down the hall, yet as unreachable as if he were on the other side of the world, she hugged the dinosaur to her as if it were Dane himself.

Of all her suites in all of Dane's homes, this was her favorite. When Dane had it remodeled for her, he'd had the contractors add a kitchenette, with a small refrigerator, a two-burner stove, and a microwave. He'd even purchased an electric kettle for her herbal tea. She could make anything she wanted.

But of course, she'd always gone downstairs for dinner, and now, with her belongings put away, she returned to the house's main level.

The door to Dane's office stood open. Unlike the

office space they'd had on the Peninsula, with an annex
for her and a waiting room outside his corner office,
this was one expanse of Persian carpet, wood paneling,
and oak bookcases. The office was large enough that
their competing phone conversations didn't drown
each other out. While Dane liked his massive oak desk,
Cammie had chosen a smaller desk and credenza set,
situating it where the late afternoon sun streamed
through the floor-to-ceiling windows.

The estate stood on a bluff overlooking the ocean.
The long, winding drive curled through the golf course
belonging to one of Dane's resorts. Although his
property was walled off, an errant golf ball occasionally
scaled the walls. The sprawling house had everything—a master chef's kitchen for Fernsby, with his
suite of rooms next to it. The formal dining room
seated twenty-four, because Fernsby thought it was a
good round number. Dane threw amazing dinners,
though often he held parties in the San Francisco flat
because it was more central to many of his business
associates. They rarely used the formal living room
except for get-togethers, but they often played chess or
gin rummy in his study or lounged in the home theater
to enjoy a classic movie or something new on a
streaming service or to binge a TV show. Dane used
the workout room daily. She did, too, but always at
different times.

A door at the end of the hall led to a shower room,

sauna, cold plunge, and spa, then out to the Olympic-size pool. When they golfed or played pickleball, they used the resort's facilities. Beyond the back gate were hiking trails through Pebble Beach and down the cliffs to the beach below. She often went out for a walk, sometimes all the way to the other end of the beach, where the Frank Lloyd Wright house stood on the bluff.

Her memories prompted her to say, "Of all the places in the world where you own real estate, this is my favorite." She gazed out at the sun sparkling on the waves, the dots of surfers riding the crests.

Dane swiveled his desk chair to look at the view. "Me too. I never get tired of looking at the ocean."

"Neither do I." But she was looking at his profile.

Turning back to her, he mused, "The San Francisco flat is kind of amazing, though, with its view of the Golden Gate and Alcatraz out in the bay."

She suddenly felt nostalgic for all his homes, places she hadn't been in more than five months. Just as Lyssa Spencer had said, the London townhouse was exquisite. The English manor house captivated her with its twenty acres of grounds. His Caribbean island was a sanctuary. But still, Pebble Beach won, hands down. This was where she felt most at home.

This was where she could heal after the long months of caring for Uncle Lochlan. After the years of watching his decline and being able to do nothing about it. This was her refuge.

Here with Dane.

He stood. "Come here. I want to show you something." He held out his hand, pulling her to the long, latticed windows.

Below them lay the pool and, beyond that, the beach and hiking trails. A rock garden filled with succulents ran beneath the windows, leading down to the pool patio.

"What?" She'd never get tired of the view, and how she'd missed it. He wanted her to see something special, but she couldn't pick out what it was in all this splendor.

Dane pointed among the succulents and rocks. "Do you see them?"

Cammie was so very aware of her hand still in Dane's warm, comforting grip. And finally she saw... something. "What are they?"

"Charlie Ballard's Zanti Misfits."

"They look like weird bugs. With big bug eyes."

Dane laughed. "That's exactly what they are. Bugs. From an old episode of *The Outer Limits*."

Cammie gasped. "Uncle Lochlan loved that show! We often watched reruns. Now I remember the Zantis." She craned her neck. "Charlie has got them down pat."

"I was going to have her make a T. Rex, but she gave me these guys instead. Rex loves barking at them."

She chuckled. "A big Tyrannosaurus Rex would have terrified him."

Squeezing her hand, he said, "That's what I finally decided."

She looked at him, smiling. "I love them."

"Thought you would."

She wondered if he'd chosen the Zanti Misfits as much for her as for Rex. Probably. It felt like she was finally home again.

"Where is he, by the way?" Rex was usually wherever they were.

Dane rolled his eyes. "Fernsby is baking."

That said it all. And now she needed to work. "Let's talk and see where we are."

Though she would have loved to stand there holding hands with him all day, it was impossible. She backed away from the window, then rounded the desk and pulled out the chair in front she always used when they discussed plans or swapped ideas. The indents in the plush Persian carpet were still there, as if Dane hadn't moved the chair in five months.

"I was able to finish most of Uncle Lochlan's estate issues. There're a couple of minor things left, but it's pretty much done."

As he took his seat, his eyes softened to a sweet blue flame. "I know how that stuff can consume you to the point that you can't even grieve. Then, all of a sudden, you wake up months later and realize you've never even cried."

"Thank you for understanding." He was thinking about his parents and the difficult estate issues he'd had to deal with. Thank goodness Uncle Lochlan's estate was so much less encumbered. If they had a different relationship, she'd have walked around the desk to hug Dane, giving him comfort, taking comfort for herself.

But they didn't have a different relationship.

He laid his hands on his desk. "That's why you should still take it easy. Don't jump into everything immediately. In fact, don't start work for a few days. Just lie by the pool, read, take long walks. You need recuperation too. This has been traumatic."

He didn't want her to come back to work? She'd thought he understood what she needed. The agony of the past months suddenly welled up in her. "I need to work. It's the only thing that helps me through the grief."

"But I can't help worrying about you."

She felt almost militant. "I'm perfectly capable of coming back as your personal assistant."

He held up his hands in surrender. "You're right. About everything. I don't know anyone else who could go through what you have and come out so well on the other side. But I won't stop you from doing what you need to do. I love all your ideas. I want to hear more about them."

His words deflated her. She actually sagged in the chair, and her grip on the armrests relaxed until her hands simply hung there. She hadn't even been aware of holding on so tightly. "I didn't mean to shout. I guess I'm still a little emotional." God, she'd almost lost it. But there was one more thing she had to add, then they never had to talk about any of this again. "I'm going to step up my payments to you for Uncle Lochlan's care."

"Cammie, you don't need to worry about paying anything back."

She held up a hand, stopping him. "You and Ava made his last years so much better than they ever could have been otherwise. I can't thank either of you enough. I need to return all that to you."

His head slightly bent, he waved a hand. "Fine. Good. I understand. But there's no time limit. You don't need to make yourself crazy taking care of it."

She shook her head, her hair falling across her face. She refused to get emotional again, so she said calmly, "I'm not being crazy about it. I just need to pay my way. I can't have this hanging over my head."

He could have said more, but instead, probably because of her earlier outburst, he nodded. "All right. Do what you have to do. I get it."

"Thank you." She appreciated his acceptance. If he'd gone on, she might have lost her cool again.

The debt was another good reason she lived in his

house; she had no rental expenses. And now every-thing she paid him could go toward the debt rather than ongoing care.

With that off her chest, she could get to the good stuff she'd been thinking about. No more dwelling on bad things. "Remember what we were discussing about Harper?"

"Sure." He nodded, his fingers steepled as he leaned back in his chair.

For a moment, she was struck by how terribly handsome he was—his dark hair, his aristocratic features, his sometimes soulful blue eyes that could read her mind. How she missed this, sitting with him, talking, even just looking at him. The sense of finally coming home stole her breath all over again.

She had to force herself back to reality. In the end, they'd postponed the video meetings with Tasha and Harper. Dane had been right to tell her to slow down with the work stuff. She'd needed to plow through the rest of the estate issues so she could come home. And it had taken her only a few more days.

Leaning forward, she crossed her knees and rested her forearms on her thighs. "Harper's been dealing with her brother's special needs for something like thirteen years. She has great expertise." Jeremy was a fine kid. She'd seen that at the soccer game. But because of his accident, he was different from other boys. That fact provided challenges for Harper.

Dane's gaze rested on her. "Isn't that why we discussed adding specialized activities at some of the resorts?"

"Yes." Her excitement grew to the point she felt jittery with it. Or maybe that was just being alone with him after so many months. "But instead of adding focused events to existing resorts, what if we created resorts designed specifically for kids with special needs?"

She'd been thinking about it for days, the idea blossoming in her mind, and now everything burst out.

"We could have classes and sports events and physical therapy and games. We can ask Harper, 'If you could have had anything you wanted while you raised Jeremy, what would it be?' There are things you and I could never even dream of. We could have activities for the parents too. Not just family activities, but things they can do on their own, like date nights. Therapy for them as well. Because it must be hard. And we could provide resources to tap into each child's unique abilities. Tasha could design special interactive games. Charlie and Rosie could give art classes. We could have shows featuring the kids' work."

Dane stared at her as if she were a mad scientist. Maybe she'd been gone so long, he'd forgotten what she looked like. Finally, head still cocked, he said, "Have I ever told you how amazing you are?"

"I—" She stopped.

"The way your mind works endlessly is fascinating. I mean, you've just been through a terrible ordeal. And yet, somehow, you're still my idea genie, coming up with incredible plans." When she opened her mouth, he held up a hand. "I know work is how you manage your grief. But I still believe that no one but you could conceive an idea like this at a time like this."

Her heart turned over and tapped out a new rhythm in her chest. "Do you really think it's a good idea?" Her voice came so softly.

His smile lit her up. "It's a freaking out-of-this-world idea. I love it. And I want to do it."

This was the kind of project she'd love to sink her teeth into—building a prototype resort from the ground up. It was important work, and she wanted to take a big role in it, shoulder more responsibility than she'd ever had—with Dane's oversight, of course.

She was eager to dive in. "Then, if you have no objection, I'll put together an idea document. We'll have something to brainstorm with and talk to Harper about."

He shook his head as if she still stunned him. "Of course."

"Unless there's something else that's more important?"

He huffed out a strange laugh, and she wondered if she was pushing too hard. But he said, "There's nothing more important. Go ahead and get your feet wet with this."

"It's a dream project. We could expand this all over the world." Her whole being felt lighter than it had in months. It was being home. It was working closely with Dane again. It was this new resort that could do so much good for so many people. "This is what all your hard work and learning have been about. Now you have the experience to build this, to do it the best way possible."

"But it was your idea," he said.

"It's *our* idea," she stressed. "Stemming from all the talks with the Mavericks and their loved ones."

She could have rubbed her hands together with glee like a little girl. All she really wanted to do right now was work on this incredible project with Dane. Yes, there were all the day-to-day tasks that would still need to be accomplished, but she thought of all the hours they'd spend, heads together, making plans, creating something miraculous.

It hit her that she longed for all those hours together a little too much. A little too desperately.

Coming off five months of family leave, that might be a very dangerous thing.

Chapter Eight

She was smart. She was courageous. She was efficient and conscientious. She was also funny under better circumstances. And she constantly surprised and amazed him. Even as Cammie worked through her uncle's estate, her beautiful mind was brainstorming, coming up with an idea so brilliant, so exciting that Dane's heart pounded in his chest.

Or maybe that was just having her sitting across from him again, her scent filling the room, filling his head, filling him up.

He'd missed her. More than he could say. And he loved that she appreciated the Zanti Misfits. They seemed a fitting homecoming.

But she stared at her hands a long moment before looking at him again, as if an errant thought had been running through her mind. "I know it's my first evening back, but it's been a long day. Would you mind if I had dinner in my room?"

"Of course not. I'll have Fernsby bring up a tray when you're ready."

"Thank you."

He sensed a vulnerability about her. As if the last five months had suddenly taken their toll. She'd been on duty with her uncle the entire time, never getting enough rest. Then she'd pushed through settling the estate in record time.

If he could have, he would have rounded his desk and pulled her into his arms.

Instead, he watched her go.

Damn the rules that kept him from holding her the way she needed to be held. That kept him from giving her the comfort he desperately wanted to supply.

They'd lived under the same roof for seven long years after she sold Lochlan's house and put the proceeds toward his care. Providing her with a suite of rooms in all his homes seemed like a win-win for both of them. He needed her. She was the order in his life and the heart in his work. When starting a new venture or project, she was instrumental in moving him to consider how he could help people. He'd come to rely on that. To rely on *her*.

That's why he'd wanted to help with Lochlan's care—to pay her back for what she'd done for him. But once the house proceeds were exhausted, she'd insisted on paying what she could, which was a good portion of her salary. Both he and Ava would willingly forgo any further payment, but accepting that wasn't in Cammie's nature.

The fact that she lived with him was an even great-er reason for the rules they'd drawn up that long-ago day. Because, damn him, he couldn't forget the satiny feel of her skin beneath his fingers, the sweet scent of her hair as he buried his face in its silkiness, the ambro-sia of her kiss.

The damn rules were the only things keeping him from marching down the hall and begging her.

Except for the fact that if he pushed, she might pack her bags and leave him.

★ ★ ★

Cammie typed feverishly long into the night, barely touching the tray of food Fernsby had brought. Rex, in his doggy bed, lifted his head every so often to gaze at her.

Since the soccer game, she'd considered the talents of all the Maverick women. This merger wasn't just about the billionaires. Their wives, fiancées, girlfriends, and family were an integral part of the Maverick group. She'd shared her thoughts with Dane, and he'd jumped on her ideas, wanting to talk to each one.

Brainstorming ideas had gotten her through those last dark days with her uncle. The video chats had kept her spirits from plummeting after he died.

Now she had work to get her through. She'd al-ready started a document, adding to it after every meeting, but tonight she dropped in all the ideas floating through her mind. And they just kept coming. God, how badly she wanted to be more than just an assistant on this new resort project. Could she actually run it? With help, yes. But that was the rub—she still needed help.

The thought didn't dampen her enthusiasm, and with every new concept, she wanted to run down the hall to Dane's room and tell him.

Which, of course, she couldn't do.

It was even harder not to think about that night. After all this time, she should barely be able to recall it. Yet she remembered each detail so vividly. His taste, his touch. The things he did with his lips, his mouth. The way he'd stolen her breath with that very first kiss.

"Stop thinking, Cammie," she growled at herself through gritted teeth. Rex popped his head up, looking around as if a real dinosaur were outside the window.

It was deep into the night, long past midnight, when she finally closed the document, the page count coming in at twenty. Rex had finally climbed onto the bed and curled into a ball, waiting for her, opening his eyes occasionally to gaze at her, pleading.

The last thing she did before shutting down her computer was to send Dane her list.

★ ★ ★

Dane looked up from his desk as she entered the office the next morning. "Lord Buttoff?"

For just a moment, she felt light and carefree. "I'm sorry. I thought that was your official title. Am I wrong?"

Laughing with her, he jumped up from the desk to grab her shoulders. "God, I love you." Humor still threaded his voice.

Until he seemed to hear the words he'd said. For a moment, they stared at each other. What the heck?

Then he rushed on. "I mean, I love your ideas. They're brilliant. Every one of them. We've got to do it all. That's what I meant."

If she didn't know better, she'd think Dane was fumbling. And Dane never fumbled. He was always smooth in business. He was smooth with women of all ages. The man was a charmer.

She didn't want to think about *why* he might have fumbled. "Of course I knew what you meant. We've been working together for twelve years. We both know the rules."

They both knew they needed those rules, because their one-night stand, even if neither of them ever said it, had been too perfect for words.

★ ★ ★

While each Maverick had his own center of operations, they occupied a shared office space in Sebastian's San Francisco headquarters for their group ventures. Will sat at the head of the conference table, surrounded by his brothers. He never thought of them as foster brothers, nor did he think of Gideon as Matt's brother-in-law or Cal as just their business manager. Well, except for that blip when he and the guys found out Cal was dating their sister. But that was only natural, right? Now they were all family.

It had been more than a month since the dinner party at Mom and Dad's, and they'd scheduled this morning's meeting to discuss possible ventures for the two groups to organize together. It was time to get things rolling. Though they'd all talked individually, Will wanted everything out in a group meeting before Dane Harrington arrived.

"He's been talking to Charlie," Sebastian said. "He wants to commission her sculptures for each of his resorts. And…" He leaned forward as if the proposal was too incredible to be believed. "He wants her to teach classes for his guests."

"He said the same to Rosie." Gideon shook his head as if it were a marvel. "He wants her to create paintings for his hotel rooms."

Matt sat back hard. "That's one hell of an undertaking. How many freaking rooms does he have in each of his resorts?"

Eyes wide with surprise, Gideon shook his head. With Gideon's being a war veteran, Will hadn't thought anything could surprise him. "Not originals. Limited-edition prints. And he wants her to put the originals in her next few shows."

"Wow," was Evan's only exclamation, but that said it for all of them.

"He wants Ari to check out the childcare accommodations at his resorts," Matt added.

"He's talked to Tasha about an interactive website." Daniel drummed his fingers on the table.

Dane and Cammie Chandler had also spoken to Harper. "I'm not sure what to make of it," Will said.

Cal leaned his elbows on the table. "He was great planning that gala with Lyssa."

"Paige had lunch with Ava Harrington," Evan divulged. "She likes her. Ava wanted to pick her brain on how to add more mental health sessions at her care facilities. Even for the families of her residents."

"I had drinks with Troy." Matt steepled his fingers. "He's got some great ideas for a new generation of workout machines. I could really get into designing that stuff."

"I've already talked to Clay about how we can combine forces—his video platform with the media I have going," Sebastian said. "And enhance both."

It was exactly what Will hoped to hear. He'd known this was the right thing to do. Otherwise, he would never have signed the contract. But it was good to know the agreement hadn't been a bunch of worthless paper. This would bring real results. Dane Harrington was a man of his word.

Sebastian said what they were all thinking. "This is freaking awesome. But what the heck, man? When are we going to do the great deals with Dane?"

"Not just this piecemeal stuff," Matt added. "But something with meat." He curled his hand into a fist.

"Something challenging," Evan added.

The timing was perfect. The idea had come to him as Harper talked about her discussions with Dane and Cammie. He tapped the end of his mechanical pencil on his notebook. "I've been giving it some thought. And here's what I think we should propose."

* * *

Dane didn't arrive alone. The ideas were mostly Cammie's, so of course she had to be there. That was never a question in his mind.

As Dane and Cammie prepared to leave for the San Francisco meeting, Fernsby had appeared. "Sir, I should go."

Dane had said as sternly as the butler himself, "Fernsby, you're not going. You're staying here to take care of Rex."

The man had stubbornly gone on. "I can make tea. And I've been baking."

That got Dane's attention. "What did you bake?"

Fernsby didn't smile. He never smiled. But his eyes glinted. "You'll find out when I bring it into the meeting."

So Fernsby had come along too.

Over the three weeks since Cammie had returned, they'd worked tirelessly on the proposal, refining each of her ideas, researching, adding details, taking to Harper and other experts. And today they would present their plan to the Mavericks.

His brothers and sisters were already approaching the Mavericks with their own ideas. Ava had lunch with Paige. Troy met with Matt. Clay had gone to Sebastian. Plans were already in motion to bring each of their specialties together. He'd talked extensively with each of them during late-night calls, discussed the details, and they'd all signed off on the first special needs resort.

Now, he and Cammie just had to convince the Mavericks. He had full confidence that Cammie could pull it off. She didn't even need him. That's how committed she was. Even if the Mavericks had no interest, the resort would happen. It was the most ambitious project of his career. And over the past three weeks, it had become the most important.

Dane had barely taken a seat facing the Mavericks, with Cammie beside him, when Fernsby rolled in his tea trolley.

"Gentlemen and lady." He nodded to Cammie. "I have tea, coffee, water, juice. What is your pleasure?"

For a long moment, the Mavericks were too stunned to answer. Then suddenly they were all calling out their orders. With each cup he served, Fernsby offered his plate of baked goods.

Of course he'd made all Dane's favorites, and without even asking, Fernsby served him a Bakewell tart, while Cammie received a butter tart.

Sebastian turned to Evan, a frown pulling at his eyebrows. "Why don't we have someone like him?" They'd all experienced Fernsby at the soccer game, but here, in the office, his service could truly be appreciated.

Will stroked his chin. "Fernsby, what can I pay you to work for me instead of Dane?"

Fernsby tipped his nose, almost as though he smelled something bad. "A very kind offer, sir. But you can't afford me."

Each of the Mavericks could afford him ten times over. But none had a comeback.

Cal bit into a Bakewell tart and groaned.

Daniel glared at him. "Jesus, you're with my sister. We don't need to hear what it's like when you're in bed."

Cal's lips twitched with a smile as he continued making what Dane considered a rather sexual noise. "I first tasted Fernsby's specialties in London," Cal said between lascivious groans. Then he smiled. "Ah, London, the best trip of my life. Changed my entire world."

Daniel damn near growled. "You're going to need

to eat that outside, then. Or I might have to beat the crap out of you. Again."

Dane hadn't been there, but he'd heard all about that infamous fight when Daniel had learned Lyssa was pregnant with Cal's baby. They weren't married. No one had even known they were seeing each other. But Dane had seen a spark between them when they visited him in London.

"Yeah," Will said. "You totally lost your mind that day, Daniel. We had to wash the blood off the deck at Mom and Dad's. And I never got to eat my steak."

"I still have the emotional scars," Cal said with a straight face.

Daniel narrowed his eyes. "You deserve them for seducing our little sister behind our backs." His face stretched in a rictus of a grin, teeth bared. "But since she adores you, I've had to be magnanimous and forgive you."

Sebastian got in on the fun. "Can we get back to important things, like how damn good these tarts are?" He turned to Fernsby. "You're freaking amazing."

Naturally, Fernsby didn't crack a smile, not even a slight lift of his eyebrows. "That's very kind of you, sir, to appreciate my baking."

Cammie glanced at Fernsby, smiling. "Fernsby has applied to *Britain's Greatest Bakers*. He's waiting to hear back."

Fernsby inclined his head slightly, as if he were

royalty. Then he bowed his way out of the room, closing the door behind him.

"I remember hearing something about that when we were in London," Cal said, indicating Dane with a jut of his chin.

"He's been trying to get on a baking show forever," Dane explained.

"He really has a shot this time." Cammie backed him up. "The tarts are amazing. The best I've tasted yet."

All the Mavericks agreed. Then Will rapped the table. "Okay, Dane. You're putting in a major effort with all our women, trying to get them to work with you. But what we want to know—" He waved a hand at his brothers. "—is when *we're* going to work a deal with you."

Chapter Nine

It was the opening Dane had been waiting for. "We have a proposal for you." He looked to Cammie, the most important team member. "Why don't you tell everyone what we've been thinking?"

"Well..." She sounded a little nervous, and Dane urged her on with a smile. "The idea came to us after talking with Harper. We'd like to create a resort for people with different abilities. Not *disabilities*, but *different* abilities," she stressed. "No matter where a person is on their path, they always have something special to offer. We want to create an environment where their specialness can blossom." She grew more eloquent as she described what was essentially her project. "We think of it along the lines of St. Jude's. None of our guests will have to pay. Everything will be fully funded by donations. It'll be a place for parents as well as children. We'll have learning, we'll have relaxation, we'll have games. We want to foster teamwork through sports, and perhaps one day a month, we'll have a big competition."

During her pause, Dane added, "The difference between us and the St. Jude's model is that our resort won't be doing research or anything medical. Everything will be therapeutic."

Cammie took over again. Damn, but she was amazing, captivating the Mavericks.

"We want them to have sun, sand, swimming, and fun, so a location near water." She put a hand to her chest, taking ownership. "I like the feel of a lakeside resort." Her confidence increased as she presented all their ideas. "We're not distinguishing by age. Some guests will be young, some in their teens, some adults. Parents and caregivers will have a place for their children or charges to go where they can all interact with each other, do fun things, like flying behind a speedboat with a parachute."

"Parasailing," Sebastian supplied for her.

She pointed a finger. "Right. This will be a place where they can live their best lives for a week or two. But we recognize that parents need to be taken care of as well. In many cases, they've been through hell, and we'll offer a host of activities to help them relax as well as their kids."

Will thumped the table and raised his hands in the air like a gold medal winner. "How did you know that's exactly what we were going to propose?"

Cammie smiled, almost shyly. "Maybe it's all coming out of the discussions that Dane and I had with your significant others. Especially Harper. She and her brother are an important part of this." She waited a moment as Will nodded.

"And you're all an important part as well." She indicated them all with a sweep of her hand. "We're going to need all of you to find ways to help fund this and to use your expertise in bringing it to fruition. Everyone here has something to offer. That's why we think it's a perfect project for this newly merged group."

Every man in the room glowed with enthusiasm. They were into this. And while Cammie gave Dane part claim to the project, it was really all her. She turned him speechless with her ability to spark the Mavericks' interest. He was so damn proud of her. She had everything together, even after the ordeal she'd been through with her uncle.

Daniel didn't need to fake his eagerness. "Lake Tahoe would be perfect for this. There are beaches for sports, the lake for swimming and kayaking, and woods for hiking. And in the winter, there's snowshoeing, skiing, and a ton of winter sports."

Holding up her hand, Cammie said, "But we wouldn't want to be right on top of the big casinos or ski resorts. Our place needs to be relatively on its own."

Daniel tapped the table. "I know the area well. Let me think about it, look around, see what I can find.

And in the meantime, we can make our plans for building."

"I'm sure we'll find the perfect place." Color bloomed in Cammie's cheeks. She was loving this—the planning, the suggestions, the buy-in.

Gideon jumped in. "This is a good use of the foundation's extra cash too."

"We've got several ongoing projects," Cal added. "But as Gideon says, we have funds that aren't allocated yet. I don't want to take away from what our veterans and foster kids need, but there is surplus."

Grinning, Gideon bopped him lightly on the arm. "We've got all these foster kids needing summer jobs, and even during holiday breaks." He looked at Dane, then Cammie. "They could be like camp counselors. It would be great experience for them. It might even help some of them find a path in life."

Under the table, Dane touched Cammie's hand. The whole was bigger than the sum of its parts, ideas coming up they hadn't even thought of on their own.

"We're glad you guys are on board," Dane said. He was as grateful to them as he was to Cammie. "This project has heart."

"You're making us look at what's needed in this world," Matt said. "And how we can use what we've been given to make it a better place to live."

"Your brothers and sisters are all on board too?" Sebastian asked.

"Absolutely." Dane tapped his temple. "Troy is already thinking about sports equipment. Gabby's planning menus."

"Don't forget Fernsby's baking." Cal chuckled, showing his priorities.

"We have you to thank for this," Will said. "Living with Jeremy, I should have seen the need long ago. But you both asked questions that made us think. It takes a team with fresh blood to look at things from a new perspective."

A team. That's what they were. Even as Dane wanted more, this was the beginning. He and his family and Cammie were the fresh blood the Mavericks needed. And vice versa.

"It's synergy," Dane said. "That's what we've got."

There were nods of agreement all around.

"We'll start talking to our contacts about donations," Evan said.

The Mavericks gave a rousing huzzah, filling the room with their voices and their enthusiasm.

With his uncanny sense of timing, Fernsby entered the room once again, his ubiquitous trolley refreshed with carafes of coffee and hot water for tea.

As the group enjoyed a celebratory round of Fernsby's goodies, someone's phone rang with a shrill rotary-phone ringtone from ages ago. All eyes went to Evan, the only one in the room who hadn't put his device on silent. As he answered, his face turned pale.

"What? But it's too early." A panicked note rose in his voice. "Okay. I'll meet you there. Have Theresa take you. Everything'll be okay." He slammed his phone down on the table with a smack that could have cracked the screen.

"Paige?" Matt asked, worry lines etching his forehead.

For a moment, Evan seemed incapable of speech. Until finally he got out the words. "She's having contractions. I have to get to the hospital. Hopefully, my mother will have driven her there by the time I arrive."

"Maybe you should call for an ambulance," Sebastian suggested.

Evan shook his head so hard his glasses wobbled. "And have Paige scold me for overreacting? No way. She'll say, very calmly, 'It's just two babies, sweetheart.'" He did a very good imitation of Paige's gentle, musical tones.

"Then have your driver take them," Matt said. "Don't make Theresa do it."

Evan's voice rose slightly, with either panic or powerlessness. "The driver is here with me."

"Guess you need to hire two drivers," Daniel said unhelpfully.

"Call Susan and Bob," Cal advised.

It was almost laughable. All these powerful men deliberating about how to get Paige Collins to the hospital.

Fernsby tapped his silver spoon against the coffee carafe, the room going as silent as a church when the priest steps up to the pulpit. "If I might interject." He didn't pause for objections. "It appears to me, sir—" He bowed slightly to Evan. "—after having met Theresa Collins at the dinner party a few weeks ago, that she's a very capable woman. I'd even go so far as to say she's unflappable. Experienced in these matters, I'm sure she will safely convey your wife to the hospital in record time."

Only Fernsby could be the voice of sanity in that room. And it worked.

Will jumped to his feet. "He's right. Now let's get the hell out of here and down to the hospital ourselves."

They raced out like a stampeding herd of horses, almost bowling Fernsby over on the way.

★ ★ ★

Dane and Camille remained in the now quiet room. "Maverick generation two-point-oh on the way," Dane said.

Camille nudged him. "Noah and Jorge are generation two-point-oh. This is generation two-point-one."

Fernsby recognized the smile lurking on Dane's lips and saw an opportunity not to be missed. "I suggest you two speed to the hospital as well. Your Maverick companions will need calming influences, so it's your duty to accompany them." He inclined his head, though he felt like cheering. "I will take care of everything on the home front, sir."

After sending them off, he looked down at Lord Rexford, sitting at attention on a chair just outside the conference room. "My dear Lord Rexford, this is an astonishingly flawless scenario. The two of them together, witnessing the birth of new babies. Oh yes, that should get at least one of them thinking."

He rubbed his hands gleefully, then patted Lord Rexford's behind, urging him off the chair.

"Even I couldn't have planned this one better." He allowed himself a smile, since only the dog was there to see.

★ ★ ★

The hospital waiting room was so packed with Mavericks and family, it was almost claustrophobic. There certainly wasn't room for anyone else. The chairs had been moved haphazardly, the magazines on the side tables splayed open, and grooves paced into the utilitarian carpet.

The Spencers had arrived soon after their sons. Cammie didn't need an introduction to recognize the matriarch of the family. Susan hugged Theresa Collins tightly. "We can't thank you enough for being there."

Theresa glowed with pride. "I was only glad I could

help. Paige didn't even tell me at first. She thought it was just a false start."

"And that's why she needed you." Susan smiled, her cap of silver hair slightly mussed, as if she'd rushed out without time to brush it. Misty-eyed, the two moms talked as if Susan were Evan's birth mother. Though Evan and Theresa had reunited, Susan was Evan's mother in all respects but blood, just as she was mother to all the Mavericks. The odd thing was that Theresa didn't seem to resent it.

Despite the tumult, Susan turned to Cammie, who was, naturally, seated next to Dane. Smiling, she headed across the waiting room. Dane was already rising to his feet, and Cammie stood with him.

"You must be Cammie Chandler." Susan took Cammie's hand in both of hers. "We're so sorry about your uncle." Her kind eyes brimmed with sympathy as Bob Spencer echoed her.

"I really appreciate that. Thank you." Cammie gave the older woman's hand a squeeze, with an added smile for Bob.

"We've heard so much about you from Dane." Susan smiled up at Dane. "Thank you both for being here today to celebrate our newest arrivals."

"We wouldn't miss it." Dane leaned down to give her a hug. All the Mavericks were prone to hugging.

Kelsey rushed in then, throwing herself at her mom, Theresa. Soon after, her twin brother, Tony, arrived—an Evan replica with the same maple-brown hair and hazel eyes, even the same smile, though he was ten years younger. Despite Evan having discovered his long-lost family only a year ago, they seemed amazingly tight-knit and completely welcomed into the Maverick fold.

Cammie and Dane took their seats again, out of the melee. Cammie leaned in to say softly, "They both seem very nice. The Spencers, I mean."

Dane nodded. "They're incredible. I wish..." He trailed off. He wished he'd had parents like them? Cammie suspected that was part of his attraction to the Mavericks—not just their business prowess, but the family as a whole.

Though individually everyone seemed to talk in hushed voices, the room felt loud. The disinfectant scent reminded Cammie of all the hours, days, and months she'd sat in her uncle's room. Yet this was so different. This was life and love and happiness.

Dane, as if sensing her thoughts, took her hand in his. "You okay?"

She didn't deny her feelings. "It's nothing like Uncle Lochlan's last days. This is—" She sighed. "It's just plain beautiful."

The sudden smile on his face would light up a stadium. "Yeah. It's a beautiful thing."

She shot him a cheeky smile. "I'd have thought you'd be squirming in your seat," she said softly so no one overheard. "I mean, it's babies, after all."

He looked down his nose with feigned affront. "I like babies."

She snorted. "You've never even been around one."

"I like them." He shrugged. "In theory."

She laughed at him.

During the wait, Cammie went out twice to a nearby café to get food for the conclave. Dane had been about to order in, but she wanted to stretch her legs. Everyone thanked her, grateful for the sandwiches and wraps, sodas, and chips she passed out.

"Too bad we don't have Fernsby as well. Or, more specifically, his tarts," Cal said.

Lyssa, leaning against him, turned dreamy. "Fernsby's tarts. The best ever. And they can lead to so many other wonderful things." She tipped her face up to kiss him.

Cammie felt a little dreamy just looking at them. She whispered into Dane's ear, "We'd better not let Gabby hear that."

Dane snickered. "Who will win their competition is one of life's greatest mysteries."

It was just after ten in the evening when the doctor came through the double doors. The whole gang, including Dane and Cammie, had stayed the entire time.

The doctor smiled widely, her dark eyes bright as

she announced, "We have two additions to your family—a boy and a girl. Mom and babies are doing well. We're just cleaning everyone up, then you can see them."

"Oh my," Theresa exclaimed, hands flying to her mouth. "That was fast. I was in labor with the twins for almost twenty-four hours."

The doctor beamed with pride. "It all went like clockwork."

Susan hugged her husband, Bob, tears streaming down her face. Kelsey and Tony hugged their mom. And the Mavericks clapped one another on the back in congratulations as if they'd all had something to do with the birthing.

Leaning into Dane, Cammie murmured, "Now the wait is over, we should take off. We all can't fit in the birthing room."

Dane held her in her seat with a look. "Not yet. I want a glimpse."

Chapter Ten

Well, well, well. The man was full of surprises.

Cammie had never known Dane to be sentimental, but he avidly watched Paige as she lay in bed, a blue-swaddled baby in her arms. Evan, the proud father, held a pink bundle, gazing down with what could only be called total adoration.

For a moment, Cammie's stomach tilted at the beautiful tableau. Not only for the Collinses and their new family, but at Dane's enchantment as he took them in. The sight brought a tear to her eye. And it made her tremble with a vivid memory of *that* night, a moment when he'd put his hand on her breast, sleekly naked, infinitely sexy, and looked up at her as if *she'd* enchanted *him*.

She zipped her memories shut. This wasn't the time or place.

Evan, or one of the Mavericks, must have pulled a few strings, because the whole clan overflowed the birthing suite, where usually only two or three visitors would be allowed. Thank goodness the room was huge. Painted a soothing powder blue, it could have housed three new mothers, but for now only Paige occupied it. Bean bags and easy chairs sat on the floor, and puffy clouds drifted across the blue ceiling.

Cammie and Dane remained on the periphery out in the hall, like twin Scrooges looking through the frost-laced panes of Bob Cratchit's house on Christmas Eve and wanting to go in.

As if he felt the same thing, Dane curled his fingers around hers. "It's unique and amazing, don't you think?"

She had to agree. "Yes." It was unique for them both.

Dane had never been around babies or children. Neither had she. This was a first. And it was awe-inspiring. But sharing this new experience, she relished the warmth of Dane's hand around hers far too much.

Bob and Susan Spencer got first crack at the new family, with hugs, kisses, tears—most of them Bob's. The man was a big softie.

As they stepped aside, Theresa moved in to tenderly kiss Evan's cheek and her tiny granddaughter's forehead, then bent to Paige and the baby in her arms.

It was so loving, Cammie felt like crying too.

Will took his turn at the bedside, smoothing a finger over the baby's hairless head. Then he turned a stern face on Evan, reminding Cammie of Fernsby. If one looked up the definition of *stern* in the dictionary, it would show a picture of Fernsby.

"You're on indefinite parental leave to be with your wife and babies," Will said. "When you're ready to come back, you let us know. But don't make it too soon."

Harper stepped to Will's side, her words for Paige. "I'm not going to let you come back too fast."

Ari, now at the bedside, Matt's arm around her, gave Paige a few instructions that were obviously for Evan too. "We're going to hold you guys to a pinkie swear that you'll take three months, maybe even six, just to be parents." She put a hand to her chest. "This bonding time is very important for the babies." Both Evan and Paige listened earnestly to her, their expert in child development.

Evan nodded resolutely. "We will. But it'll be hard not to be a part of this family."

Sebastian snorted a laugh. "Just because you're not working doesn't mean you're getting out of coming to the barbecues. And dinners. And whatever other events we feel like throwing. You just won't be working yourself to the bone. You'll be looking out for your family."

Evan bowed his head in agreement.

Rosie stepped in to kiss each newborn on the forehead, then placed a loving kiss on Paige's cheek. "Take this time," she said. "They grow up so fast." Then she looked at Evan. "The business will be here when you come back."

Paige wiped away a tear. "You're right. All of you. Thank you."

The rest of the women, as if they were of one mind, gathered round Paige. Ari put out her pinkie finger. "Pinkie swear." All of them hooked pinkies in a circle. "We want you to take care of yourself while you're caring for your babies. Anything you need, we're here for you."

Paige rubbed away another tear. "Thank you. I love you all so much."

Then Susan took over. "We'll let you get some rest now. It's been a long day." She glanced across the bed to Evan, and even from the doorway, Cammie recognized her joy and love. "And a long day for you too." She gave Evan a loving smile.

The Mavericks separated into couples then, and Cammie had a feeling the pregnant ladies would receive tender foot rubs tonight. It was so sweet— Gideon kissing the top of Rosie's head, Matt with his hand on Ari's burgeoning belly, Cal with a sweeping gaze of love over Lyssa's features. Noah held his hand out to Ari, looking up at her with the love only a seven-year-old child could feel. Gideon hefted a sleepy Jorge into his arms and gathered Rosie's hand in his. Charlie laid her head on Sebastian's shoulder, Daniel nuzzled Tasha's hair, and Will wrapped an arm around Harper.

Then Jeremy raised his voice above all the others.

"Nobody told me the babies' names."

A chorus of laughter filled the room because none of them had thought to ask.

Evan kissed the baby wrapped in pink. "This is Savannah."

Paige resettled the baby in her arms. "And this is Keegan."

Cammie whispered into Dane's ear, "Welcome, Maverick generation two-point-one."

★ ★ ★

The silence in the car as they drove felt comfortable, especially as Cammie's scent filled the air. For the first time since she'd come back—or maybe the second, third, or fourth time—Dane acknowledged how much he'd missed her.

Their working relationship had always been exceptional. She ran his life smoothly. Even more, her brilliant ideas fueled his work. They fueled *him*. Thus the need for the rules. And the reason that, even as he lay only steps away from her at any of the houses or flats or condos they shared, he never actually crawled into her bed.

And he wouldn't now. But still, this five-month ordeal had gotten under his skin. Just as that tender scene in Paige's birthing suite had been a topsy-turvy moment. In the past, he'd offhandedly thought babies were cute and children could be adorable. But witnessing the love lighting up that room, the joy of each and every man, the sweetness of the women, Dane felt his innards slip-sliding. Seeing the pride on Evan's face as he'd looked at his newborns and the reverence with which he'd gazed at his wife, as if she was the first woman ever to have given birth, Dane's priorities had turned into a mishmash. His heart had flipped over in his chest at the gooey, love-swept glances among all of them in that room, knowing in his gut they would return home tonight to reaffirm their love.

He wanted what these Mavericks had. He'd mused over it at the soccer game, and at the signing dinner, he'd gazed at Susan and Bob and the clan they'd brought together. He wanted his family to experience the same phenomenon.

Cammie touched his hand. "You're so quiet." Her soft laughter caressed him. "Did seeing the new babies scare you to death?"

Dane couldn't laugh. He could only answer truthfully. Even if he held back the genuine depth of his feeling. "I have to admit I was a little jealous."

Her touch vanished like a phantom into the night. "Jealous? But you haven't had a serious relationship since I've known you."

He shrugged. "Maybe I've just never found the right woman."

He'd dated, but they'd been more like flings than relationships. No woman had erased the memory of that one night with Cammie. Was that what he was searching for? A woman who could make him forget how amazing that night had been? A woman who could surpass it?

"I like them as a family," he tried to explain. "They're a powerful force because they've created such a cohesive unit."

"But so have you. With Ava and Troy and Clay and Gabby."

He shook his head slowly, barreling down the highway toward Pebble Beach, toward the home he shared with her. He had only one answer to offer. "We don't have anyone like Susan and Bob Spencer. We never had an example of how it should be between a couple who totally love each other. Who want to raise a family together." Parents who didn't leave and who didn't feel their children's love was a burden.

She sat silently for a long moment, as if she had to recall the scene in the hospital room—Susan, Bob, the love, the tears, the joy. "I get it. It's like me and Uncle Lochlan. We were so close, and I loved him so much. But I still miss my parents. I miss my mom even more now that I'm grown up."

Dane no longer missed his parents. But he missed what he'd never had—parents like Susan and Bob.

Then she added breathlessly, "That's why you wanted this merger. It's more than just the business ventures. Even more than the respect you have for them. It's Susan and Bob and the family they've created."

He couldn't quite admit that to her. Not now. He was still too raw with the emotions that swamped him as he'd watched that special family in that joyous room with those beautiful and much-wanted new babies.

He told Cammie the first lie he ever had. "I'm really not sure. I need to think about it more."

That part, at least, was true. He had to sit with these feelings.

And with the new feelings Cammie's return had brought up in him.

★ ★ ★

The weekly family barbecue was held at Sebastian Montgomery's Hayward Hills estate. Charlie Ballard's fabulous metalwork was all over the property— burbling fountains, wind spinners, a magnificent blue crane standing in a pond, sculptures of woodland animals, mythical creatures, and ancient beasts, some large and in-your-face, some small and barely visible unless you looked carefully.

The family gathered around the terraced pool deck out back. It was amazing that these rich, powerful men still held weekly barbecues with their family. They were like normal people rather than billionaires who could have rented an entire country club and catered the whole affair. It was this side of the Mavericks that drew Dane, Cammie knew, even if he hadn't fully admitted it.

Since the babies were only two weeks old, Paige and Evan had asked everyone to wash their hands. Once that was done, the bundles of joy were passed around like they were the most miraculous babies anyone had ever known.

This family barbecue was different, since all the Harringtons had been invited—*family* being the operative word. Sadly, only Ava and Gabby could make it this time, while Troy and Clay had jetted off to events they couldn't miss.

Cammie smiled to herself, because they weren't exactly jet-setters. The two were always working on new deals. Troy was giving the keynote at a conference for young athletes. As an influencer, he was often a guest speaker, not just because of the company he'd started, but for the Olympic gold medals he'd won diving. He never missed an opportunity to encourage fledgling athletes. Clay, of course, was off looking for new talent he could introduce to his exclusive video platform and for sponsors and patrons of the arts.

Flagstone terraces led down to a sparkling infinity pool, and the scent of barbecuing meat wafted in the air. Will and Sebastian manned the grill, the other Mavericks watching the proceedings and making snide comments about the quality of the cooks.

Dressed in shorts and deck shoes, Dane stood with

them, drinking a beer, laughing, and getting in a few good-natured digs too.

His tanned, muscular legs drew Cammie's glance despite herself.

Noah, Jeremy, and Jorge raced back and forth on the grass, playing with the dogs. Tasha and Daniel had rescued shepherd-mix puppies abandoned in the woods near Tahoe's Fallen Leaf Lake. Tasha had kept one, the only female, whom she'd named Darla, while the two males, Flash and Duke, had gone to live with Noah and Jeremy, respectively. Though the dogs were about a year old now, they still hadn't grown into their gangly paws, and they rolled around on the grass, play-fighting like three-month-old puppies. T. Rex, of course, had to be right in there, rolling with the big dogs. Since, of course, he believed he was a big dog.

Fernsby hadn't joined the festivities today. He was supposedly working on another masterpiece for when he secured a spot on *Britain's Greatest Bakers*, something that would wow the judges. Something that was sure to surpass anything Clyde's butler, Digbert, could make. The baking rivalry between the two butlers was legendary, almost as legendary as the one between Fernsby and Gabby.

Sitting on a lounger, Cammie sipped a margarita and listened to the ladies' conversations around her. Gabby, wearing a flowered tankini, stretched out in the sun, her eyes closed, drinking in the spring sunshine.

Ava, who'd positioned herself so that only her legs below her one-piece were in the sun, kept up with the women's running commentary, nursing her margarita.

Mid-April could be rainy in the Bay Area, but today, nature provided a lovely sunny day. Half the women wore swimsuits, the other half shorts, but Cammie, having dressed at Pebble Beach where it was cooler, had chosen light leggings. Though it wasn't hot, merely warm, she sat in the shade now, watching as Savannah, Paige's little pink bundle, was passed from arm to arm, receiving kisses and hugs while she slept peacefully.

Under a big umbrella on the opposite side of the pool, the two grandmothers, Susan and Theresa, cooed over a burrito-style blue bundle, sweet little Keegan. With arthritically gnarled fingers, Francine Ballard chucked the baby under the chin. She sat on her walker, decorated with pink and blue crêpe paper wrapped around its handles and down the bars leading to its wheels. The sight sent a pang through Cammie. She wished Uncle Lochlan could have known Francine. She was a beautiful soul, always smiling despite her infirmities.

She tuned in to the conversation around her as Paige said, "Bob and Susan are so involved. It's been a blessing." She patted Lyssa's arm. "They've practically moved in with us."

"But didn't you hire a nanny?" Ari asked, her head

tipped to the side, probably wondering how she would manage when her new baby arrived.

"We did." Paige shrugged. "But Susan just seems to know everything."

Lyssa added, "She truly does."

Gazing across the flagstones at the men crowded around the barbecue, Bob Spencer included, Paige smiled. "Bob is adorable with the babies. He seems to find them endlessly fascinating, like they're some mystical miracle he's never seen before." She shared a meaningful look with Lyssa. "You'd think he'd never had children of his own."

The ladies laughed together, obviously knowing Bob much better than Cammie did.

Even as they all talked, Dane separated himself from the men and headed to the table where Susan, Theresa, and Francine fussed over the baby. He smiled, then chuckled as he caressed a soft baby cheek. The women seemed as spellbound by him as they were by the sleeping child. He made them laugh, he made them blush, and he charmed them. But that was Dane. He could charm anyone.

Then, in the most amazing gesture, he held out his hands to Susan, and she lifted the baby into his waiting arms.

Cammie marveled at the tenderness softening all the aristocratic planes of Dane's face. Just as on that day at the hospital, his curiosity and attentiveness surprised her. As he held Keegan in his arms, rocking slightly side to side, she swore he was a natural. As if he could be a father. It was usually women who got the urge to have a child, but looking at Dane now, it seemed as if he might actually be thinking about fatherhood himself.

In that moment, the adorable baby in his arms, Dane looked up at her. And smiled.

Cammie's heart kicked over in her chest. What had he said in the car? That with all his dating, he hadn't found the right woman? Maybe he was ready to find that woman now. It seemed impossible, yet the evidence was right before her eyes. How good he looked cuddling the baby so tenderly. How manly. How utterly endearing. She couldn't help smiling back at him.

Though she would have gone on watching forever, Gideon joined them, holding out his arms, and Dane handed over the child. Was that reluctance on his face? The way he looked at the baby boy almost with longing?

Or maybe she was imagining it, and Dane was just being polite.

Yet she couldn't forget that image of tiny Keegan in Dane's powerful arms.

Chapter Eleven

"What'll you ladies have? We've got hamburgers, hot dogs, and ribs," Sebastian called, filling a platter with meat. "And for you, Gabby, there's a vegan patty, along with a gluten-free bun."

Gabby sat up, sliding her legs off the lounger, and raised her hand. "You guys are fantastic. Thank you. But can I have one rib too?"

Utter silence fell over the pool deck. The only sounds were the children and dogs playing on the lawn.

"But—" Ari sputtered. Then she dropped her voice to a whisper. "The ribs aren't vegan. They're meat." She almost bared her teeth as she said the word.

Gabby smiled, answering her in the same whisper, loud enough for all the women nearby to hear. "I know." Then she grinned. "I'm vegan most of the time. But once in a while, I can't resist a barbecued rib. Even if I have a stomachache the next day."

Ava laughed. "You're only doing it because Fernsby's not here to see you."

Gabby shook her finger at Ava. "Don't you tell him. He'll think he's won the war." She raised her voice. "And don't you tell Fernsby either, Dane."

Dane put an offended hand to his gorgeous chest and mouthed, *Who, me?*

Cammie had very occasionally seen Gabby indulge. And only when Fernsby wasn't nearby.

A few minutes were spent by everyone picking and pouring condiments, adding potato salad and green salad, then taking their seats again to enjoy the barbecue. Cammie couldn't resist a rib either, and it was definitely yummy.

She licked her fingers clean one by one—because, really, a napkin never worked—and looked up to find Dane's eyes on her from his perch on the edge of the picnic table by the grill. He raised an eyebrow. She raised one back at him. Then he held up a margarita glass, tipping it side to side, asking if she wanted another. She shook her head. When he held up a plate with a hot dog, she shook her head again. He shrugged and took a big bite, closing his eyes and making faces as if it were the absolute best thing ever. She laughed.

They could say so much without a single word.

Ava's voice tore her away from Dane's antics. "I'm so happy for all of you," Ava gushed, her hands outstretched, her empty plate now on the table beside her.

She was always enthusiastic, her gestures expansive. Cammie could see her confidently taking charge of a boardroom full of men just as easily as she wore the eye-catching royal blue one-piece that wowed unattached men. Today, she'd pulled the waves of her thick hair, the color of dark cherries, high on her head in case she decided to swim.

"But I'm not jealous," Ava said airily, a glitter in her amber eyes. "I wrote off relationships a long time ago."

Engrossed in watching Dane, Cammie must have missed a major part of the conversation, because she had no idea how it had reached this point.

Harper, leaning forward with curiosity, asked Ava, "So you're not looking for love?"

As she shook her head, Ava's hair glinted in the sun. "It's worked out so well for you all. I mean, look at your guys." She waved a hand at the male tableau zealously manning the barbecue as more meat sputtered and spat. "They're a dazzling bunch." Then she smiled gently with either sadness or relief. "But love has never worked out for me. I didn't make good choices in men." She shuddered dramatically. "So I'm done. And I'm totally okay with that."

Though Cammie had known Ava Harrington for twelve years, they'd never shared confidences about relationships. And Cammie had only a couple of past relationships that were serious enough to even talk about. She had no clue about Ava's bad choices. But she did wonder if Ava was protesting a little too much, as though she wasn't as okay with it as she said.

But the ladies really got into the discussion. "Yeah," Charlie agreed. "Men can totally suck." She looked at Sebastian, though he obviously didn't suck at all.

Ari laughed. "And we certainly don't want you to think that everything was a bed of roses with this lot." She hooked a thumb over her shoulder at the barbecue crowd.

Cammie longed to hear their stories. She wanted so much to know them better.

"I mean it," Ari insisted. "Matt was so overprotective of Noah that he watched me like a hawk in case I did anything wrong."

Tasha rolled her eyes. "And they're all so bossy."

"You should have been there when Daniel tried to knock Cal's block off after he found out we were dating." Lyssa heaved a huge sigh in Daniel's direction.

Rosie added dryly, "I believe there was something about Daniel also finding out you were going to have Cal's baby…?"

Lyssa flapped her hand casually in the air. "Okay, there was that."

"I had to whack some sense into Daniel for that one," Tasha revealed with a disgusted shake of her head. "He couldn't accept you were a grown woman and not just his little sister anymore."

"I've got you all beat," Paige said, her smile almost smug. "Because Evan was married to my sister. I think you'll all agree it was a total disaster for both of them."

"I hate to speak ill of anyone," Harper said, spreading her fingers. "But your sister…" She left it hanging, and all the women seemed to know exactly what she hadn't said.

There must be a heck of a story there, but Cammie wasn't comfortable enough to ask.

"But look at you two now." Rosie's dark eyes twinkled. "Two adorable babies. And everything worked out beautifully."

Paige looked at her husband with the other Mavericks. "Yeah," she said with a tender smile. "It's all worked out so perfectly."

Even after hearing their stories, Ava crossed her legs on the lounge chair, her arms folded over her chest, a smile that could have been a grimace on her face. "But you all picked men with potential. While my decision-making has been extraordinarily bad."

Cammie hoped she'd go on. Ava had been so good to her. Maybe Cammie could help her by being a good listener. Except that she might be required to reveal her own secrets… and *her* mistakes took the cake. She could only imagine the look on Ava's face—on all the women's faces—if she were to say, *My biggest mistake was a one-night stand with your brother right before my job interview with him.* It wouldn't matter to them that she hadn't known who he was when she'd slept with him. In fact, that might be worse.

Closing her eyes for the briefest moment, she could

almost feel his touch on her skin, the softness of his hair beneath her fingers, the caress of his lips on her throat, her breasts, her belly. Everywhere.

Lord, that night had been the absolute best. Even if it was a total screwup.

But Dane wasn't her only screwup. She'd made two other extremely bad choices, far worse than what she'd done with Dane, and like Ava, she was never letting that happen again. Though Dane was the only worthwhile one in the bunch, she'd had to let him go for Uncle Lochlan's sake. The job with Dane was her and Uncle Lochlan's lifeline. As glorious as that night with Dane had been, as incredible as the memories still were, she would never have sacrificed Uncle Lochlan's well-being.

Besides, both she and Dane had dated other people. Clearly, if they were meant to be, they'd never have dated anyone at all. And since she'd fallen for another guy as hard as she had, even after Dane, he couldn't be the one. No, she simply sucked at picking men, as badly as Ava claimed she did. *Sometimes you just aren't enough for the man you yearn for, and it never turns out the way you hope it will.*

Ava kicked Gabby's foot where she lay on her lounger. "What about you, darling sister? You're awfully quiet there." Ava gave her a dastardly smile. "Let's hear all your secrets."

Gabby smiled and drew her thumb and forefinger

across her lips, zipping them shut.

Which made all the ladies laugh.

Kelsey swayed back and forth, Savannah sighing sweetly in her arms. "Oh my gosh, I think she's smiling."

"I'm pretty sure that's just gas," Paige said dryly.

"Then I guess that means I need another margarita," Kelsey said with a laugh, handing Savannah to Cammie.

For a moment, she felt paralyzed. Gideon wandered over, Keegan in his arms, and brushed a kiss against Rosie's ear. Matt came with him, standing behind Ari's chair, his hand on her shoulder, her hair, her arm.

Evan arrived right behind them. "Like, would it be possible to hold one of my kids for a minute?"

Kelsey, who hadn't yet left for her margarita refresh, said, "No, you can't. Stop asking and go away." With so many Mavericks around, the joke was that Paige and Evan never got to hold their own children.

Chucking Savannah under the chin, Kelsey grinned up at her older brother. "Don't you think they look just like Tony and me?"

Holding Savannah, Cammie couldn't see any resemblance at all. But then, she couldn't see Evan or Paige in the babies either.

Kelsey threw an arm around Evan's shoulders. "Come on, big brother, you can get me a margarita."

With Savannah in her arms, Cammie couldn't seem to let go, couldn't pass the baby on to Tasha beside her. She'd never thought about being a mother. Her whole life had been consumed by Uncle Lochlan and her job. And Dane.

He'd joined the kids on the grass, where Rex was getting bossy with the big dogs. Picking up a soccer ball, Dane spun it on his finger, enticing Jorge and Noah into learning how to play soccer.

Gideon handed Keegan off to Rosie. "I'd better get over there and teach Jorge how to play the game. Or he'll just learn the Harrington way."

Ava shot him with a finger gun. "You wish."

Gabby laughed. "Maybe Ava and I need to show them how to do things the right way."

Matt held up his fingers in the sign of the cross. "Hell, no. We're not letting you two near them."

With a snort, Ava said, "You're just afraid they'll learn so many hot moves they'll start beating you."

Matt grabbed Evan's arm. "We need to take charge."

And the whole troop of Mavericks descended upon the field.

"They'll never get over it." Charlie laughed. "Almost getting beat down by two women."

All the ladies laughed knowingly.

Bob headed out to the grass, too, and Susan called, "Just be careful of your back, Bob. And wear your sunscreen."

Holding the sweet-smelling Savannah in her arms, Cammie watched as the men played with the boys.

Dane hunkered down to their level, explaining something about the game, the two boys listening avidly. Then he stood, dribbled the ball between his feet. Even from her lounger by the pool, Cammie heard Jorge say, "Let me try," closely followed by Noah's, "Me too. I want to pass the ball to Jorge."

"They're both so lovable." Gabby pulled her silky blond hair on top of her head, holding it there for a moment to cool off her neck.

Both Rosie and Ari smiled.

But Cammie thought the truly lovable one was Dane.

He played with the boys, the Mavericks joining in, all of them just a bunch of big kids. Sometimes he stood on the sidelines, gabbing with one or two of the guys. He was so natural with everyone. Then they'd all rush back into the fray.

Savannah made a sound, and as Cammie looked down, she was sure that was a smile, not just gas. The baby was so tiny and so beautiful. She smelled like sweet milk and baby wash. Something clenched deep inside her, and a barely discernible need began to grow. It wasn't just about the baby. It was more. It was this life she saw before her, a life that all these Mavericks had. Love, camaraderie, the ability to share all this love with one another.

Without thinking, she raised her gaze to Dane. All the guys were getting in their two cents, teaching Jorge and Noah this move and that play. But it was Dane the two boys looked to, Dane they listened to, perhaps because he was the new man in their sphere. He taught them with patience, gave them his undivided attention. As though he were a father.

He was so good with animals, babies, and small children.

And she wanted that. Maybe because she was alone now, because she'd lost Uncle Lochlan, because he no longer needed her, she had a sudden vision of a future she'd never before imagined. The truth was, she wanted the Maverick life. She wanted marriage and love and babies.

God help her, she wanted that life with Dane.

Breathing in the sweet baby scent, she wondered if she'd been lying to herself. She'd tried to be with other men. She'd even found a special man and told herself he was the one. But maybe that was just another lie she'd made up. Maybe it was the only way she could keep her hands off Dane. And keep her heart safe.

Dane raced down the field with the boys, shouting encouragement, clapping his hands, urging them on.

The Mavericks were out there, but all she saw was Dane. It didn't matter that she could never have him. It didn't matter that she sustained herself with memories of their one night, of his kiss, his taste, his touch. It didn't matter that she sucked at choosing men, same as Ava. She knew all the reasons she and Dane couldn't be together.

And it was twelve years too late anyway. Whatever happened that night was so far in the past that, in Dane's mind, it could be only a distant memory. She couldn't risk losing the life she'd made for herself. She couldn't risk another change after losing Uncle Lochlan. She couldn't risk the possibility of losing Dane as her best friend. That's what he was—her very best friend in all the world now that her uncle was gone. Even as she craved the lives of these wonderful Maverick ladies, she couldn't risk losing what she already had.

It was safer to stay where she was, with the perfect working relationship, the perfect friendship.

All she could do was watch Dane on the grass with the boys. All she could let herself have were memories of his kiss, of his hands trailing her skin, of his male scent filling her head, and his body filling her up. That would have to sustain her.

But as she held the darling baby in her arms, as she bent to kiss the sweetly scented skin, she simply could not stop her gaze from drifting to Dane once more. He seemed to be having the time of his life with the two boys, and fear curled in her belly. Fear of the day when he realized how much he wanted to be a father. Fear of the day he'd go in search of the perfect woman to be the mother of his children. Fear that woman could never be her.

It all hit her in a single sucker punch—the baby in her arms, Dane doing fatherly things with two little boys, the memories of their one night, the loss of what might have been. If she'd been alone, she'd have curled into a tight ball, terrified of her future.

Instead, she stood too fast, feeling a wave of dizziness, suddenly afraid for the child she held. Pasting a ridiculously cheerful smile on her face that felt like a caricature of her real self, she thrust the child at Paige. "You should get to hold your baby too. We've been monopolizing the twins."

Paige took Savannah happily as all the women gathered round, smiling and clueless as to why Cammie had to surrender the tiny pink bundle. Paige kissed her child's smooth cheek, closed her eyes, and breathed in deeply of that sweet baby scent.

It was almost Cammie's undoing. She didn't dare cast another glance in Dane's direction. All she could do was run for the house, where she could hide inside, take deep breaths—or scream and cry—until she found herself again.

Chapter Twelve

Dane was aware of Cammie every moment, even as he showed the boys how to dribble the ball, as he ran with them, encouraged them, even as he stood on the sidelines watching them scramble for the ball. Maverick generation two-point-oh.

Still keeping her in his sights, he said to Matt and Gideon, "You've got a couple of future powerhouse players there."

Matt laughed. "We have to bring out the younger generation to have any chance of beating your sisters."

Gideon folded his arms, gazing at the boys. "Yeah, your sisters are unbelievable."

"A more ruthless couple of players I've never known," Matt agreed, still grinning.

"They started really young. Gabby played in middle school. We all helped her train." He breathed in deeply, his eye on Cammie holding one of the babies. The pink swaddle must be Savannah. And Cammie looked so damn good.

He wondered if her job had been holding her back

from her true calling—being a mother. Or maybe it was all the years of caring for Lochlan, when she couldn't dream of anything else.

With Sebastian close behind him, Will joined them just in time to ask, "That was after your parents died, right?"

Dane nodded, turning once more to watch Jorge and Noah, with Cal and Daniel calling instructions and Bob imparting words of wisdom. "It was more than just training for Gabby. I guess you could say that's how we all vented our feelings. And there was a helluva lot to vent after our parents died."

"We all grieve in different ways," Will said. "What-ever works."

Dane couldn't say why, but something broke loose then, a tiny piece of himself. Maybe it was watching the boys. Maybe it had been feeling the delicate weight of a child in his arms. Or maybe, most likely, it was the sight of Cammie holding a baby as if motherhood was the only thing she'd ever wanted. And never had.

"Ava and I were still in college when the avalanche killed our parents." It had been an avalanche in so many ways. "She was a freshman, and I was a junior. I wanted to be a veterinarian," he said with a wry smile. "But we both had to drop out." He hardly remembered those days, except for his love of animals. As a teen, he'd volunteered at an animal rescue, fostering injured birds, squirrels, a skunk, and once even a rattlesnake who'd lost its rattle.

"Man, that's really tough, losing your parents as well as having to give up your dream," Gideon said. The man was probably remembering all his losses before he'd finally found his sister, Ari, again. And then Rosie.

Will slapped Dane on the back. "So you actually raised your whole family as well."

Dane shook his head, glancing at the group of women by the pool, Ava talking animatedly, her hands sweeping through the air as if she was making a proclamation, Gabby tranquilly basking in the sun, eyes closed but taking it all in. And Cammie, who listened. She always listened, gathering information, a quiet voice and a thrilling mind.

He told the guys the truth. "Ava did far more than me. She's really smart. She got her healthcare management degree in night school while she worked full time at a nursing home. We made it through, and yeah, we did it together, but I never would've held up without Ava."

And he would never have found his focus if it hadn't been for Cammie.

"It's the women in our lives who keep us sane." Sebastian threw a glance at Charlie, then jutted his chin toward Susan. "Without them, we'd be nothing."

The herd of Mavericks surrounding Dane erupted in a loud huzzah of agreement.

Dane had to add, "Your mom is awesome."

Then he ran back in to help the boys, feeling almost as if he were fleeing the revealing moment on the sidelines. He'd never divulged so much to anyone in his life. Except Cammie and his own family.

But that's what Mavericks did. They talked. They shared. They confided.

What if he confided how badly he wanted his assistant back in his bed? How he dreamed of her at night? How he closed his eyes, and her scent filled him up? How he still felt the softness of her hair against his fingers, the taste of her on his tongue, the silken tightness of her body around him?

Somehow his need had amplified with Lochlan's passing. As if now there was nothing truly holding them back. Even the rules seemed superfluous. They'd been there to protect her job, mostly for Lochlan's sake.

Or, hell, maybe it was just the fact that she'd been gone for five months, and he'd missed her.

Cammie had never given him a single signal that she wanted more. If they got too close, if there was a moment when sexual tension seemed to vibrate in the air around them, if he looked at her mouth and thought about leaning close enough to kiss her, there were the rules. And he would never do one damn thing to ruin the relationship they had or make her run away. Having her in his life was more important than a single night in her bed.

But now, the beautiful sight of her with a baby in her arms terrified him.

She'd had a couple of close calls with men—at least one he knew of for sure. Or maybe it was more accurate to say it had been a close call for *him*. In the end, though, none of her relationships had lasted. And as badly as he wanted her to have the life she deserved, he'd never been so damned glad of anything in his life.

But how could he compete with a woman's desire to have a child?

"Da-ane," Noah cried, turning his name into two syllables. "You missed the ball."

Sure enough, Dane had let the ball roll right on by.

"Sorry, guys, let me get it." He ran for the ball, kicking it back to the two boys. Then, inevitably, inexorably, Cammie drew his gaze once more.

She stood, handing the baby to Paige. Even as she smiled, Cammie turned and walked up to the house. Maybe he was the only one who saw that by the time she reached the three top steps, she was running.

How thoughtless he'd been. He hadn't even considered how hard it would be for her to see this big, beautiful family and not think of how she'd just lost her uncle. Damn, he was an insensitive idiot.

He called to the boys, "Okay, you two keep practicing with that ball. I'll be back in just a sec."

He tried not to run off the field, but as he closed in

on Matt, he said softly, "I just saw Cammie go inside. I think she might be feeling bad about her uncle. I'll just check it out."

Matt rested a hand on his shoulder. "You're the best damn boss I've ever known." Then he looked at his wife, her hand on her pregnant belly, and he smiled softly. "Except maybe for me when it comes to Noah's nanny."

All Dane could think about was getting to Cammie.

* * *

Cammie stood for a long moment in the hallway powder room. She patted her cheeks, checking the mirror to make sure there was no sign of tear tracks. She hadn't exactly cried. Her eyes were just a little misty and her nose a little runny. But she was fine now. In control of herself again.

An outside door slammed, and self-consciousness flushed her cheeks. How long had she been gone?

She opened the bathroom door.

Dane was in the hall. "You okay?" His voice was raspy with something she couldn't define.

Before she could open her mouth to say she was fine—even if she wasn't—he enveloped her in his powerful arms.

Lord help her, he felt so good she wanted to weep.

"I saw you rush inside." His breath against her ear sent a delicious shiver traveling down her spine.

"Maybe bringing you here was too soon," he murmured against her hair. "You're still mourning your uncle. I'm so sorry. I didn't even think of that. I just thought it would be good for you to get out and have a fun afternoon by the pool."

She couldn't tell him this had nothing to do with Uncle Lochlan. She still missed him. She always would. But she couldn't tell Dane that her emotions had been all about imagining the child she held in her arms was his, a child they'd made together. As she'd stood in the bathroom, mist in her eyes, she'd envisioned walking down the aisle and taking his hand.

She could never tell him that. She couldn't tell him she wanted so much more than just being his PA. She had no idea how she could ever get it, and yet, she didn't know how to go on without it.

The thought just made her hug him even tighter. Until she could feel the beat of his heart as if it were her own.

He rubbed her back, whispered soothing words in her ear. She could barely hear them as hopelessness washed over her. He was holding her only because he was a compassionate man providing comfort to an employee who'd recently lost her uncle. Literally, he hadn't made a move in twelve years. Maybe he didn't think that night had been as good as she remembered it.

A terrible thought struck her.

If he was as into me as I am now willing to admit I'm into him, he would have made a move long ago.

She'd been overwhelmed with concern for her uncle, taking care of him, making sure the last years of his life were as good as she could make them. But Dane had no such compunction. If he'd wanted her at all, wouldn't he have shown her in some way? There'd been moments when she'd felt the tension, the need, the desire. When everything in the room had stilled and they'd leaned a little too close, and she'd thought maybe... But it never happened. And then she'd remember the rules. He'd never even tried to break them.

It could mean only one thing. That Dane *wasn't* into her.

She hadn't made a move either, true, but she had big reasons. Other than keeping his work life on track, what reason did Dane have? Just the women he liked to date.

At that thought, she wanted to slip out of his arms, but Dane held her tight.

It had been so long since she'd been held like this—his arms enveloping her, his back strong against her fingers, his heart beating against her ear, his deliciously musky male scent making her dizzy. She couldn't bear to move. Couldn't bear to push him away.

Yet her mind drifted back to all his women over the years. She'd died a little inside every time. She'd waited, even prayed, for each relationship to end, as awful as that was. She truly wanted him to be happy. She'd consoled herself with the thought that he hadn't seemed overjoyed to be with any of them. And she'd dated, too, had even had two serious relationships, one before Dane, one after. But now she knew deep in her heart, deep in her soul, that neither had been the one. When Arlo Doyle had cheated on her—how long ago had it been? Seven years. It said a lot that she had to think about how long. She could see now that her despair had been all about the fact that Arlo had lied, not that he might have been the man she would spend the rest of her life with.

Because there had never been anyone for her but Dane.

That made her want to cry again, real tears this time, not just misty eyes.

One tiny sob, little more than a hiccup, escaped her.

Dane's hold on her grew only tighter, overwhelming, tempting. She never wanted it to end.

* * *

Every part of Dane's body lit up with the feel of her in his arms. More than his next breath, more than his next heartbeat, more than the rush of blood through his veins, he wanted to kiss her.

And that made him the world's biggest ass. He was

supposed to be consoling her, not relishing the feel of her body against his, her scent swirling around his head, her breasts against his chest.

For God's sake, she'd just lost her uncle. Yet here he was getting horny all over her when she was still grieving.

Somehow it was like the day he'd gone ballistic on Troy for asking her out. He'd actually wanted to pound his fist into his own brother's face. That's how crazy he'd been. How totally inappropriate. Just like now.

Luckily, no one had ever mentioned the Troy incident again, though he was aware it had become family legend, the one and only time their big brother had lost it. The problem was, Dane did things without thinking where Cammie was concerned. Thank God his family hadn't understood the real reason.

But if he thought of her in another man's arms the way he was holding her now, he'd go crazy. He admitted to having one or two daydreams of pounding on a few of the jerks she'd dated. Especially the last one, seven years ago. He'd wanted to wipe the floor with that ass and throw him out with the trash. How dare the man hurt Cammie?

But he hadn't beaten up anyone. He'd pretended he didn't know the full extent of her heartbreak. Because he knew the rules. And if he broke them, he could lose her.

But holding her like this, feeling every inch of her against him, he knew without a doubt that this was where his mind and his body wanted to be. Just like that night twelve years ago…

She lay beneath him as he tasted her like she was the sweetest ambrosia. She was more beautiful than any woman he'd ever seen. Her hair was like silk, her skin like satin, and her taste like fire. She moaned as he pushed her to the peak. He wanted her right there, right on the edge, trembling, begging him with her sighs and her moans and her cries. And only then would he take her fully, burying himself inside her, staying there endlessly…

Before he could kiss her in the here and now, before he could taste her the way he craved—so badly his guts ached with the need—Cammie stepped away, blowing the daydream to bits.

Chapter Thirteen

During the days after the barbecue, Cammie did her best to shake off her thoughts and feelings. To ignore how badly she'd wanted Dane to kiss her right in the middle of that beautiful hug. Otherwise, wanting something she could never have would make her crazy. Her desire would drive her to despair. And she absolutely would not be that kind of person. She wouldn't spend her life mooning over something out of her reach.

She'd learned that lesson when her parents died. No matter how much she hoped and prayed, they never came back.

The new resort project provided the perfect panacea. Especially when, a week later, she and Dane were seated side by side at the conference table in the Pebble Beach office, going over her endless lists.

He sat back abruptly, folding his arms over his broad chest—an action so tempting she had to look away. "You've got fabulous ideas. But we need to figure out how to get from idea stage to completed project. Let's fly to the island, where there won't be any distractions. We'll spend a couple of days throwing out ideas and brainstorming the whole thing."

Outside the office's floor-to-ceiling windows, the ocean lay before them, the morning fog finally burning off and the sun sparkling on the waves. Though spring had rolled in, it was still cool, and a dip in the ocean would require putting on a wetsuit. Dane's Caribbean island was exactly what she needed—warm waters and hot sand, where she could lounge around in only a sundress all day. They could even lie on the beach while they brainstormed, recording their discussions on her phone for later transcription.

"Brilliant," she said.

It would be the first time the two of them had been alone in a very long time. Then she had to laugh at herself. They wouldn't be alone. Fernsby went every-where with them. And she wouldn't think about Dane sleeping on the other side of the lanai. Just like she didn't think about him sleeping down the hall right now in the big house. She hadn't allowed herself those thoughts since the barbecue. That way lay heartache.

Instead, she thought almost constantly about the resort. She loved everything they'd come up with. Could she handle managing the project? Yes, maybe she could, even if she had to ask for Dane's help, since he'd done this so many times. She'd even relish the chance, though she wasn't quite ready to jump in without backup.

But there was plenty of time to think about that. They were still in the planning stage. She picked up her phone and scrolled through her contacts as she spoke. "I'll make arrangements with your pilot. When do you want to leave?"

Dane grinned as if they were going on a romantic holiday for two. Which, of course, they weren't. "ASAP."

After informing Dane's pilot, she called Fernsby about food preparations.

Dane's island was one of the many specks of land dotting the Caribbean. Too small for a resort, its amenities consisted of two huts on opposite sides of the island. One served as the living quarters, with three bedrooms and a common area, including the gorgeous lanai overlooking the beach and the ocean, with a marvelous view of the sunset. The second hut contained the kitchen and a living area where Fernsby stayed, doing all the cooking and bringing food over in a golf cart.

He could have stayed in the main house, but the first time Dane offered that, Fernsby had looked down his nose and drawled, "I prefer my privacy, sir."

Cammie had never actually seen his room in the cookhouse, as they called it, but knowing Fernsby, it would be laid out with precision.

The island wasn't large enough for a runway, so a

helicopter flew them over from Martinique, where the plane had landed.

As always, Fernsby efficiently handled the distribution of goods and suitcases to the two huts, then doled out instructions. "I will prepare food for you for the week, sir, and bring it over later today." He set T. Rex's carrier in the golf cart.

Cammie held out a hand. "You can leave him here."

Her words were met with a frosty admonition. "Camille, you two are here to work. I'll take the little tyke with me since he can be such a nuisance."

Rex wasn't a nuisance at all. But with the quarter mile between the two huts, Fernsby would miss the dog. Even if he would never say so.

The weather was glorious, the sun warm but not too hot. The ocean air wafted through her room as she unpacked, the constant rhythm of the waves a balm to her soul.

Before leaving home, she'd arranged for a cleaning service to open up the island house, put fresh linens on the beds, and dust. No one had been here in all the months of her family leave.

Outside her room, the screened-in porch wrapped around the house. She could leave the two sets of French doors open all night long if she chose. She laid her teal T. Rex against the pillows. As odd as it might be, she always packed the dinosaur. Because its teal color made her happy. Because it reminded her of Dane.

His room was far closer here than in the big house in Pebble Beach. It would be easy to step outside her French doors and walk the length of the veranda to where his doors, too, would be open to the night air.

And Fernsby was on the other side of the island.

Of course she wouldn't do it. She never had. She never would.

God, how she dreamed of it, though. She wanted it more than ever.

But knowing now how badly she wanted love and a life together to blossom between them, a rejection if she made a move would make the loss only more poignant.

Unbearable.

★ ★ ★

Half an hour later, Cammie pulled a sundress over her head, the stretchy smocked bodice fitting tightly over her chest. Sundresses and bathing suits were all she wore on the island. Dane liked his board shorts, his long legs tanned and muscled. And when he threw his shirt off for a swim? She had to count her breaths so she wouldn't hyperventilate.

Dane was already pouring champagne when she stepped out of her room straight into the living room.

"I don't think I can work if you give me champagne," she said as he handed her a glass.

"We worked the entire flight. Now we need a break. We can start again tomorrow." He tapped his glass to hers with the tinkle of crystal.

Fernsby arrived only minutes later, his golf cart laden with food he unloaded into the small kitchen's refrigerator.

Dane stared in wonder. "Did you make all that this afternoon?"

With a hint of disdain, Fernsby said, "I am always prepared, sir." He pointed to the fridge. "You'll have cold salmon on a bed of asparagus, green salads, fruit salads. You'll also find a fish pie with instructions on how to reheat it."

Cammie's mouth watered. She loved Fernsby's fish pie.

"There's also shepherd's pie, cold cuts for lunches, and a selection of fruit for breakfast." He clapped his hands. "If you need anything, please do call. Otherwise, just work away to your *hearts'*," he said with emphasis, "desire." Then he stretched his lips in what could pass for a smile, at least for Fernsby, who never smiled.

"Fernsby, you are brilliant," Dane said.

"Of course I am, sir."

"There's enough food here to feed an army, let alone two people." Dane put a hand to his chest. "So why don't you just take some time off, for however long we're here. You can come up with more recipes for the baking competition that will pound Digbert into the sand."

Fernsby drawled, "You're so kind, sir. But that man doesn't give me a single worry. He uses *frozen pastry*, for God's sake." Then he trundled off in his golf cart.

"How does he do that?" Cammie asked with wonder. "Taking care of everything with barely a moment's notice?" She smiled, then huffed out a laugh. "He really needs to write a book. *How Life Should Be Lived According to Fernsby.*"

Dane added dryly, "Don't mention it, or he'll start writing it while we're on the island."

She put a hand on her waist and cocked her hip. "Tell me, do you know anything about his life before he came to work for you?"

They both looked at the dust settling in Fernsby's wake. "I thought about putting a private investigator on him. But then I tossed the idea. It's better that Fernsby remains a mystery."

She had to agree.

★ ★ ★

They'd worked straight through for two days, to their hearts' desire, as Fernsby put it, and they'd accomplished so much. Today, the morning dawned bright and beautiful. Dane had a need for something different, perhaps a round of golf on the nine-hole course he'd had built on the island.

So far, spring had been rather cool in the Bay Area, and Dane relished the heat of the Caribbean. He hadn't come here while Cammie was on family leave. Somehow the sea and the sun were so much more relaxing when she was with him.

He'd lain awake last night with more of his crazy thoughts, like padding along the lanai to her French doors. They'd be standing open. Cammie loved the scent of the ocean and the breeze that blew through during the night. He thought incessantly of blowing through the doors himself, just like the breeze. The thought had been so inviting that his body clenched tight. She was so close. And yet, so far away, as the saying went.

His fantasies seemed so much more potent after that hug in Sebastian Montgomery's hallway, after the crazy need to kiss her almost got the better of him.

With thoughts like that running rampant through his nights, maybe coming to the island hadn't been the best idea. Especially with Fernsby a quarter mile away. Because now nothing stood between them.

Nothing except the rules.

For two days, he'd repeated that to himself. *Remember the rules.* Even if he'd started to hate them.

But as much as they kept her safe, they kept him safe too. Kept him from making a mistake, kept him from pushing her away by asking for more than she could give.

Over a breakfast of toast and fruit, he suggested, "Let's play a round of golf." It had nothing to do with how much he liked watching her swing a golf club in those sexy little sundresses of hers. Or they could go down to the beach, where he liked watching her in those sexy swimsuits just as much.

But then he'd have to slap himself for his thoughts.

Those errant thoughts were also why he used the Pebble Beach home gym at a different time than she did. Watching her in her tight leggings and skimpy workout tops drove him just a little bit mad.

"Great idea." Cammie gave a little fist pump. "I haven't golfed in months." Then she added with a smile, "We always do our best brainstorming while I'm beating you."

"Beating me?" he scoffed. "We'll see about that."

Even as *he* was beating *her*, she'd have her recorder going, and the brainstorming transcript would magically appear a few hours later.

A most irreverent thought occurred to him. What if he touched her? What if he kissed her? What if it was all on that recording?

The idea made him smile. Even as it heated him up.

Of course it was just another of his many daydreams.

The island wasn't big enough for eighteen holes, but Dane had eked out enough land for nine. Right after breakfast, they hit the course and tossed around ideas.

"I like Daniel's idea of finding something in Tahoe," she said behind him as he lined up his ball. "We'll have the sand for volleyball games and the lake right there for swimming. And what do you think about putting in a nine-hole golf course as well?"

"I love the way you think," Dane agreed as he whacked his ball and overshot the hole by a wide margin. His mind wasn't on this game, but on that long-ago golf game. Twelve years ago, to be exact.

He'd gone out that day to hit a few balls and ease the tension out of his muscles. He'd needed to get away from his office mess. Where better to go than the golf course he owned, especially since he had a condo there where he could shower after the game? He hadn't known who she was when he'd spotted her. He'd been playing alone. She'd played alone too. Then they'd been playing together. He'd been about to introduce himself when she'd held up her hand. "No names," she'd said in the sexiest damn voice that seemed to curl around his insides. "That way, I'll feel more comfortable playing cutthroat."

No names. A mystery woman.

And cutthroat she'd been. So had he, even as he drove himself crazy every time he got near her. He remembered the way she smelled, some citrusy scent that mesmerized him. Just the way her fruity scent mesmerized him now, like the fresh mangoes they'd had for breakfast.

With his very first sight of her, his heart had tried to beat itself right out of his chest.

"And we'll offer all the necessary facilities, a physical therapy room with all the equipment, as well as providing therapists," she was saying.

But he was thinking how physical that game had become. He couldn't tear his eyes away from the way her body moved. He'd damn near salivated. That little wiggle when she stood in front of the ball lining up her shot. The graceful movements of every muscle as she swung. How badly he wanted to put his hands on her and feel her body's moves with each swing.

"Do you think we should have a big hall with family-style dining—long tables where everyone sits together?" She stopped for a moment to look at him, flushing as if his thoughts were written all over his face. Just like they had been that day. She rushed on, "Or maybe we should have more intimate dining. Tables for two and four or six, where people can talk more easily than in a big group."

That word. *Intimate*. He thought of how intimate they'd gotten after that golf game. Even as he knew he shouldn't think about it at all. Even as it did things to his body in this moment.

"We should have both," he said. He wanted both, business and pleasure. With her.

"Yeah." She nodded, turning back to the ball. "We need both."

He never should have hugged her at Sebastian's house. Now his body remembered the feel of her against him. While she was grieving for her uncle, he'd been having lustful thoughts, making him a complete ass. Even as he admitted that, he couldn't stop looking at her in that too sexy sundress, couldn't stop thinking about touching her, kissing her.

Just the way he'd been thinking that day during their first sexy, mind-blowing golf game.

* * *

She couldn't concentrate. Her thoughts were scattered all over the place. She was throwing out ideas that were already on their list, for Pete's sake. They were supposed to be talking logistics—geology reports, engineering drawings, how to start building. But her mind wouldn't work properly. It was how close he stood, how good he smelled, how hard his muscles were as he swung.

Just like that other golf game.

She tried to sound coherent. "We need a full gym and workout area. And a massage therapy room." Her nerves were jumping. Every time they'd played golf since that day, her body had tingled with the memory of that night. Her body tingled now with the memory of his touch, his kiss, his scent.

"We need a pickleball court too," he said.

She laughed, the sound a little strangled. "Of course we need a pickleball court."

She remembered how he'd stood there that day, setting up for a shot, the sun making his hair gleam blue-black, his body so tempting she'd wanted to lick him like an ice cream cone. She'd been at the golf course only because Clyde had said her jitters were making him edgy. He'd told her to get some exercise to burn off all that nervous energy. She'd had that interview the next day with one of Clyde's associates, whom she'd never met. And Clyde had made her swear she wouldn't research the man beforehand. That had been a big mistake.

But Clyde had insisted, "I don't want you to have any preconceptions." Despite Clyde having told her the job was in the bag—he'd obviously been singing her praises—she couldn't count on anything. And she'd gone out to the golf course to play and relax.

Then *he* had come along, a man so handsome, so sexy that she'd forgotten all her nerves about the job interview. In fact, she'd forgotten the interview completely. There'd only been him.

She'd challenged him with that no-names thing and playing cutthroat. She just hadn't imagined exactly what *cutthroat* meant. He'd made wisecracks, sidling close to her, saying things like, "Do you really want to take your shot that way? Maybe you should try it this way." Then he'd stand right behind her, less than a breath of air between them, and guide her hands on the club. His sexy, slightly sweaty male scent had made her dizzy. It had been so hard not to let him throw her off her game. Hot and cold shivers had run up and down her spine. At some point, she'd leaned back, felt him against her, all of him.

The game—and the games—continued, touches that weren't necessary, his breath against her hair as he whispered how good her stroke was, what a good grip she had on the shaft of her club, all those innuendoes making her crazy as much as they made her laugh. Everything was so much sexier without names. He was a seductive stranger she'd never have to see again.

"We should have single rooms as well as family cottages," she said, her voice too sexy, too husky as her memories made her hot and bothered, ready to turn around and jump him. Just the way she'd wanted to that day. "And we should also have dorm rooms the kids can share, as if they're at school."

Did she even make sense anymore?

Yet everything had seemed to make so much sense that day. He'd enchanted her with his touches, his whispers, his hard body, his sexual innuendos. And when she'd won the game—had he let her win? She'd never asked—he'd said, "This calls for champagne." He'd had a condo right on the golf course and *not* taking up his offer had never been an option. She would have followed him anywhere.

His taste had been exquisite, his lovemaking so beautiful it still made her ache late at night. He'd made her forget the lover who'd broken her heart as if the man had never existed.

"We need to have the best chef," he said.

She laughed. "You're always thinking about food." The champagne and appetizers had been exquisite that night. And he'd been exquisite, knowing exactly how to touch her.

"I'm always thinking about life's pleasures." His smile reached deep down inside her to all those memories, to all that pleasure he'd given her, to the taste of him on her tongue, the feel of him inside her.

She'd never known such dazzling sensations as those he'd given her that night.

What would have happened if she hadn't walked into the interview the next morning and discovered that Dane Harrington, her potential new employer, was the very man who'd made such beautiful love to her the night before?

Chapter Fourteen

Pleasure. "We want our guests to have the best of everything," Dane insisted.

He realized now that she was the best he'd ever had. Her taste had made his mind reel, her skin had been as soft as rose petals, and the lyrical sounds of her ecstasy still played in his mind every night.

He found himself close to her now—close enough to sense the heat of her body, the sweetness of her shampoo, the citrus of the lotion she always wore. "We need to offer leisure time for the parents, like a couple's massage followed by a romantic candlelit dinner in their suite. So they can learn how to be lovers again." He painted the romantic picture he dreamed of with her.

She smelled so damn good. He shouldn't want this. He shouldn't need this. It could be so bad for them.

But it could be so damned good.

He put his finger beneath her chin and tipped it up, forcing her to look at him. "What do you think?" His voice was so low it couldn't even be called a whisper.

Her eyes were wide, her breath coming fast, and her scent carried the sexual musk of that night. Even as his mind shouted a warning—*bad idea alert!*—his body and his heart didn't care.

She was so close. Her lips were so pretty and plump, begging for his kiss.

With just the tip of his finger beneath her chin, he touched his lips to hers. The sweetest, lightest touch.

She made a sound, almost a moan.

He trailed the tip of his tongue along the seam of her lips. Tasted her. Tempted her. Just the way he had that night. With the tiniest gasp of air, her lips parted for him.

Nothing had ever been so good as when his mouth closed over hers. When her tongue touched his, and the kiss became a slow, sweet devouring of each other. Delicious little moans rose up her throat, sounds of pleasure that were as sweet as her taste. He wanted to haul her against him, feel her body plastered to his. And yet, he wanted this, just her lips, her mouth, her tongue, her taste still filled with the luscious fruit they'd eaten that morning.

★ ★ ★

She wanted to curl her arms around his neck and climb his body until she could wrap her legs around his hips, to hold him there, tight against her, the feel of him hard against her core. He tasted like heaven. He tasted like the sweetest treat she'd ever known. He tasted of desire and sexy, steamy nights.

He tasted of twelve years of craving.

And he tasted of rules that shouldn't be broken, of everything she wanted and everything she couldn't have.

As if he'd stolen every last breath from her, she had to step back just to drag in a lungful of air before she drowned in him.

They were both breathing hard.

She'd been so deep in those memories of that day. When there'd been no need to resist. When there'd been no need for rules. When there'd been nothing but the feel of him, the taste of him, the scent of him.

But that day had been left behind long ago.

★ ★ ★

He wanted her. He also knew how easily he could push her away forever. Needing something or someone this much always brought disappointment.

But he had to fix it. Right now. Before she left him because he'd overstepped. "I'm so sorry. That was totally inappropriate."

She rolled her lips together, swallowed, her eyes too wide, too stark. Finally, she said, "I'm sorry too. It breaks all the rules."

Who had thought up their idiotic rules? Was it him? Was it her? But the rules were the reason the two of them had been able to work together for so long in the most symbiotic relationship he'd ever known.

She spoke again, saying things he didn't want to hear but needed to anyway. "Our rules matter. We can't change them now, especially not when we're in the midst of the most important project of our careers."

He wanted to argue. Something in him said the rules just didn't ring true anymore. She'd needed the job to give her the wherewithal to care for Lochlan.

But Lochlan was no longer here.

Didn't that mean the reason for the rules no longer existed?

"I mean, we can't throw it all out now." Was that desperation in her voice? "I mean, it would be throwing away everything we've worked so hard for."

Would it be so bad to let themselves go?

"I mean, the rules enabled me to help my uncle. And they made everything about our relationship work. I mean…" She finally stopped.

I mean. She kept saying that, as if she was trying to convince herself as much as him. And he saw then, without a doubt, that if he pushed, she absolutely would run. She needed her rules. As sweet as that kiss had been, the rules were truly what kept them together. And if he blew them up, he might blow up his life and this crucial relationship.

You always want too much from people, Dane.

Even as his throat wanted to close around the words, he had to force them out. "You're right. You're right about everything."

In a voice that threatened to tear them apart, she said, "We've been here for three days, and we've got a ton of material. Why don't we head home, where I can collate all of it and put together our presentation for the Mavericks?"

Metaphorically, she was running, even if he hadn't destroyed the rules.

★ ★ ★

How many times did she need to go over all the reasons why an affair with Dane was a really bad idea? Over and over, obviously.

Even that didn't work when she thought about his lips on hers, his taste filling her mouth, filling her entire being. His scent was like a drug to her senses. No man had ever been as potent for her. Even as she packed her bag, alone in her room, the scent of him still mesmerized her, and his kiss still steamed her up.

So she *had* to go through all her reasons. Again.

It would end badly.

They would lose their friendship.

She would lose her job.

Nothing would ever be the same between them once it was over.

Her life would change irrevocably, and she

couldn't stand another change. Not now. Not right after losing Uncle Lochlan.

But still, she couldn't help craving one more kiss, one more night, one more moment of pleasure.

A pair of silk panties in her hands, she had the most awful thought. Dane hadn't even fought her when she'd said they shouldn't forget the rules. And he'd been the first to apologize. *So why did he kiss me in the first place?*

On the heels of that, another horrible thought rammed its way in. Was *she* the one who'd kissed him first? Was that why he'd immediately apologized? Oh God, she couldn't remember how it happened.

She could only remember wanting him, being in his arms, kissing him.

It was only a kiss, yet it tore her apart. Without Dane, without this job, she had nothing. She didn't even have her uncle anymore.

No, the best thing for her was to forget about that kiss, forget about that long-ago night, forget about him with the kids at the barbecue, with a baby in his arms. She might want all that, and she might want it with Dane, but it was never going to happen. At least it wouldn't happen the way she wanted it.

And her beautiful, comfortable, secure life could turn into a hot mess.

* * *

While they waited in Martinique for his pilot to ready the jet, Dane set up the Maverick meeting in San Francisco for the next morning. "Are you sure we're ready?" he'd asked Cammie as she busied herself on her laptop.

"I'm sure we will be," she'd said without looking up.

He had nothing else to do. Because Cammie wasn't speaking to him. Not in an angry, *I never want to speak to you again* way. Cammie wasn't like that. This was more of an *I can't believe I kissed you and I don't know what to do about it* way.

He was just as shell-shocked.

That kiss reminded him of every single moment they'd spent in his condo on the golf course that night. Not that he'd ever forgotten a single moment. But now the memories were fresh with the taste of her, the scent of her, his need for her.

He just wasn't sure what to do that wouldn't ruin the good thing they already had.

But he had the hours of the flight to think about it.

And to think about her.

★ ★ ★

They flew home overnight, working some of the time, sleeping some of the time. After preparing a special treat for the morning's Maverick meeting—the plane had a sufficient galley kitchen—Fernsby watched

Dane's and Camille's every waking moment with a hawk's eyes.

Of course they didn't notice his scrutiny; they were too busy ignoring each other. *What's up with that?* he thought, just like an American.

But he wasn't American. He was British. The British were always more reserved, especially when they were being devious. And he was totally (another Americanism) devious.

Something had happened on that island. SOME-THING BIG. He thought the words in huge capital letters.

He could have clapped with glee, but of course he didn't. Things were finally moving in the right direction. FINALLY. Again in huge capital letters.

He'd brought food to the island, much of it already prepared, so they'd have all the meals they needed and could just forget he was there.

But something hadn't worked the way he'd planned.

"Just get on with it, you two," he muttered under his breath. He wanted to rail at them. But he'd just have to work harder. A good butler's work was never done.

Then a brilliant plan came to him, which was not unusual. Quite often, he was filled with brilliant plans. He was a mastermind, if he did say so himself.

He almost wanted to buff his fingernails on his lapel. Because this was one of his most brilliant ideas yet. And it would work.

★ ★ ★

It was almost the end of April, and the Mavericks were eager to hear Dane and Cammie's plans for the resort. They all wanted to get a move on. So the following morning, Will and his best friends and brothers sat around the big conference table for the meeting. All of them except Evan. Will knew Evan would never last three months, never mind six, but at least he was taking the time now to bond with his children.

Matt was telling the story, with wide gestures and a resounding voice, of how he'd taken Ari and Noah to see the babies. "I swear, Mom and Dad made an edict that Evan and Paige needed a date night." He dropped his voice as if they were in a conspiracy. "Secretly, I think Paige was horrified at leaving the babies alone for one evening. After all, they're only a month old." He laughed. "But you know Mom. She told them they needed to reconnect over more than being peed on and changing dirty diapers."

Of course that's how Mom and Dad would be, the ultimate grandma and grandpa. They were in seventh heaven over the twins, as well as the three new babies on the way.

Will had a sudden vision of Harper, hands on her belly that was huge with his child. He wanted it. Badly.

He just wasn't sure the time was right for her. But when it was, he'd be overjoyed.

"And I swear," Matt went on, unusually long-winded, "Paige was all, 'But-but-but...'" He smiled. "And Mom simply held up her hands, saying, 'It's nonnegotiable, and I don't want to hear any excuses.' You should've seen Mom. And you can't argue with her, because she's always right!" Every Maverick at the table chuckled. They knew their mother well.

So true. Mom had known Harper was right for him, and she hadn't allowed him to make a mistake that would scare away the love of his life. Will would be forever grateful for that.

The conference room door burst open. Dane should have been there, but instead, Will—and all his brothers—were delightfully surprised to see Fernsby rolling in his tea trolley with another mind-boggling delicacy. The man must spend every waking moment in the kitchen.

Cammie Chandler and Dane followed, but not a single Maverick cared about them.

"Do you travel with that trolley, Fernsby?" Will asked.

The man looked down his nose. "Of course, sir. A butler is always prepared. I keep it in the trunk of the car, which we left at the airport."

Then he began pouring coffee and dishing out another of his creations.

Around a mouthful of delicious cake covered in warm custard called a jam roly-poly, Sebastian said, "Okay, so is there a butler registry, like Butler-dot-com or something, where we can find someone just like you?"

Dane laughed. "There's no one like Fernsby."

Fernsby, with as straight a face as ever could be, said, "There's no one on this planet who can handle bosses who are too big for their britches the way I can."

Each and every Maverick laughed himself sick. Fernsby was so right—they were all too big for their britches, as their mom often told them.

Mom and Fernsby would get along great.

★ ★ ★

Cammie ran through the slide deck demonstrating their ideas, from a pickleball court to basketball hoops to activity rooms, along with art classes for painting to metalwork, and even a dance studio. Her tummy had done flipflops on the drive from the airport when Dane had said he wanted her to take the lead, claiming most of the ideas were hers.

And now she found she couldn't look at him. As if one look would make her stumble.

Or remind her of that island kiss, and then she'd become completely flustered.

She concentrated on the conference room full of

Mavericks, all seated at the big table, their arms folded. The blinds behind them were pulled to cut the glare on the large display screen from the sun shining through the windows overlooking San Francisco Bay. She was glad they'd dressed informally, making her feel better about the fact that she and Dane still wore casual clothes. When they'd been heading to the Caribbean, she hadn't thought to take business attire to change into.

As she clicked through the last slide, Sebastian breathed in deeply, letting it out in a long sigh. "Don't you think we're asking a lot of these kids—dancing, painting, metalworking?" He might have been wondering how much time Charlie would have to devote to teaching special kids how to create art out of scrap.

But Cammie had an answer. "Our guests will rise to the level of their capabilities. We talked to Harper." She glanced at Will. "She feels that these kids need to be given all the opportunities their contemporaries have available to them."

Daniel looked at the practical side. "So how much land do you think you'll need for this, if we're building from the ground up?"

Cammie nodded, grateful for the question. She wanted these men to know she'd thought of everything. "We don't necessarily need to build from the ground up. We want to be in Tahoe—that was a great suggestion, thank you." She tipped her head to Daniel, giving credit where credit was due. "But as the Maverick Group is committed to its environmental policies, there are a few long-vacant old resorts or casinos with lakefront property that might work, with existing roads, power, and water." She clicked to a slide with a chart showing square footage for every activity area they'd talked about adding to the resort. "If we can do it all on the same level, the footprint could be a lot. But there's no reason we can't have a multilevel facility and still have room for outdoor activities. Our main objective is to be on the waterfront with the forest at the back, making hiking trails available to our guests."

"What about skiing in the winter?" Matt wanted to know.

"Rather than having our own slopes, we could work out deals with ski resorts for day trips."

Matt nodded his approval.

"So how much money do we need to start?" Gideon asked.

Cammie didn't hesitate. She felt good about the material, confident in her presentation. "The lowball figure would be two hundred million to start, if we do this in stages. But to do it right, we need at least five hundred million."

Not a single Maverick choked or guffawed or batted an eyelash, not even Cal, who was the Mavericks' business manager. With the billionaires, it could be all pie-in-the-sky, but Cal was down to earth. "We'll sure as hell have our work cut out for us." He paused, looking at the square footage slide a long moment. "But it's doable."

Cammie smiled and finally looked at Dane. She saw pride gleaming in his eyes. Little did he know it had taken every ounce of confidence she possessed to run the meeting. But she'd really done it.

"We've already started opening doors," she told them. "We left a message with Clyde Westerbourne to see how he can help."

Cal whistled. "Westerbourne. Great man. He helped us with Gideon's foundation."

"And I'm sure he'll want to help with this too." Then she added smoothly, "We'd welcome any additional ideas or comments you have. This is a group project. We need your input."

Will sat back in his chair, holding a pen between his fingertips. "I believe I speak for all of us. You've done the work." He flashed his gaze around the room, and the Mavericks let him be their mouthpiece. "And we like all of it. If we have something to add, we'll let you know, but you've got an amazing start here. Obviously, there'll be massive fundraising for this. But you two have such a mind meld, we don't want to get in your way."

"Cal and I will look at how the foundation can help," Gideon said. "But you know you can call on us if you need anything."

She wanted to clap. She wanted to cry. They'd done it. The Mavericks were in. And finally, she could look at Dane again.

She felt that mind meld, as if they didn't need words.

And it told her he was extremely proud of her.

/

Chapter Fifteen

Dane had planned on three days to go through the entire project with the Mavericks, to discuss it, take suggestions, make changes, think it over, but the group had decided in less than two hours. It wasn't even much past eleven a.m. The whole thing was kind of crazy.

But then, it wasn't crazy at all. Cammie had done an exceptional job, polishing their presentation on the overnight flight from the Caribbean. He'd gotten some good shut-eye, but he wasn't sure how long she'd slept, though it had certainly been long enough for her to be sharp and ready for whatever the Mavericks threw at her.

That was why she hadn't spoken to him much on the flight—because she'd been working, perfecting.

It couldn't have had anything to do with that kiss.

"Great presentation," Will said, rising to shake Cammie's hand, then Dane's.

Fernsby's trolley was empty. Ah yes, that was probably why the Mavericks were letting them go: The cake was gone.

Back at the car in the parking garage, Dane had left the air on—the car had a special climate control—since Rex was sleeping inside.

Fernsby stored his foldable tea trolley in the trunk and turned, regarding them with his staid British façade. "I've flown halfway around the globe with you today, sir." Did he even recognize what a huge exaggeration that was? But Dane didn't stop him. "So please don't ask me to drive another three hours down to Pebble Beach. I need my rest." He sniffed loudly as if Dane should have known this. "I'll take the dog to the flat with me while you two play tourist for the rest of the day."

Fernsby didn't fool him. He adored the dog, and taking Rex was no hardship. Both he and Cammie had seen Fernsby sneaking dog treats to Rex, though the butler claimed it was Dane who gave out way too many.

Cammie jumped in. "We can't play tourist. We've got a lot of work to do."

Fernsby eyed her with a look that could have flayed the flesh from a lesser human's bones. His voice when he answered held its usual stern tone, though slightly more tender, perhaps because of Cammie's loss. "My dear Camille," he said softly. "You two have worked like dogs," he said with an exaggerated drawl, "for the past three days. You must take some recuperation time."

When Cammie opened her mouth, he wagged a finger. "You are still grieving, my dear." Was that compassion in Fernsby's eyes? "Make no mistake about that. And now I am ordering you to go out and enjoy the most beautiful city on earth."

"I thought London was the most beautiful city on earth," Cammie said, not exactly arguing with him.

Fernsby looked at her as if she were incredibly misguided. "Home is where the heart is," he said simply. With that, he crammed his tall frame into the car, slammed the door, turned on the engine, and expertly backed out of the parking spot at high speed.

Thank God the two of them weren't still standing by the trunk. In a flash, Fernsby and the car were a distant memory.

"He's so bossy," she said, hands on her hips.

Dane merely smiled. By some miracle, he had exactly what he wanted—free time with Cammie. Taking her elbow, he guided her to the carpark stairs. "Let's get a coffee and talk about what we'd like to do today. After all, Fernsby gave us an order."

She harrumphed like an old lady. And Dane smiled deep down inside.

* * *

They found a little café just outside the garage entrance, and the scent of freshly ground coffee almost made her swoon.

She staked out a table while Dane ordered espresso for himself and a latte for her. He always knew exactly what she wanted. She watched him charm the barista, laugh with the other customers, and make the young woman in line behind him look to see if he wore a wedding ring.

He was just so... likable. Sexy. Drool-worthy. And the perfect boss.

But right now, she wanted to squeal her delight like a child who'd just won a stuffed animal at a carnival. She couldn't have been happier with how well the meeting had gone. She'd answered every question as if she knew what she was talking about. Which she did. She'd put together the slides, found example photos, worked out square footage, looked at cost estimates. The Mavericks hadn't looked to Dane for answers. They'd listened to *her*. And now she overflowed with triumph.

The feeling was momentous. As she'd talked, she'd realized she wanted this project with every fiber of her being. It was the project of a lifetime.

She could do it. Sure, her nerves could get the better of her every once in a while. But she'd worked with Dane on so many projects. She had all the contacts they needed. He came to her often enough, asking who they should call about this and who they needed for that. If she let this project slip through her fingers because of a few nerves, she'd regret it forever.

She wouldn't let fear get the better of her.

When he finally returned to their table, setting the perfect latte in front of her and pulling his seat close to hers, she managed to say the words she absolutely had to.

"You know I love working with you, Dane. It's been totally great."

Something like panic flared in his eyes, and he pressed her hand tightly. For a man who always knew the right words, Dane actually stammered. "No, wait—please, let me—"

She cut him off. "Just hear me out, okay?" She pushed through her nerves, pushed through her memories of all the bad days with her uncle, pushed through the grief and the moments where she'd felt powerless to help him. "I've been your assistant for twelve years." She pressed her lips together when unbidden tears wanted to rush to her eyes. Maybe it was her uncle. Maybe it was all those good years with Dane. Or maybe it was the night that started it all.

Dane grabbed her hand, held on a little too tightly. "Cammie, please."

She reclaimed her hand to say what she had to. "I'm ready for a promotion. I don't want to be just an assistant on this project. I want to manage it."

He sat back, hand dropping to his lap, staring at her as if she'd never shown him this side of herself before.

Maybe she hadn't.

Then he puffed out a snort. "Now why the hell didn't I think of that?" He shook his head, something like wonder widening his eyes. "Of course you'll do the best job. Everything we talked about in that meeting was your idea." He tapped his temple. "In fact, I think the original idea was yours."

She couldn't remember anymore. It didn't matter. Because, miracle of miracles, he'd agreed. "I might need some help." She was stepping out of her comfort zone, but she needed to do this. "But I'm ready to try it."

He pointed his finger at her nose. "You're my idea genius." *Genius.* Before she'd always been his idea *genie*, as if what they did together was magic. But now she was already promoted. To *genius.*

"You can bounce things off me," he said. "Just the way I bounce things off you. But you can do this."

She might never be one hundred percent in control of her nervousness. But was anyone—except Dane? She'd settle for ninety-nine. "Thank you. We'll absolutely do our normal idea exchange."

They always would, because she would never let anything get in the way of what they had together.

★ ★ ★

Cammie left to use the powder room.

That moment had stretched on endlessly, when

he'd believed she was going to quit. Her beloved uncle was no longer her responsibility. Which meant she didn't need this job, because she could now work anywhere. The rules he'd always thought protected her had protected him from losing her. And now, she didn't need either anymore—not the job, not the rules. And not him.

But his heart rate was under control once more. He could breathe again. Cammie wasn't leaving.

Dane wished he could be his own punching bag. How stupid could a man be?

Cammie had worked for him for twelve years without a single promotion. And because he was thoughtless and selfish, he'd been holding her back all along. He'd kept her in the place he wanted her to be instead of helping her get to the place she needed to be. She was his idea *genius*, not his genie, as if she conjured things out of smoke. She was so intelligent, so competent. She even told him when he was going in the wrong direction, sometimes knowing it before he did. She was his right-hand woman, not just his girl Friday. She wasn't a *girl* at all, but a resourceful, thoughtful, caring, loyal woman.

And he was an ass for not giving her this chance before.

The moment she returned to the table, he took her hand. "I apologize."

"For what?" she asked, as if she couldn't see how

he'd held her back.

"I've given you raises, but I should've realized that wasn't enough. You've always taken on more responsibility, doing whatever new task I asked of you. We just never acknowledged it. You've always directed my projects. And I've always listened to you."

She shook her head, staring him down. "Don't rewrite history, Dane." Then she patted his hand as if it were Rex's head. "This is different. This is me calling the shots. I've never asked to do that before. But I want it now. So please don't apologize. You had no idea it was important to me, because I didn't even know I wanted it. Maybe I had to get through the ordeal with Uncle Lochlan." She shrugged. "But now I know what I want. And thank you for the promotion." She put her hand to her heart. "Thank you so much."

"Of course you'll get a raise commensurate with your new title of project manager."

"Thank you." She didn't turn him down. He wouldn't have let her.

He still could have smacked himself. Why hadn't Fernsby forced him to open his eyes? "You need to know I'm in awe of you. And I can't wait to see everything you come up with along the way. Because it will all be astounding."

Her smile turned him inside out. He should have done this years ago. Just so she'd smile at him exactly that way.

★ ★ ★

Cammie's cheeks flushed at his praise. Something wanted to bubble up inside her. Excitement. Maybe even joy. Certainly pride. Because Dane hadn't *given* her the promotion. She'd *asked* for it. She'd taken her own personal bull by the horns and wrestled it to the ground, telling Dane what she should have told him years ago. She wanted a project, and what better project than a resort for special needs kids? It was almost like a calling. And she was going to do the absolute best job ever.

But she smiled so Dane wouldn't know the overwhelming effect his words had. "Now that's out of the way, let's talk about our plans for the day. We've always done our best brainstorming while we're outdoors—golfing, hiking in Pebble Beach, or wherever."

Just as she had on the island, she remembered that fateful golf game. All their golf games. But she also remembered the long hikes when she'd felt so in tune with Dane. A walk around San Francisco would be the next best thing.

"Why don't we go to the windmills in Golden Gate Park?" she suggested. "It's the perfect time of year for the tulips." She chuckled at herself. "I always seem to think about visiting the windmills when the tulips are out of season."

"Deal." Their coffees finished, they headed out, and Dane pulled her hand around his crooked elbow. "I'm glad we both wore our walking shoes."

Since Fernsby had taken the car back to the flat, Cammie booked an Uber.

They were picked up by a massive SUV. Once they were ensconced in the back seat, she enjoyed the drive across San Francisco, with a brief detour around Alamo Square and the Painted Ladies, those gorgeous Victorian houses, then through Golden Gate Park past the Botanical Gardens.

They climbed out of the car to find the tulips still blooming in the Queen Wilhelmina Garden at the Dutch Windmill. Hand over her mouth to cover her gasp, she clutched Dane's arm. "Have you ever seen anything more beautiful?"

Looking at her, he said softly, "Yes, I have."

For a moment, she was struck speechless. But of course he wasn't talking about her. He might not even have meant a woman. He was probably thinking of Kew Gardens in London or the Tuileries in Paris or a Pebble Beach sunset.

The tulips flowered in a burst of color—red, yellow, white, pink—all against the backdrop of the Dutch Windmill.

"Let's sit," she said. She would beg if she had to. "And just contemplate."

They found a bench amid the flowers, the perfume

of sweet, growing things filling the air. "Doesn't it make you feel serene?"

In the oddest gesture, Dane laced his fingers through hers and held her hand. Usually, it was a squeeze or a touch, but he didn't let go. "It's the perfect place for reflection."

Cammie dropped her voice to a low note. "Thank you for coming here with me."

She'd been pushy about the promotion, but he'd acquiesced with such chivalry, taking blame for never before giving her a project to manage. But how could he have known when she'd never said what she wanted?

He smiled down at her. "Fernsby damn near ordered us to go out and enjoy the day. So I say no work, no brainstorming, just enjoying. What else can we do when Fernsby lays down the law?"

Her heart fluttered at his touch, his smile, and the thought of a day just being with him. But she giggled. "He just wanted to practice baking for the show without us hanging around."

Dane laughed with her. "So true."

Once they had their fill of the sweet air, Dane stood, pulling her with him. "There's a place I'd like to go. It's maybe a mile and a half walk. But I haven't been there in years, and I'd like to see it again."

She tipped her head, having no idea what he could be talking about.

"It's called Portals of the Past. I'll tell you about it when we get there. You game?"

Lord, to be with him, she was game for anything. Thank goodness she wasn't wearing heels.

They strolled the sidewalk, few cars passing them. The more popular part of Golden Gate Park was on the other side of Nineteenth Avenue with the Japanese Tea Garden, the Academy of Sciences, and the de Young Museum. They didn't talk about the job or the resort, or even her uncle's passing.

Instead, falling into the smile on his beautiful lips, she waited for something... momentous.

Dane asked, "When you were a little girl, did you wear your hair in pigtails or braids?"

Chapter Sixteen

Cammie laughed so hard she had to put her hand over her mouth. "Neither. With my red hair…" She flicked her curls. "I would have looked like Pippi Longstocking."

He blinked. "Who's Pippi Longstocking?"

The inane conversation was delightful, even making her heart flutter. "She was the nine-year-old heroine in a series of children's books I used to read when I was a kid." Then she turned the questioning back on him. "What about you when you were a little boy?"

With a straight face, he said, "My hair wasn't long enough for pigtails or braids."

She slapped at him playfully. "I didn't mean your hair. What did you like to do?"

He held her hand as they walked, nonchalantly, almost as if he didn't notice what he was doing. But she felt the warmth of his palm and the strength in his grip. "I was all about animals. I had a pony. Later on, a horse. And if there was ever an injured animal out there, I found it." He tapped his chest as if he was proud. "And made sure I healed it. Then I released it back into the wild," he added with a flourish.

She knew he'd wanted to be a vet, that he'd been in his third year of college, with veterinary school in mind. He'd never made it.

"What was your favorite pet?"

He tipped his face skyward. "There are so many to choose from. I had a wild turkey with an injured leg. I found her when I was hiking and walked right into a flock of wild turkeys with all these chicks. Turkey chicks are called poults—and they were so damned cute." His eyes shone when he looked at her. "She was their heroine, hobbling off in the opposite direction, squawking and shrieking, trying to draw me away from the poults while the other female led them to safety. She thought I was some sort of predator, and I admired her heroism."

When he looked down at her, she could almost see the little boy in his face, the young child chasing after a turkey so he could heal her leg.

"I caught her, took her home. I thought I could fix her." His voice rose as if he still remembered his hopefulness. "But she'd been born with a deformed leg. She liked to wander around the yard, even though my parents complained—at least when they were home—about the poop on the grass."

"Did you at least clean up the poop?"

His eyes still glittering, he shook his head. "You can't just clean up turkey poop, let me tell you, especially when the whole flock joined her. Now that really drove everyone crazy. But she was great, even ate out of my hand."

"What did you name her?"

"Stumpy."

She stopped in the middle of the sidewalk. "Stumpy? That's just plain mean."

Dane's smile shone down on her, as warm as the sun on the top of her head. "She always came when I called, so she must have liked it."

"You're terrible," she complained, walking again. "What happened to her?"

He shrugged. "One day, the whole flock just moved on. I'm not sure why. Could have been a predator that drove them away."

"Did you miss her?"

"For a while." He sighed. "I hoped she'd come back. But she never did. Sometimes you just have to accept that the things you love don't always come back to you."

She thought how incredibly sad that was.

But then Dane smiled. "I figured she'd gone on to enjoy life elsewhere. That's what I hoped for all the animals and birds I rescued. That they moved on to a better life. If I didn't do that, it would have been too depressing."

She suddenly wanted to hug him. Because, really, how many men could there be who just wanted their protégés to move on to a better life?

Just like her, with the way he'd so readily agreed to give her the project and a promotion. But that was Dane.

They reached Lloyd Lake, where Dane stopped at a spot with a clear sight line across the water. With him standing behind her, his body close enough for her to feel his heat against her back, his whisper sent a sweet little quiver down her spine.

"Over there." He pointed. "See it?"

The structure reminded her of a columned doorway from Roman times, standing by itself on the other side of the lake as if it might lead to another world.

Dane murmured, "It was the front entry to railroad tycoon Alban Towne's Nob Hill mansion. It's all that was left after the 1906 earthquake. Just the entryway. It was moved here as a reminder of all that was lost that fateful day in San Francisco, when our fair city burned to the ground after the great earthquake."

She felt his heat everywhere along her skin, the timbre of his voice resonating deep inside her. She wanted to lean back, to lay her head on his shoulder and look at him. But all she could do was whisper, "It's beautiful."

"You've never seen it before?"

She shook her head, her hair brushing his cheek.

"Never heard of it." It wasn't far from the soccer field where they'd played the game that Sunday in January.

"You said the tulip garden was serene. I feel that here, like it's a peaceful place." His breath washed over her ear as he chuckled. "Except Pebble Beach, of course, when we're hiking in the woods."

On a spring weekday, just the two of them were at the lake, and the beauty and harmony enveloped them. The intimacy of his body so close and his breath in her hair shot tingles to all her erogenous zones.

"Thank you for showing me this."

"Thank you for showing me the tulips. Sometimes we forget to stop and smell the flowers."

She couldn't even laugh at the cliché. The moment was too perfect. And she nodded against him, reluctant to step away. If only they could stay this way forever.

How long they gazed at the portal she couldn't say. A path led around the lake, and they could have walked through the columns, but somehow the memorial was best seen from afar, as if you could step through into the San Francisco of the early 1900s. Getting too close would ruin the effect.

"Where to now?" he finally asked, even as she remained mesmerized by his nearness.

To his bed, she thought. It was the only place she really wanted to be.

But it was the only place she could never be. Not ever again.

"We should ride a cable car." The words almost burst from her, as if she needed the clickety-clack of a cable car and the laughter of other people to burst the bubble in which they stood.

She called another Uber. It dropped them off a couple of blocks from the cable car turnaround near Union Square so they didn't have to wait in the long line with the other tourists. And soon they swung up onto the running board of an overpacked car, Cammie's heart in her throat when she thought her foot might slip. Dane was right there, helping her grab a pole and paying the fare in exact change when the conductor came by. They went up, up, up the monumental hills of San Francisco, turned left on California and then right on Hyde, the car swaying as she held on tight. At the top of Lombard Street, the crookedest street in the world, the crush of bodies eased as many of the passengers jumped off for their turn to walk down among the blooming hydrangeas.

Dane pulled her inside, where it was still standing room only. "Unless you want to get off here and walk down Lombard."

She shook her head. He was so close behind her she didn't want to move, not even an inch. "I've done that. Let's ride all the way to Ghirardelli Square."

"Sounds good to me." His breath whispered across her hair. The cable car's jolt as it took off again pressed her against him. And somehow she just stayed there.

Even above the clank and clang of the car, she was sure she heard him breathe deeply, as though he was sniffing her hair. His heat caressed her spine, sending more tingles through her, all the way to her fingers and toes. And other parts.

It was crazy. It was unprofessional. And it was exhilarating.

★ ★ ★

Dane breathed her in as if she were a life-giving elixir. Allowing the cable car's gripman behind him plenty of room to work the manual brakes, he used it as an excuse to hold her close. And he felt her everywhere.

It was enough to make a man want unthinkable things.

With her body flush against him, he could let his imagination run wild. He could imagine hauling her high against his body until she wrapped her legs around him. Until he pressed her against the office wall. Or laid her out on his desk.

Dane knew he'd truly gone crazy when he imagined kissing her right here on the cable car. Imagined undoing her blouse and tasting her. Imagined taking a seat and pulling her down to straddle him.

Hell if he wasn't fully, temptingly aroused when they stepped off the cable car near Ghirardelli Square. How many blocks had that been from Lombard? Five, maybe. He wished the ride had been longer.

"Where to now?" His voice almost cracked.

She looked at him, her gaze dreamy. If he didn't know better, he'd think she felt the same agonizing need that he did. But of course she didn't. Cammie was always in control.

Except for that one night twelve years ago.

She grabbed his hand and pulled him, walking backward. "I want an ice cream sundae at Ghirardelli Square."

He would have given her anything she asked for.

They shared a banana split with butter pecan, cookie dough, and rocky road ice cream, lots of chocolate sauce, whipped cream, nuts, and sprinkles on top.

Who could have known that sharing a sundae would be so sexy? The cramped table forced them to sit close, the sundae between them, with only one spoon. Had he failed to ask for two spoons on purpose? He couldn't say. But they worked their way through the ice cream with him feeding her a spoonful, then taking one of his own. He was so pathetic he actually relished the lingering taste of her on the spoon.

"Good?" he asked. Hell, it was better than good. It was freaking awesome.

Her pupils were wide, as if he'd stolen her breath, as if he'd stolen a kiss.

"It's so good."

He felt her breathlessness deep inside.

Giving her the last bite, he watched her lick the

spoon clean. How he wanted to lick her just that way, wanted to feel her tremble with desire.

The way he trembled with desire at this very moment.

When they were done, he grabbed her hand. "That was dessert, but we definitely need a starter." They dodged tourists on the sidewalk down to Fisherman's Wharf, where he bought her clam chowder in a bread bowl.

"One spoon again?" she asked.

He couldn't let her know how badly he had designs on her. This day was for fun and games, but if she thought any of it was real, she might balk.

"They only gave me one. Here, take a bite." He fed her again, and she groaned at the clam chowder's creaminess. He opened the bag of oyster crackers and held it out. "You need a chaser." After pouring a few into her hand, he watched her suck them down.

His insides tensed.

He kept on feeding her, wanting her, kept on remembering that kiss on the island, remembering the golf game and that night in his condo. He was close to losing his mind. If he went on tempting himself this way, he'd lose it completely.

And he could very well lose her.

With the chowder bowl empty, they were heading to Pier 39 when she suddenly dug in her heels and pointed. "We need a balloon animal."

Her hand in his, the two of them watched as a clown sitting on a camp stool blew up balloons, twisted them into shapes, and handed them to little kids walking by.

Chuckling, Dane murmured into her sweetly fragrant hair, "You want one of those?"

When she nodded, Dane stepped up to the man. "Can you make a dachshund?"

The man rolled his eyes beneath his white face paint and oversized fake lips. Then he blew hard on the balloon, twisting, shaping, laughing, smiling. And finally, he held out a dachshund balloon on his palm.

"For a very pretty lady." He handed it to Cammie.

Her smile grew like a flower opening. "Thank you. I love it."

Without a thought, Dane tipped the man a fifty. If he'd had a hundred, he'd have given him that, too, just for the smile the clown had put on her face.

He held her hand as they wandered Pier 39, shared a shrimp cocktail, and stopped to watch the seals.

Then Cammie found it. Though it wasn't a pet shop, it sold dog toys. Her eyes shone so brightly, he could have kissed her right then.

She held out a... thing.

He looked at it for a long moment. "What is it?"

She laughed. He loved it when she laughed at him. "It's a log," she said with exaggerated slowness. "With chipmunks inside."

Her words didn't make sense. Until she shook the thing and stuffed chipmunks fell out all over the floor.

Dane couldn't help laughing as she gathered up the little creatures, stuffing them back inside.

"Rex will go wild, shaking out all the chipmunks and chasing them," she said, demonstrating, hands on both ends so nothing fell out.

He could see her playing with the dog. How she loved that dachshund. He did too. And he loved that T. Rex was theirs together.

She looked at him pointedly, her face tipped up. "Rex absolutely must have this."

Dane reached for it. "I'll get it."

She hugged the chipmunk log to her chest. "No. I'll get it."

"But this is my trip. I'll buy it."

She glowered at him. "But if you do, it's not my gift to Rex."

"It doesn't really matter who pays for it—it's from both of us."

"You don't get it."

He opened his mouth, ready to argue with her, but before he could utter another word, she slapped her hand over his lips, shutting him up.

An electric shock zipped through him. He wanted to lick her palm, wanted to grab her and lick way more than that.

But Cammie yanked back before he could get his

tongue between his lips.

Her eyes were wide, her face a grimace, as if she'd been scorched by boiling water.

And maybe she had.

Certainly, he'd been scorched.

Chapter Seventeen

Cammie could barely speak. She could barely even think. She still felt his lips on her palm. Had he licked her?

No, that was just her imagination.

Yet an electric current had rushed through her, so powerful that if she hadn't been stunned, she might have thrown herself into his arms and kissed him.

It was the only thing on earth she wanted to do.

Even twenty minutes later, when they'd made it back to the cable car turnaround near Ghirardelli Square, Cammie was still reeling from that almost... She didn't know what to call it. Not a kiss; it was just his mouth under her hand. But it was *something*. Something delicious and sexy.

Something she needed to forget.

It had been such a fabulous day. First, the meeting with the Mavericks, then mustering the courage to ask to be project manager. Then she'd been swept away by the beauty of the gardens and the park, mesmerized by the cable car ride and Dane feeding her the banana split and clam chowder, the seals, the view of the Golden Gate Bridge and Alcatraz on a sunny day.

Being with him made it sublime.

He stopped before entering the line waiting for the next cable car. "Let's do something to celebrate everything we've accomplished."

"That's what we've been doing all day."

He shook his head, looking at her as if she had no imagination. "We were playing tourist. Now we need something truly special."

"Like what?" Her heart beat faster, as if it expected something amazing.

Dane took out his phone, checking the time. Then he smiled. "It's close to dinnertime. Let's go back to the flat and ask Fernsby to make us the most delectable meal. We'll let him choose. In fact, I'll call him right now so he can start preparing. What do you think?"

It was the crowning touch to a flawless day. "That's brilliant. No restaurant chef can make anything better than Fernsby can."

Dane raised an eyebrow and made a mock choking sound in his throat. "Now that will go to his head."

Laughing, Cammie said, "He's the one who told me that." Then she looked at the cable car line. It wasn't as long as the one at Powell and Market, but they still might not make it onto the next car. "Let's walk. It's only a mile or so, right?"

Dane looked up, and up and up. Somewhere up

there was Nob Hill. "We'll certainly work up an appetite. Let's do it." Then he grinned. "Even if you are crazy."

Cammie wanted to be crazy. With him. They were both in good shape. While she'd been caring for her uncle, taking a break for a walk had kept her sanity intact. "Don't tell me you're afraid of a few hills," she scoffed.

Dane could never turn down a challenge. "You're on."

They climbed at a measured pace, never rushing, not trying to outdo each other, just taking the hills one step at a time. Just before Lombard Street, a cable car clanked down the hill, its bell ringing. Another came up filled with passengers from the turnaround. Cammie waved, and the gripman rang his bell.

The route wasn't all straight up. Sometimes they had a respite, but after all their long hikes, neither she nor Dane was breathing terribly hard when they finally reached his flat on Nob Hill. It comprised the entire top floor of one of San Francisco's beautiful old buildings that had been rebuilt right after the 1906 earthquake.

Though not the biggest in San Francisco, what the flat lacked in size it made up for in sheer beauty, everything constructed with precision. But that didn't mean it was minuscule. Dane had remodeled after purchasing it, creating three suites, one for each of them—Dane, Cammie, and, of course, Fernsby, whose rooms were next to the chef's kitchen he'd had a big hand in designing. In addition, there was a great room, dining room, guest bathroom, and an office large enough for their two desks.

Cammie had discovered the flat and supervised the remodeling and decorating. With the world's biggest Rolodex—no longer the old-fashioned mechanical kind, but an app—she'd tapped into some great resources and brilliant artisans. Since Dane always paid well, many of the workmen had willingly slipped their project in between others. Decorating appealed to her, and she'd made several suggestions for his resorts, as well as decorating all his other houses. The London townhouse and the countryside manor, however, had been perfect just the way they were, with the exception of the kitchens, which they'd modernized for Fernsby.

Beyond the massive great-room windows lay Alcatraz and the Golden Gate, Sausalito and Tiburon, the sun sparkling on the bay. Each of Dane's homes had its own unique beauty that called to her. But for a city view, nothing surpassed that of the San Francisco flat.

The patter of doggy nails on the hardwood floor signaled Rex's imminent arrival. He dashed into the room, followed by Fernsby.

"Here, you give it to Rex." Dane handed her the bag with her balloon and the chipmunks, which he'd carried all the way up the hill.

When she threw the log for the dog, she smiled at

Dane. "I told you he'd love it."

Rex pounced, shook the toy viciously, and the chipmunks flew every which way.

"Good Lord," Fernsby drawled. "What on earth is that?"

"Rex's new toy," Dane supplied.

"And just who is going to clean up the mess, sir?" Fernsby asked as Rex tore into a chipmunk and sent its stuffing flying.

"Well, that didn't last long," Dane noted.

Cammie huffed at them both. "He's got nine more chipmunks."

Fernsby merely blinked, slowly, with great meaning, which could have been either, *That's nine more chipmunk innards I'll have to clean up* or *It's your mess, you clean it up*. Then he said in the driest of voices, "As instructed, I've prepared a celebratory feast for you. You'll find it up on the terrace, where you can enjoy the sunset."

She couldn't wait to see what he'd come up with.

★ ★ ★

Cammie gasped as she stepped out on the rooftop terrace.

The sound hit Dane like her hand over his mouth had in the store. And he wanted to lick her.

He had no choice, of course, but to maintain control.

She laughed, a beautiful musical sound that wrapped around him.

Yeah, he really should have licked her.

He thought the gorgeous sunset through the glass had grabbed her attention. Then Dane saw it—a hot tub where no tub had been before. With a soaker tub in his suite, he'd never felt the need for a hot tub.

But suddenly, Fernsby had created a need. Dane wanted nothing more than to lounge in that tub with Cammie.

Two tables sat on either side, each filled with goodies, from bruschetta to shrimp rolls, seafood mushroom caps to pâté-stuffed phyllo kisses, antipasto skewers to crab cakes with mango relish. Fairy lights strung around the terrace winked on, illuminating the sparkling bottle already chilling in the champagne bucket, two glasses beside it.

Fernsby stood impassively by the terrace door as if he didn't even recognize the impressiveness of what he'd done.

Dane gestured at the hot tub. "Did you forklift this thing up here?"

In a voice as cool as his features, Fernsby said, "You needn't worry yourself about how I did it, sir. Just enjoy the fact that I was able to."

He'd even laid out their swimsuits on a lounge chair, two rolled towels beside them.

Cammie put her hands on her hips. "That's why

you didn't want to drive back to Pebble Beach. And why you wanted us out of the way today."

Was that a flicker of humor in Fernsby's eyes? Of course not. Fernsby was the antonym of humor.

"Let me just say, sir," Fernsby intoned like the talking head on a news program, "I've watched you two work yourselves silly, and I've concocted some special treats for you." Fernsby had obviously been working on this long before Dane called him. "Now enjoy the sunset, sir, drink the champagne, eat those scrumptious hors d'oeuvres over which I slaved all afternoon, and enjoy that hot tub. I'll take care of the dog." He gathered Rex under his arm, the little dog covered in chipmunk fluff, and marched through the terrace door, closing it behind him and leaving Dane alone on the roof with Cammie.

"Only Fernsby could get a hot tub up here." Cammie inhaled deeply, exhaling with wonder.

Dane was still shaking his head. "I could drag him back here to tell me how he did it."

Cammie pressed her lips together. "He'll never tell." Then she smiled. "And it's more fun if we don't know."

Then she grabbed her suit off the lounge chair. "I'll just put this on while you pop the cork." She gave him a cheeky grin. "I want to sit in that tub and watch the sunset with champagne in my hand and one of Fernsby's treats in my mouth."

Of course that made him look at her mouth. And one glance made him think of all the things he'd like to do with that beautiful mouth.

But she was already out of reach.

Dane stripped down right there on the deck. Unless a plane flew overhead, no one would see him. He pulled his trunks on, then pushed the button to retract the glass roof, opening the hot tub to the sky and the stars that would soon pop out. Then he did exactly as she'd told him, pouring champagne, adding three raspberries to each flute from the small bowl Fernsby had left.

She stole his breath when she returned in a slim black one-piece that hugged her stunning curves, a keyhole gold buckle between her breasts and a plunging back that revealed every beautiful inch of skin right down to the base of her spine.

He drooled, wanting to kiss her right there in that keyhole.

Instead, he handed her a glass of champagne. After thanking him, she climbed into the two-person tub. Priceless. They'd have to sit facing each other, their bodies almost touching. Leaning over the side, she grabbed one of Fernsby's shrimp puffs and popped it in her mouth, closed her eyes, and savored the delicacy, damn near moaning over it.

The sounds she made could drive a man crazy.

Opening her eyes, she looked at him without a single clue as to what she'd just done to him.

He had to sink beneath the water before she noticed.

"That sunset is amazing." With the hot tub positioned so they could both see the view over the bay— Fernsby thought of everything—Cammie pointed with her glass out the terrace windows, where the sun streaked stunning colors across the sky.

"Gorgeous." But he was looking at her.

With a satisfied sigh, she smiled. "I'm addicted to Fernsby's treats." She patted her stomach. "At some point, I'm going to have to back off, or my figure will soon be dealing with the consequences."

What the hell was she talking about? Without thinking, he blurted, "Are you kidding? You have the most perfect body I've ever seen."

Her beautiful jade eyes went wide. "Really?" Then she blushed. "Thank you. That's really nice of you to say." She paused two seconds, as if she actually had to think about what she was saying, and whispered, "Right back at ya." Then she sank into the water up to her chin as if afraid of her own words.

He hadn't meant to say it. It was one thing to compliment a woman on a new dress or a different hairstyle, but you simply couldn't talk about your employee's body. Not ever. You weren't even supposed to *look*. Of course, he'd been looking for years; he couldn't help himself. But he'd never let her catch him at it.

And what he'd really wanted to say was that she had the hottest body ever. Twelve years ago, she'd made him breathless, made him drool, made him hard. He'd delighted in every facet of this beautiful woman. But now, at thirty-four, she was even more striking than the day he'd met her. Because now he *knew* her—the sharpness of her mind, the sweetness of her character, the beauty of her soul.

Holding her glass above the bubbling water, she said, "You know how it is when you're over thirty and everything starts to sag, and you go, wow, I'm getting older?"

"Are you crazy? You're even more perfect than the day I met you."

Suddenly, as though she couldn't take another compliment without shrieking and jumping out of the tub, she changed the conversation entirely. "I can't believe Fernsby actually found a two-seater tub."

The tub was exactly right, but he said, "It had to be a two-seater. How else could he have hoisted it up here?"

Their body heat ratcheted up the water temperature. Their legs touched briefly, his thigh to her calf. He wanted to run his hand all the way up. But she jerked away as though he'd burned her. Maybe he had. He was certainly on fire.

Instead of sipping her champagne, she gulped it.

Then she leaned over for a phyllo kiss, giving him a view of her swimsuit's plunging back.

Matching her move for move, he stretched for a mushroom cap. And that brought him in contact with her leg again, her warm, fragrant skin skimming his.

He could have laughed at himself, getting intensely worked up over her leg. But she had beautiful legs, her calves toned from all the hiking, her muscles lean. His lusty thoughts almost made him choke on Fernsby's scrumptious mushroom.

He was glad for the jets stirring the water so she couldn't see him beneath the surface. She'd probably jump out in shock.

As if she needed to keep things on an even keel—and they might have been getting out of hand—she said, "I've always appreciated the work you've done. But this resort we're putting together, it will help so many in the future. Special children who are really in need, as well as their parents and caregivers. I've never been more proud of you than I am right now."

He gazed at her steadily, letting his eyes roam her striking features, her lush lips, her silky red-gold hair pulled into a knot on top of her head. "You took the words right out of my mouth. Only you could put all your heart and soul into managing this project."

Cammie put her heart and soul into everything she did, from decorating his homes, to running his life, to caring for her uncle. He'd already proven he was a mess without her.

She was everything, and he was pretty damn sure she didn't even know it.

Before he could think how ill-advised it might be, he leaned forward to wrap his hand around her nape. Then slowly, giving her every chance to stop him, he pulled her close. The island kiss had been spectacular but brief. This kiss was openmouthed, sweet with champagne and raspberries and her. Their tongues played hide-and-seek, and their bodies drifted together. He kissed her until their breaths became one, until their heartbeats raced at the same pace.

She put her hands on his shoulders and floated over him as he leaned back against the tub, their bodies caressing, their skin hot. He took her mouth as if he'd been starved for her. With a teasing bite on her lip, he drew her in, delving deep, his tongue sliding along hers. She came down on him, parting her legs, straddling him until he felt her everywhere. If he'd thought he'd known heaven before, he'd been wrong. Because *this* was heaven.

This was what he'd dreamed of night after night, knowing she was just down the hall. Knowing she was off-limits. Until this moment. When she was everything he could ever want in his arms.

Her skin was like satin, her taste like the finest champagne, her thighs taut and inviting. Sliding his hands down her sides, he wanted nothing more than to tear off the sexy swimsuit. Tracing his fingers across her back, he held her closer, closer as he slipped his fingers down to the base of her spine, touching her there, feeling her quiver against him, her legs tightening around him.

She pulled away to whisper against his lips, "Rules."

Putting a hand to the back of her head, he murmured, "What rules?"

He wanted to break every single one. Now. Wanted to feast on her skin, her breasts, every part of her.

Her voice tantalized him. "We're being so naughty."

The word made him crazy. "Say that again. It's so damned sexy and hot."

She whispered, "Naughty."

He might have exploded right then. He might have pushed her up on the side of the tub and tasted her. He might have done every single naughty, rule-breaking thing he'd thought of for so long. Everything he'd denied himself.

But her phone rang.

At first, he thought it had to be a dream. No, a nightmare.

But the phone kept ringing.

Then she pushed away from him, her eyes wide, perhaps even frightened. "It's Clyde."

"We've been waiting over a week to hear from

him." They'd called Clyde first, even before presenting to the Mavericks.

Her voice grew tremulous. "What if he needs help?"

Dane's worry ratcheted up, just as Cammie's did. He truly liked the old man. "You'd better get it."

Yet he mourned the loss of this moment between them. There might never be another.

Chapter Eighteen

What was going on with Clyde?

Cammie didn't have time to think about what she and Dane had been doing in the hot tub. Not now. Because that was Clyde's special ringtone. His butler, Digbert, usually made any calls, then transferred after she answered. But Clyde himself was calling. Something had to be wrong.

After climbing out of the tub, she dripped water across the deck as she ran for her phone on the lounge chair. Even after twelve years, she was still close to the old man. She flew out to see him every six months or so. He was like another uncle. And she was a surrogate daughter, since he'd never had kids. They often talked on the phone, but never this late, considering the three-hour time difference. He should have been in bed by now. Worry churned her stomach.

"Clyde?" She heard the anxiety in her own voice. "How are you doing? Is everything okay?"

"Of course it is, dear." He harrumphed with irritation. "Everything's fine. I'm going to live forever. Do you think I'm an old man?" His British accent hadn't faded, though he'd left the UK years ago.

"No, no, no. I never think of you that way."

Dane climbed out of the water, sleek and beautiful, grabbing the two towels and wrapping one around his waist, hiding every inch of beautiful skin.

She sagged onto the lounge chair, still dizzy with worry even as it waned, and mouthed to Dane, *He's okay.*

Dane draped the towel over her shoulders. She'd grown cold in just a minute or two.

Only now could she think about what almost happened in that tub. How amazing his taste was after all these years, the feel of his skin against hers, his hands on her, his lips taking hers. It was as if they'd time-traveled back to that night in his condo on the golf course.

She would have done anything with him in that hot tub. She *had* done everything with him all those years ago.

But Clyde was talking. She had to pretend that everything was perfectly normal, and she hadn't been sitting on Dane's lap only moments before, the hard feel of him between her legs.

"I'm sorry it took me so long to get back to you about your new project," Clyde said.

She and Dane had briefed him, letting him know they were looking for sponsors as well as donations.

"It's only been a week. We didn't expect you to have an immediate answer." She looked at Dane as he sat down next to her on the lounge chair. "Dane's right here. Let me put you on speaker."

"I told you I'd get back to you after I'd thought it over. And I've concluded it's a brilliant project, and I absolutely need to be a part of it." Relief flooded her. Clyde was in. That was a huge boon, since he had an enormous pool of contacts.

"Thank you, Clyde. We're so glad."

"I've been making calls," he went on. "And I haven't heard a single no yet."

"That's amazing news."

She glanced at Dane, whose smile beamed across his entire face. "As always, Clyde, you're a powerhouse. Thank you."

"I take it you're close to breaking ground for the resort?"

Dane jutted his chin at her, indicating that it was her project and her answer to give.

"We're looking for just the right property." Or she would be, as soon as they got back to Pebble Beach.

"Brilliant. I have yeses to the tune of two hundred million already."

Cammie gasped. That was her lowball figure just to start. "Clyde, you are the absolute best."

"I know," he said without an inflection of either humor or humility. "But I do miss seeing you. I hope you can come out soon."

Guilt hit her that she and Dane had just been in the Caribbean, and she hadn't even flown over to see Clyde. She hadn't seen him since the summer, before she'd taken the leave of absence. Of course, Clyde had understood, since they'd talked extensively about her uncle's condition. But she still hadn't arranged to see him.

The worst was that she didn't know when she could get out there again now that she was running the new project.

Dane came to her rescue. "We're going to come see you, Clyde, don't you worry. If you can let us nail down the property and get things rolling, we'll be out for a visit."

Clyde gave a guttural laugh. "Good. I see I'm guilting you into a trip." Then he added more seriously, "I know you're both busy. Just know you have a standing invitation."

"Thanks for understanding, Clyde. We appreciate it," Dane told him.

Cammie's guilt eased slightly. Clyde claimed he would live forever, but she knew time would catch up to him. She vowed to make it out to see him as soon as they had a property secured.

After they'd said their goodbyes and she'd pushed the End button, Dane touched her arm. "You don't need to feel guilty."

"We were just in the Caribbean, and I didn't even think," she berated herself.

"Neither did I. But we had other things on our minds."

Oh yes, she had. That kiss.

"We'll see him in a very short while, like I said. Let's just get a site deal going." He squeezed her hand, his touch reminding her of everything they'd done in the hot tub.

And she couldn't help an irreverent thought. Clyde really was the best, and she was so happy he'd called, but did he have to call *right* at that moment? Couldn't he have called two hours earlier? Yes, there were all the rules they shouldn't break, rules that kept them safe for twelve years, just like she'd told Dane on the island.

But oh, how badly she'd wanted to get naughty with him. In those few sexy, amazing moments in the hot tub, she hadn't cared about the consequences. It was obvious Dane wanted the same thing.

Just as she'd felt when she watched him at the barbecue, with the children and the babies, she wanted *everything*.

Even if she knew how terribly wrong it could all go.

Maybe the person she really had to fight wasn't Dane, but herself.

Of course she didn't want her heart broken. She couldn't let their relationship change when it wouldn't be for the better. As much as she wanted that dream of love and family, she couldn't trust that she'd get it. She couldn't ruin everything they already had.

Even as badly as she wanted him.

★ ★ ★

Clyde was bringing them two hundred million for the resort. Dane couldn't shake that off. But couldn't the news have waited until tomorrow? Couldn't the Fates let them have tonight?

They would have broken all the rules. And he would have convinced her there was no reason to leave him because of it.

Cammie stuffed her arms into the robe, courtesy of Fernsby, that Dane held out for her and belted it tightly, letting the towel fall to the decking.

He pulled on his own robe. The champagne sat forgotten by the hot tub, the bubbles gone flat. Just the way he felt.

But he couldn't let what happened in the hot tub pass. Everything he wanted had bubbled over. He'd let loose. He couldn't rein any of it in again.

"We need to talk," he said with an authority he hoped she'd listen to.

She forestalled anything else he might have said, rushing her words. "What just happened in the hot tub shouldn't have happened. We both know it would have been a mistake."

"It's not a mistake," he insisted, even if he feared it was. Without the rules, and despite the new project, she still might decide it was time to hit the road. Especially now that Lochlan was no longer holding her here.

She shook her head, wet tendrils of hair escaping her topknot and sticking to her cheeks. "Twelve years ago, we were right to make rules. We're just going to have to get a handle on this. No more hot tubs."

"What about golf games? I seem to remember a kiss during a golf game too."

He was baiting her, he admitted it. But he wanted something more from her than a flat no.

Her nostrils flared and her lips thinned, as if there were so many thoughts whizzing around in her head that she didn't know what to do with them. "Maybe we shouldn't play golf either."

Now, that was going too far.

"No," he said, his voice emphatic. "I remember how good it was the first time. And I still want you now." He didn't talk about feelings. Feelings could scare her off. But the chemistry between them was undeniable.

She stepped back, putting physical distance between them as well as emotional. "We've always agreed that was a mistake. And we're not going to make another."

He wanted to grab her shoulders, get right down in

her face and say, *Screw that.* After that kiss on the island, that sweet, sexy kiss that could have become so much more, even then he'd agreed about the rules. But no longer. Not after he'd felt how much she wanted him in that hot tub. Not after how badly he wanted her. Had always wanted her.

And now he was torn between losing her and wanting her.

His desire for her won.

"No," he said, claiming the step she'd put between them, her scent ratcheting up his emotions, his need. "I won't pretend it didn't happen. I won't say it was a mistake. On the contrary, that night was the best damned thing I've ever known. And I don't know why the hell we've had to wait twelve long years to do it again."

She stared at him for a long, agonizing moment while his guts twisted into a tight coil. That day at the barbecue, when he'd held her in his arms, he'd known then how much he wanted her, yet he'd still been pretending that all he could do was offer her comfort.

But he had so much more to give her. So he whispered, "I can make you feel so good."

That's when she ran.

★ ★ ★

Turning so fast on the deck she almost slipped, she felt him reaching out. If he touched her, she was a goner.

That day at Sebastian's, when Dane had wrapped his arms around her and held her close to his heart, she'd wanted to kiss him. But her desire for him had been a force inside her for so much longer than that. She'd wanted another night like the first. Dreamed about it.

But that was just fantasy.

And suddenly, because he didn't care about the ramifications, Dane wanted to change their status quo. *I know how this will go down. You can want something so badly you ache with need, but when you finally get it, it never works out the way you want.*

He wanted to give her pleasure, to have sex with her, and yes, it would be out of this world. But then what would happen when she wanted more than pleasure?

She tried so hard not to slam the door of her bedroom, but once inside, she couldn't help herself. She locked it. Because Dane wanted to talk. And talking would lead to so much more. Because she simply didn't have the willpower to resist him—and, worse, to resist herself.

She slid down the locked door until her butt hit the floor.

He wanted her. He couldn't know what those words did to her, how much she wanted to throw herself at him and say, *Yes, yes, yes, I want it all.*

But he hadn't said he loved her. He hadn't even

said he wanted a relationship. He'd said nothing of marriage, home, babies—all the things she'd realized she wanted desperately that day as she'd watched him with Savannah and Keegan, with Jorge and Noah.

It was so easy for a man to want a woman, but wanting didn't mean a relationship and love. How many women had Dane drifted through? He dated for a few weeks, sometimes even a couple of months, then moved on. He wasn't callous; he didn't *want* to hurt anyone. She was sure he was upfront that he didn't want a serious relationship. She was pretty sure he'd never been in love, not even before she'd met him.

She'd thought she was in love twice, yet in the end, both men hadn't felt the same. She couldn't make another bad decision, especially not with Dane. He was her livelihood. Even more, he was her best friend. Now that her uncle was gone, he was the closest person in the world to her.

Climbing into his bed would ruin everything because she wouldn't accept anything less than love the next time around. And if she put her heart on the line, he could crush her with only a few agonizing words.

She could never tell him how she felt. She could never ask for what she wanted. She couldn't even ask him what he was offering. Because if she asked for specifics, he would tell her he wanted a hot and heavy sexual relationship.

And that would absolutely kill her.

★ ★ ★

Dane followed her to her room, only to hear the lock click on her bedroom door. As if she were afraid of him.

All he wanted to do was make her feel good. He wanted to hold her in his arms, wake up beside her in the morning, open his eyes and see her face next to his.

But she'd run from him. Just the way he'd feared.

Maybe he'd jumped into the conversation too quickly. Tomorrow might have made more sense, when they'd both calmed down, and she'd had a chance to think about what she really wanted.

He could only hope it was him.

He dumped the robe in his room and pulled on sweats, then wandered along to the kitchen. He should tell Fernsby they hadn't eaten all the food. Fernsby could pack it up. Or eat it himself.

He stared at the door to Fernsby's suite just off the kitchen, exactly where the man had designated it should be. With a sitting room, bedroom, and bathroom, the suite also acted as an office, where Fernsby could sit at his desk to take care of the household accounts. Dane trusted him implicitly.

Fernsby had been with him for close to fifteen years, since the first resort. They knew each other's character, each other's foibles. But they never really talked on a personal level. He knew little about the man's past. And he would never ask Fernsby for details. A man had to *offer* his past, and once given, it couldn't be taken for granted.

If Dane had ever gone to Fernsby about any of the women he'd dated, Fernsby would have looked down his nose and sternly said, *I'm your butler, sir, not your therapist.*

But these were desperate times. As much as his brothers and sisters were his best friends, as much as they were a team—not just in soccer but in life—he couldn't talk to any of them about this. If he'd been at a Maverick barbecue, he might have turned to Susan Spencer, but he couldn't wait even a week for the next one.

Before he could talk himself out of it, he knocked on Fernsby's door.

The man opened it still wearing his bespoke suit, even at this late hour. His face remained expressionless, though the number of times Dane had knocked on his door could be counted on one hand.

Dane finally spoke. "I need help."

Fernsby stepped back and waved his hand expansively, entreating Dane to enter. "Tell me what I can do, sir. And I will do it."

Yet Dane could almost feel Fernsby rolling his eyes. Except that rolling his eyes was beneath him.

So he said it. Because Fernsby was the only one who knew Cammie almost as well as Dane did. "I need advice." He breathed in. Then practically spat out the words as he exhaled. "Cammie and I shared a kiss on the island."

Was that a twinkle in Fernsby's eyes? He had to be mistaken. Fernsby absolutely did not twinkle.

Dane admitted the whole truth. "Then we kissed in the hot tub." Damn, this was humiliating. But Cammie was worth any humiliation. "Actually, it was far more than a kiss. It was romantic—the stars overhead, the bubbling water, the champagne, the feast you pre-pared."

Shockingly, he swore that Fernsby's eyes *did* twin-kle.

Suddenly, he got it. "Damn it, you were setting us up." He pointed at Fernsby. "In fact, you've been trying to set us up for twelve years, haven't you?" He threw his hands in the air, circled the room, and came back to Fernsby once more. "I can't believe I didn't see it."

If ever there was a poker face, Fernsby wore it now. "I can neither confirm nor deny, sir."

He didn't need to admit it. That twinkle Dane had never seen before confirmed it all.

But now Dane had Fernsby right where he wanted him. "You need to help me. Because I'm afraid I'm going to screw up the best thing that's ever happened to me." He added, more emphatically, "I absolutely can't screw this up."

Fernsby, never one to swear, muttered, "Crikey," in an East End accent Dane had never heard before. "I'm afraid you're already screwing this up, sir," he added with a completely straight face, as if he hadn't just insulted his boss.

Although Dane sometimes wondered who was the boss and who was the employee, since Fernsby usually did whatever he wanted.

"Thank you very much, Fernsby," he said dryly, almost as dryly as Fernsby would say it himself. "I'm well aware that my romantic skills are rather lacking."

"Lacking?" Fernsby croaked, one eyebrow raised. "Shall we say *nonexistent*, sir?"

Dane harrumphed like Fernsby often did himself. "I'll admit I haven't had many examples." His parents certainly hadn't taught him anything about love, except to make him realize he wasn't going to get it and should certainly stop expecting it.

"Shall we say no *good* examples?" Fernsby belatedly added, "Sir."

"True," Dane had to concede. "I'm not sure I know how to romance a woman. Especially not Cammie." The women he'd dated hadn't required romance. And he wasn't sure he could give Cammie the romance she deserved. "There're her emotions to worry about." He absolutely didn't want to hurt her. "I'm not equipped with the proper skills." And he did not mean sexually.

Fernsby, once again the staunch and proper butler,

said in his highly cultured British voice, "I'm very glad you came to me, sir. I will help you." That stretching of his lips couldn't possibly be a smile. "This is the task I've waited years to perform." He held up a hand. "Leave it to me, sir. I know exactly what to do." He narrowed his eyes. "You just need to say yes to anything I propose."

Fernsby might do anything he wanted to do, but he'd never before ordered Dane to do his bidding. This, however, was a special case.

Dane said, "On any other subject, I'd tell you to go pound sand. But this is about Cammie. If you think you can find a way to make her mine, I'll do whatever you suggest."

★ ★ ★

Fernsby closed the door. Then he did a little jig. He never jigged in front of anyone. But this deserved two jigs.

He was quite aware that Dane hadn't said he was in love with Cammie. But Fernsby had known the man's feelings for years. How those two hadn't figured it out themselves was beyond him.

Yet Fernsby well knew that Dane hadn't mentioned *love*, using the euphemism of *romance* instead, because he was afraid of it. Because he didn't believe he possessed the skills to love Camille the way she deserved. After learning how his parents had abandoned their children to a series of nannies and flown off to God only knew where, Fernsby had realized long ago that *none* of the Harringtons had a clue about love or how to be good examples of it.

Thus, Dane had always held himself aloof from love. After fifteen years, Fernsby knew it all. There wasn't a single time Dane had left for an evening out with a female companion that he hadn't claimed the date was no big deal. It wasn't only because of Camille either. Dane Harrington was afraid to open himself up to love. Afraid it wouldn't be reciprocated.

It was Fernsby's job to show his employer that he needn't be frightened of love, especially when it came to Camille.

He rubbed his hands together with glee. Because what he'd told Dane was the absolute truth. This was the job he'd been waiting for all his life.

And he never failed.

Well, perhaps once.

But he certainly wouldn't this time.

Chapter Nineteen

Seated at his desk in Pebble Beach only two days later while Cammie was out for a walk with Rex, Dane beckoned Fernsby in when he knocked on the door-jamb. "What can I do for you, Fernsby?"

Impassive as always, Fernsby said, "It's not what you can do for me, sir, but what I can do for you."

He paused for effect, forcing Dane to ask, "And what is that?"

"I've heard back from *Britain's Greatest Bakers*, and I've made it through the first round." Fernsby seemed neither elated nor downcast. As always, he showed no emotion at all.

Dane wanted to clap, but instead he merely said, "Congratulations, Fernsby."

"Thank you, sir." His butler went on, "They need to see how I appear on camera, so they've asked to interview me."

Dane wasn't sure how this was something Fernsby could do for him. Rather, it was the other way around. "So you need a couple of days off?"

Fernsby stared him down for a very long moment, then drawled, "They want to see me in England, sir. And Bradford Park is only a ten-mile drive from the site of this season's competition. Therefore, I respectfully request that we spend a few days there for my interviews and screen tests."

"Of course." Dane waved his hand, giving imperious permission. "Stay at the manor house. Take whatever time you need. I know how important this is to you. But I'm not sure why I need to go along." He tipped his head slightly in question.

Fernsby let out a long-suffering sigh. "Sir, I require that you and Camille travel with me. I'm going to be doing interviews, a lot of them. I'll be talking with producers." He widened his eyes fractionally. "In fact, I'll rarely be at the house." He allowed a very pregnant pause.

Until Dane saw the light and lowered his voice, even though Cammie wasn't home. "This is part of the plan to help me with Cammie, isn't it? But I'm still not getting how the manor house will help."

Fernsby squeezed his eyes shut and pinched the bridge of his nose. "Did I not say, sir, that I will rarely be at Bradford Park?" He waited for Dane's lightbulb to actually turn on.

Dane should have gotten it the moment Fernsby had said he wanted both Dane and Cammie to fly to England. It was just that this was so unlike his staid butler. But he'd asked for help, and Fernsby was throwing him the bone he needed. Plus, Cammie loved the manor, loved the long walks, loved to tease him about his title, Lord Fuzzybottom or Lord Bumstead, or any of the silly names she made up.

"Fernsby, you're a genius. A few days at the manor will be perfect."

Fernsby winked, startling Dane still further. "I'm leaving it up to you, sir, to do the rest. I know you can. Because when you set your mind to something, especially if it's your heart's desire, you always make it happen. And I do believe Camille is your heart's desire."

Dane couldn't say why the words shocked him more than Fernsby's wink. Heart's desire? It was such a powerful image. He desired Cammie, had since the day he'd first seen her on the golf course.

Cammie was always the one to make sure he added heart to his projects. As though he had no heart at all. Yet his heart always beat faster when she was around. His mind and body craved more. And yes, his heart did as well. So much more.

Which was actually quite terrifying.

What if he laid everything before her—and it scared her off?

And yet… he couldn't go on with her only as his assistant. Or his project manager. Not even as his best friend. He wanted her. His heart wanted her.

Even as Dane reeled inside, Fernsby said, "Have no fear, sir. Everything you need will be at your fingertips. Because I've been planning this moment for twelve very long years." He stared down his long nose at Dane. "And trust me when I say, I've already prepared for the things you don't even know you're going to want or need."

But had he prepared Dane for his heart's desire?

Dane could only hope he had and that he showed not an ounce of his trepidation. "Why do you think I've kept you around for so long? You always know what I need before I know I need it."

Fernsby's expression was suddenly as satisfied as a cat who'd just wheedled a handful of treats when it wasn't even dinnertime. "I have faith in you, sir." As the man disappeared around the doorjamb, his voice floated back to Dane. "Get 'er done, sir," he added like a rodeo star.

Dane wondered if a paranormal entity had taken over Fernsby's body.

When Cammie bounded into the room only a short time later, still wearing her hiking clothes, she flashed him a grin. "What's up with Fernsby?"

He told her the partial truth. "He's made it past the baking show's first round. Now they want to do interviews and screen tests. I'm afraid we need to go to Bradford Park. The show will be filming only a few miles away, and he needs our moral support."

Cammie clapped her hands. "This is so exciting." Her eyes were bright as she bounced on the balls of her feet. "I *knew* they'd pick him. He'll totally ace any interviews and screen tests. And then he's going to win."

"Since he is the quintessential British butler, they'll love him."

But he couldn't forget everything else Fernsby had said. *His heart's desire.*

She was beautiful and smart. She was dedicated and kindhearted. She was loyal. She was his best friend. He'd never known a more caring woman in his life.

He felt the phantom touch of her fingers on his cheek, the imagined sweetness of her kiss on his lips. Now that he'd tasted her again and felt the thrum of her body against his, there was no way he could go back.

He had to have her as more than his project manager, more even than his best friend. But how to tell her? He couldn't ask Fernsby for the right words. That was too much. He'd just have to tell her the unvarnished truth, that he wanted her, that he cared about her, that they'd be good together, that they could make a relationship work. No over-the-top declarations like he'd die if he didn't make her his. Nothing that would send her running straight back to the airport.

He'd tone everything down, tread lightly. Be calm, cool, and collected. Yeah.

Even if he felt like he'd go stark raving mad if he didn't make her his right this moment.

★ ★ ★

He'd gotten them to Bradford Park. Fernsby felt like doing another jig. Of course he wouldn't, not with his patron and the lovely Camille standing before him.

"I will leave you both now," he said formally. "I must go forth and battle for top dog over that person who shall remain unnamed." Digbert might be butler for the inestimable Mr. Westerbourne, but Fernsby would still wipe the kitchen floor with him.

She knew exactly of whom he spoke as a battle light glowed in Camille's eyes. "I can't believe *he* made it into this round too. You're going to trounce him."

She was a feisty one, always ready to go to war for the ones she loved.

Fernsby drawled in his most unaffected voice, "Rest assured, Camille, I've got him. You can count on that." He stretched his lips as if they might want to smile.

"Digbert is going down," she said, pounding her fist into her palm. Then her eyes widened, and she put a hand over her mouth. "Oops. I said the unmentionable name."

Fernsby nodded his forgiveness. He was sure the only reason his nemesis, Clyde Westerbourne's ignominious butler, had entered the contest was because he knew how badly Fernsby wanted to win. Digbert was that kind of dastardly villain.

Dane appeared to stifle a laugh. "He certainly doesn't bake as well as you do."

Fernsby almost snorted, refraining only at the last moment. "That's never been a question."

"And you're much more congenial than he is," Camille added.

Fernsby was well aware he didn't have a congenial bone in his body. That was part of his charm. "Have no fear, dear lady, I will win." He would fight to his dying breath to make sure Digbert didn't best him.

But there was so much more on the line than Digbert, more even than winning a baking contest. There was Camille and Dane's happiness. He had it all set up—the best champagne, the most delicious food, all Dane's and Camille's favorites, and beautiful flowers gracing the table. He'd turned the house into a romantic getaway for two.

Dane wanted this despite any fears he might have. Sadly, they were two people who couldn't see what was right in front of their faces, let alone written in the stars. So this was up to Fernsby. And with the romantic stage he'd set, they would have to succumb.

He knew it in his gut just as strongly as he knew Digbert hadn't a prayer of beating him.

Getting these two together was truly his life's work.

Suitcase in hand, he stood in the flagstone entrance hall and said severely, "Please don't forget to feed the dog while I'm gone." Then he left them to it.

He was right that Dane and Camille were meant to be. Because he was Fernsby. And he was right about everything.

★ ★ ★

Cammie wasn't tired, since she'd slept well during the flight. But she was starving after the drive to the manor. "Fernsby said he left food. What do you think it is?"

"Let's check out the dining room." Dane held out his hand. "Shall I escort you, my dear?" he asked in a fair imitation of Fernsby.

As her stomach rumbled, she couldn't resist. Especially when Dane laughed. His laughter was like sweet wine in her blood.

Champagne chilled in a silver bucket, and flowers bloomed in a magnificent centerpiece. The sideboard was laid with an array of delicacies—tender slices of roast beef and Yorkshire pudding with gravy, roasted vegetables and perfectly crisped potatoes. And, of course, there was an English trifle for dessert, topped with a mountain of whipped cream.

"Oh my God, my favorite," she gasped. "I missed the roast beef and Yorkshire pudding at the signing party, and I haven't had it since last year. How did he do all this?" Awe dripped from her voice. "He was on the plane with us the whole time."

Dane was already popping the champagne cork and expertly pouring two flutes. "He must have made calls with very explicit instructions on exactly what he wanted and how it was to be prepared."

Handing her a glass, he raised his own in a toast. "To us."

It hit her then. "This smacks of romance." She put a hand on her hip. "Did you put Fernsby up to this, Lord Badboy?"

He smiled. "I may resemble that."

She spoke in her sternest voice, though she would never be able to emulate Fernsby properly. "We talked about this in San Francisco. We have our rules."

"I heard all your reasons why we still need the rules." Dane raised an eyebrow. "But I've changed my mind."

This was bad, really bad. He could make her lower all her defenses. And then her heart could very well be crushed. "But you can't change your mind. All my reasons are still valid."

He pulled out her chair, then snugged her closer to the table when she sat.

If her stomach hadn't rumbled again, she might have jumped right back up and run out of the room.

"Are they?" he asked softly. Then he took her plate and began to fill it at the sideboard. "Let's put that to the test."

She was terrified to ask how.

He gave her a bit of everything she most desired—slices of rare roast beef, a gravy-laden Yorkshire, vegetables, and mouthwatering roast potatoes. As he set the plate in front of her, she couldn't help breathing in the heavenly aromas, somehow breathing in his scent as well.

He plated roast beef and Yorkshire pudding for himself, and the moment he sat, she dove into hers, because, honestly, she couldn't wait.

"You're totally right. This is a very romantic setting." He waved a hand over the table. "Delectable food, good champagne, beautiful flowers. We're all alone." He smiled roguishly. "I just made my move. But I'm not going to haul you close and kiss you again."

She couldn't help but wish he would.

He held her gaze like a hypnotist, stealing her ability to look away. "And since I already know we're meant to be together…" He raised his glass. "The next move is yours."

If this was a contest, she couldn't let Dane win. Her heart was at stake. "My move isn't coming. I won't give up the perfect relationship we've had all this time for a romance that will potentially fail and ruin everything."

There. She'd said it. Even as her heart cried out

with how badly she wanted what he offered, she couldn't go through another heartache. Especially not a heartache over Dane.

He calmly cut into his tender beef, chewed, swallowed, his eyes on her the entire time. Until finally, he said, "I'm not willing to risk failure either. But since I know we won't fail, I also know there's no risk." He speared a forkful of Yorkshire pudding dripping with gravy. "I have feelings for you, feelings that haven't gone away for twelve years. I know we need to be together. And I know we can make a relationship work."

He wasn't talking about *just* sex. They knew each other too well for it to be only about sex. Of course he had feelings. But he hadn't said *love*. Instead, he'd used the word *relationship*. But a relationship could mean so many things. *Feelings* and *relationship* didn't necessarily add up to love. It certainly didn't mean marriage. It couldn't even be called permanent.

Besides, they already had a relationship that worked.

She could sleep with the billionaire. She could revel in his attention. But it would all come tumbling down eventually. It was the age-old story of the secretary having a fling with her boss. And who ended up out in the cold? Always the secretary.

Dane had made this switch so fast, after only a couple of sexy, heated kisses in a hot tub. He wasn't a bad man; he was full of integrity. But when Dane Harrington wanted something, he went for it. And when the initial drive was satisfied, he moved on to the next project. She didn't want to be the next project he left behind.

She didn't want a broken heart.

She didn't want to lose the only thing that had any meaning in her life—her relationship with Dane, just the way it was. No changes, no deviations. It was better to keep the beautiful thing she knew rather than risk everything on a fleeting affair, no matter how dazzling, that couldn't last.

Chapter Twenty

Since I already know we're meant to be together, the next move is yours.

Dane waited for her to say yes. But everything she felt was written in the strained lines of her lovely face. She didn't believe a relationship with him could work.

He wasn't even sure himself. Could anyone be sure? Until he'd met Susan and Bob Spencer, he hadn't believed it was a possibility.

The only thing he knew for certain was that he couldn't go on with Cammie the same way he had for twelve years. But what if he pushed too hard and ended up pushing her away? If he confessed all his feelings, that meant he was asking her to declare herself too. Then the pressure was on. Essentially, he'd be putting his heart in her hands, and she'd be expected to do something with it.

That very expectation could make her run.

He'd thought about this all the way to England, picked apart his feelings, his thoughts, his heart. It wasn't that he feared for his own heart. His fears were all about putting pressure and expectations on her.

After the hot tub, he'd admitted that first time with her had been the best damned night ever. And he'd just admitted his feelings had never gone away. He'd even admitted Fernsby was right, that she was his heart's desire.

He couldn't say *nothing*.

Finally, he whispered, over tender roast beef, over mouthwatering Yorkshire pudding, over trifle and flowers and champagne, "Tell me why you think it won't work."

* * *

The compassion in his voice brought her close to tears.

Cammie had never talked with him about her love life, but even though they hadn't discussed it, he knew of one bad relationship she'd had. He couldn't know, however, what had happened when she'd been Clyde's assistant.

There were men who lied to women to get what they wanted. Dane, of course, had never been that type. He'd always built her up, telling her what a great job she did, how she organized his life, how he'd be nothing without her. She was his idea genius.

And he was as honest as they came.

But she knew men who thought nothing of spinning a web of lies, or of the devastation they left behind. Maybe in telling Dane her story, he would understand why she couldn't go through it all again with him.

"I made two big mistakes." The trifle sat untouched in her bowl. "The first time was when I'd worked with Clyde for about three years." She sighed, looking up at the ceiling a moment. "And Rufus Mayhew came into our lives. I was twenty-one, still living at home and looking after my uncle, since he was in the early stages then. Between work and Uncle Lochlan, I hadn't dated much." Actually, she hadn't dated at all.

Toying with her cloth napkin, she wished it were paper. Then she'd have the satisfaction of tearing it to shreds. But even if she couldn't look at him, she owed Dane her story. "He was beautiful. I was innocent. I had no idea what men were like. He took me to the best restaurants, bought me wonderful gifts. He was older, and he was magnetic." She'd cared so much, and it hurt to think about how naïve she'd been.

Dane's eyes were flinty in the candlelight. If Rufus had been standing there, he'd have punched him in the nose, she was sure. Yet something more lurked in his gaze—perhaps an ache, though for what exactly, she couldn't tell.

She had to clear her throat. "I fell for him completely. If he'd asked me to marry him right then, I would have handed in my notice to Clyde and said yes." She closed her eyes, put her hands to her flaming cheeks, her skin hot against her fingers. "He didn't start pumping me for information until about two months into our relationship. I had no idea what he was doing. He said he just wanted to know about everything I did during the day so he could feel like he was with me when I was working. And he helped me with Uncle Lochlan, coming to the house, playing card games with us. He seemed so kind, so caring. I had no idea that all he wanted was information about Clyde. Things he could use to make money off him."

She was so ashamed, she wanted to cry.

Dane laid his hand over hers on the table. "It wasn't your fault. He took advantage. He stole your innocence. You're not to blame."

She whispered, "Yes, he stole my innocence." And then she admitted, "In every possible way."

The hard glint in Dane's eyes turned into a burning flame. Like a gallant knight, he'd have thrown Rufus out on his butt. After running him through with his sword.

But she had yet to admit her full culpability. "One day, a deal of Clyde's went south. Someone had gotten wind of what he'd planned and stepped in to subvert him, obviously taking the profits for themselves."

Dane squeezed her hand so tightly it would have been painful if it were anyone else's touch. "It. Wasn't. Your. Fault," he said succinctly, each word its own sentence.

"I was so excited for Clyde's big deal." The words

seemed to rush out of her then. "It was going to be wonderful. And Clyde was so thrilled." She stopped, held her breath, then finally made herself add, "And I told Rufus about it."

"Even then, you still didn't get it, did you?" Dane said softly. "You were still innocent. You had no idea there were people like that in the world."

She sighed. "I didn't have a clue." It shamed her even now to think about what she'd done. "When I was in Clyde's office, and he was railing that no one knew about the deal except him and his lawyers, I suddenly saw it. *I* knew about the deal." She put a hand to her chest. "And Rufus knew because I told him." Her soul felt like a bleak landscape as she remembered that day, realizing Rufus had used her information against them. "I had to admit to Clyde what I did." She swallowed hard. "He didn't even yell at me. He just said that when we're young, it's hard to know who to trust and who not to."

"Did Clyde ever do an investigation?" That's what Dane would have done.

"He found a shell company that eventually led back to Rufus Mayhew." That was her shame. And her broken heart.

A menacing growl rose up Dane's throat. "I hope Clyde crushed him." But even as he fisted one hand, he stroked her knuckles gently with the other.

But her story wasn't over. "I realized right then I

had terrible taste in men, and that no matter what, they would find a way to screw me over in the end."

Except Dane. He'd never screwed anyone over.

"Then I met you on the golf course. And we... you know." She shrugged painfully. Though it had been only one night, she'd once again chosen the wrong man. Even if she hadn't known it. Her shock the next day when she'd found out he was the man she was interviewing with had been like a body blow she couldn't recover from. "But Clyde was leaving, and I desperately needed the job to support my uncle."

"That's why we needed the rules, wasn't it?" Dane said for her. He sounded almost as sad as she'd felt that day.

"It was clear I was so bad at choosing who I slept with that my judgment couldn't be trusted."

"But what we did was amazing." His gentle declaration was both poignant and sweet, thrilling her and saddening her at the same time. He traced a finger across her knuckles. "There was nothing bad or wrong about it. It wasn't a mistake."

"I know it wasn't wrong. And you weren't one of my bad mistakes." She shook her head. "But it was never going to work out either."

Now that she'd revealed her first shameful secret, why bother holding back the rest? "I dated after that, but if anyone got serious, I cut them off." She slashed a hand through the air. "Just in case I was making another bad decision. I swear, I never told anyone anything about your business."

He sat back, his dark brows scrunching together. "How could you think I'd ever believe you would? I trust you absolutely."

"Even now? After what I did for Rufus?"

"You were the innocent. You didn't do it *for* him. He was the monster who *used* you." He balled his fist. "If he were here…" He let the sentence hang. Then he whispered, "You said you made two big mistakes. Tell me about the other guy."

"It was five years into working for you," she said, so softly he leaned in close to hear.

Five years after *their* night. Five years of their rules. Five years of watching him date so many other women.

It cut her every time she'd set up a dinner date for him or sent roses to another of his ladies. She'd torn herself apart wondering if this one could be *the one*. But she'd chosen the job and her uncle over anything she could have had with Dane. She'd made the irrevocable decision the day she'd walked in to discover that her prospective employer was the man she'd slept with the night before. The man she would have to work for. The man who was a hot property to every woman who came sniffing around.

And especially to her.

So she'd ordered the gifts and made the reservations and wrapped herself in cellophane so tight nothing could puncture her.

And she'd been doing that for twelve years.

★ ★ ★

Dane's heart tied itself into knots. She'd bared her soul to him, and he knew what that cost her. In so many ways, she was a very private person. He'd never known about Rufus Mayhew. Clyde had never said a word. Perhaps Clyde had thought Dane wouldn't hire her if he knew. But he would never hold an innocent young woman's mistake against her, especially when Dane knew how very much Clyde trusted her.

Clyde obviously knew she'd never make the same mistake again. But she'd learned so much more. She'd learned not to trust at all.

If she'd never met Rufus Mayhew, would things have been different twelve years ago? Would they have made the same rules the next morning? Or would they have thrown out the rule book completely?

But Mayhew had happened, and Cammie had received an almost mortal wound. Yet she'd recovered. And she'd remained strong.

She'd said it was five years after coming to work for him before she allowed herself to fall for another man. That would have been before she'd moved Lochlan and sold the house.

Five years. Which made it seven years since the

Rufus Mayhew debacle. Didn't they say things turned in seven-year cycles?

And now it had been another seven years.

She'd never told Dane about this second man, but he'd known something was up. He'd become used to reaching her almost immediately whenever he needed her, even in off hours, but she'd stopped picking up the phone right away. Sometimes she'd even had to call him back. She'd dressed up a bit more, wearing slightly more low-cut blouses—nothing untoward. Her skirts, though still circumspect, had been a little tighter, showing off her curves. Curves he couldn't help salivating over. She'd worn a little more makeup, and her lipstick had become bolder.

Now she told him the whole story. "He was actually a very nice guy. Arlo Doyle. He'd worked for Uncle Lochlan before my uncle had to retire. Arlo came to the house one day, and Uncle Lochlan lit up. He talked as if nothing was wrong—not a single sign of dementia." She looked at Dane. "You remember how bad he got seven years ago, when I had to put him in memory care?"

Dane nodded. He remembered so well her trauma over the decision.

"But he was himself again. The uncle I used to know. For days afterward, he remembered everything they'd talked about even though Arlo had been there only a couple of hours. I actually thought I must have imagined the shift in him, that he couldn't be as bad as I thought."

"I understand completely. I had a similar day with my grandfather."

An old school chum of his grandfather's had come to visit. The man had known him before the war, before he'd changed. And for that one day, Grandpa had been a completely different man—the man he must have been when Dane's grandmother married him, when he'd been fresh out of college, with hopes and dreams the war had yet to destroy.

Dane still treasured that glimpse of the grandfather he'd never known.

Cammie nodded. "I thought I could make the phenomenon happen again, so I invited Arlo over." She closed her eyes, and Dane reached for her hand once more. "But I couldn't duplicate it," she whispered.

He stroked her warm skin before he withdrew and let her go on.

"Uncle Lochlan liked Arlo so much. And I thought he was sweet. Then he asked me out. I said yes. I didn't intend for it to get serious." She blinked away what might have been a tear, so it didn't fall. "He told me right away that he was separated, not divorced yet, but that he'd left his wife a few months before. I appreciated his honesty. And he was so good to me. We laughed together. We watched movies together. He liked all the old classics the way I do. We went to that old theater on University Avenue in Palo Alto, the Stanford, where they played classic movies, and we saw *Meet Me in St. Louis*. Margaret O'Brien, who played the little sister, gave a talk before the movie. It was amazing. We had pizza afterward."

His heart flipped over, and he had to admit he was jealous. Binge-watching classic movies was their thing. And he was incredibly sad that he hadn't been the one to take her to see Margaret O'Brien and *Meet Me in St. Louis*.

She shrugged. "Anyway." And she left it at that.

He wanted to see her laugh. But they had to get through this. He didn't ask if she'd slept with this Arlo. He accepted that she had. And he didn't rage inwardly, since he'd skated through his always brief relationships.

She pressed her lips together for a moment, before she finally got out, "Then he told me his wife wanted to patch things up. And that she was pregnant."

Her words tore a hole in the pit of his stomach. "I'm so sorry."

Even now, she straightened her shoulders. "I kept my dignity. I didn't cry. I was very proud of myself," she said with the barest of smiles. "I told him, 'Go back to your wife for the sake of the child.'" She waved a hand as if she were shooing a phantom away. "'And if you need a good family therapist, I'll find you the best one. I'm good at finding what people need.'"

That's what Cammie always did—found exactly

what a man needed right when he needed it.

"It was a thousand times worse than Mayhew, wasn't it?" he said, not wanting to hurt her, but realizing she needed to get it all out, that she wanted him to understand why it could never work between them.

"You see, she was only three months pregnant. And we'd been dating for five." She swallowed. "Which meant he'd slept with her while he was with me. He'd been playing both ends. Maybe he hadn't meant to." She shrugged her shoulders as if giving Doyle the benefit of the doubt even now. "But it made me realize I wasn't—" She paused.

He knew exactly what she'd been about to say. "But you *are* good enough. He was a two-timing ass."

Her eyes were bleak. She was back in that moment, feeling the pain all over again. The first guy she loved had only wanted her for Clyde's contacts and his business acumen. He was a leech, a thief. The next guy had been on the rebound. He might not have meant to screw her over, but he had. And in between, there was Dane himself, seducing her on a golf course, taking her back to his condo, and making love to her that very night. Rushing her. Pushing her.

And the next morning, allowing her to make up all the rules that would keep them apart for twelve years.

He should have told her right then how he felt— though truthfully, he hadn't known the extent of it.

But he wouldn't believe it was too late.

"Remember when you brought me those flowers?" she asked.

He nodded.

"You knew how hurt I was even though I tried to hide it from you."

"I knew. And I hurt here." He put his hand over his heart. "So badly for you."

"Then you brought T. Rex into our lives." She sniffed. Though no tear tracks traced her cheeks, he knew she was crying inside. "I'd just come out of the office restroom, where I'd been crying, when you walked in with a big box and two coffees from the corner café." She laughed, though it was shaky. "And you said some lady outside the coffee shop was giving away puppies."

He smiled with the memory. "I couldn't resist those sad puppy-dog eyes." Just as he couldn't resist Cammie. He'd known something was terribly wrong, and he'd been pretty sure it involved a man. He'd have done anything to make her feel better.

Her laughter came stronger now. "Then you said I'd need to help you figure out what to call him. And how to get him in and out of other countries when you traveled so you wouldn't have to leave him behind." Her eyes shone with her laughter, and he felt his heart beat normally again. "You gave me a task to take my mind off the bad stuff."

She reached for him then, laying her hand over his.

"Every time I think of how sweet you were that day, it makes me cry all over again. And you bought me that stuffed T. Rex after we named our puppy."

"You've still got him too." Dane had seen the puffy thing on her bed. It had been such a small thing to do, yet it made her smile. Even then, he'd wanted to make her smile.

She put her fingers to the corners of her eyes to wipe up the tears. And Rex chose that moment to pop up from beneath the table and put his paws on her thigh. Cammie tugged him onto her lap, and he curled into a ball, the way he always did when he thought she was sad. The way he had when she'd come home after her uncle died. The way he had that very first day when Dane brought the puppy into the office.

Dane told her what was in his heart. "I've always known when you needed me, even if you tried to pretend you didn't."

After a deep breath, she said, "It's the same for me."

He turned his hand over in hers and held on. He wanted to be right where the little dachshund was, his head cradled in her lap, her fingers running through his hair.

But he'd told her he would wait for her to make the next move, and if nothing else, he was a man of his word.

He knew, even if she didn't, that her revelations

were a huge step for her. And for him. She'd kept this locked inside. And he'd never asked, though he'd known she'd been terribly hurt. She'd put herself out there, only to prove she wasn't good enough and that her judgment sucked. At least, that's what she'd told herself.

He understood now why it had been so important to her to ask for that promotion. It wasn't just about being more involved or wanting more responsibility. It was about her self-esteem, about finding the courage to ask for what she wanted. And she'd done it.

He wanted to pummel those two jerks into the ground for the way they'd treated her, but he was so damn glad the relationships hadn't worked. He would never do the same to her. He couldn't push her. He couldn't put expectations on her. He couldn't take control away from her.

Nor could they let things go on the way they had for the last twelve years. He had to be as honest as she had been. They both had their fears. And they both needed to move past them.

"Thank you for telling me all this. I understand so much better now." He wanted to pull her into his arms, but the time wasn't right. "We made up the rules that day in my office, and we've lived by them ever since." He waited until she looked at him again. "But those rules don't apply anymore. We need to throw them out. We need to change everything. We need more." He stood, stopped by her chair, put his hand on her cheek. "It's been a long travel day. Let's sleep on it." He kissed her forehead and whispered close to her ear, "I hope you'll dream of me."

He'd dream of her. He always had. He always would.

★ ★ ★

The sound of his footsteps faded as Rex snuggled into her lap. She'd thought Dane had been in the dark about her affair with Arlo until that big vase of flowers had appeared on her desk. She remembered asking, "Who are these from?" She'd brushed aside the leaves. "There's no card."

Dane had stood before her with not so much as a smirk on his face and said, "You must have a secret admirer."

But she'd known it was him. He'd never taken credit for any of the nice things he'd done for her. For how he'd helped her uncle. Even in giving her the promotion when she asked for it, he'd blamed himself for not having promoted her long ago.

Maybe that day, as she'd cried her eyes out in the bathroom, she hadn't been crying so much for Arlo and the way it ended, but for the way Dane had always seen inside her, even the things she hid from him. Maybe she'd been crying out of gratitude and longing and a sense of regret. What if, the moment she'd walked into his office the morning after the golf game and seen the man of her dreams, she'd told him right then she couldn't work for him because she wanted to be in his life as far more than an assistant?

If she'd found the courage to ask for what she wanted all those years ago, what might have been?

Chapter Twenty-One

True to his word, Dane left her alone. After sipping the last of the champagne in her glass, Cammie picked up Rex. He hadn't moved except to lift his head when Dane left the room.

She carried the dog up the wide manor staircase to the first landing, where a portrait of some naval hero took pride of place on the wall. There the stairs separated, going up each side. She took the right-hand stairway, heading to her room. She kept clothes and other necessities at the manor and hadn't brought much with her. At the top, her door stood open.

She had a fleeting wish that Dane would be waiting inside.

But when she stepped across the threshold, the room was empty. After she set Rex on the bed, he curled into a ball, falling asleep right away. He would stay there all night as if guarding her, where he could jump up at a moment's notice.

In the bathroom, she wiped away her makeup and the residue of the long day.

A voice inside told her the truth. *Dane always comes to me when I really need him.*

When Arlo betrayed her, Dane had recognized her distress and surprised her with flowers, then the cutest puppy in the world.

Now that she thought about it, he had the office space on the Peninsula because of her. He would have been more centrally located for business if he'd been in the city. But he'd chosen that location so she wouldn't have a long commute and could drive home quickly if her uncle needed her. Right after she'd put her uncle in memory care and sold the house, Dane had given up that office. Then he'd offered her a place in each of his homes—always a massive suite that was as big as an apartment. He'd helped her pay for her uncle's care.

He'd done so many kind and thoughtful things for her, many of which she hadn't even recognized. When she'd called him with the news that her uncle was near the end, he'd rushed to her side without hesitation. He'd stayed with her, held her, comforted her.

She pulled her flannel pajamas from the bureau. Even though it was early May, English nights could be cool. She climbed into bed, then tugged the covers to her chin. Wrapping her arms around the stuffed dinosaur—of course she'd brought it with her—she hugged it as if it were Dane, while Rex curled into the crook at the backs of her knees.

So many times, Dane had gone above and beyond

for her. He was her best friend, always there. At the barbecue, he'd noticed she was feeling bad and followed her into the house. He'd held her so tenderly, never asking a thing from her. Her grief at the time had been all about him, about realizing what she wanted from him, about knowing what she'd never have. But he'd thought she was grieving for her uncle, and he'd held her.

He said they could make a relationship work. But they had such a good working relationship now. She lay in bed, not thinking about that night or how beautifully he'd made love to her, but about the intervening years.

And she saw everything he hadn't said. He hadn't said he loved her, yet she could see now he'd actually told her in a zillion different ways. Even if he didn't realize it himself. She couldn't live without him. She needed his big, beautiful hugs and his steady reassurance that told her how special she was to him.

She could go on being afraid that it might end badly. That she wasn't good enough.

But what if their relationship *wasn't* damaged? What if he *could* love her?

Lying in her lonely bed, she spoke aloud. "We've both been such dummies."

And she left T. Rex sleeping peacefully.

★ ★ ★

Dane paced the room, strategizing like an army general. "By God, I will not fail at this. She will be mine, and I'll be hers."

He wanted nothing more than to race down the hall and knock on her bedroom door. To make love to her the way he'd thought about all the years they'd lived under the same roof, and even before. To feel her skin beneath his fingertips, her lips against his, her body taking him to all the places he'd dreamed of.

But she needed to make the next move. He knew in his gut it was the only way it could work. He could knock on her door, and she'd probably let him in. She'd probably even let him make love to her again if he pushed.

But that would be her *letting* him. Him *pushing* her. Instead of her wanting it as urgently as he did. And choosing what she wanted.

He was thinking so hard he almost didn't hear the soft knock. Then he thought it had to be his imagination. But who wouldn't let his fantasy walk right through the door? He hurried to answer it.

She wore the most adorable flannel pajamas with polar bears all over them. They made him want to gather her up and kiss her senseless.

But she was already talking. Even as badly as he wanted to shower her with kisses, he needed to hear every word.

"You've been my whole world for so many years,"

she told him, her eyes wide, their soft jade color darkened almost to emerald.

His body wanted to burst into flames. His heart wanted to soar into the night.

"In every way but one." Her gaze traced the contours of his face. "And I'm ready—really, really ready—to fix that." After only one step into his room, she added, "You're the missing piece of my puzzle."

If a heart could burst wide open and spill over the floor at her feet, his did right then.

He got everything she was saying, totally. She'd thought of him for the past twelve years, just as he'd dreamed of her. She hadn't said she loved him. He couldn't say he loved her. But he could show her in every way possible.

He grabbed her up in his arms, holding her tight. His hands on her rear, she hooked her legs around his waist, and he whispered, "You have no idea how many nights I've dreamed of this."

She bent her head for a kiss so gentle and so sweet, it felt like butterfly wings caressing him. Then she opened her mouth and delved deep into his inner being. A wealth of emotion, so much bigger than anything he'd ever felt in his life, welled up inside him. And he took her mouth as if he'd never kissed anyone before, as if she was the only one he'd ever kiss again.

Memories were supposedly so much more poignant than reality. You built them up in your mind, turned them into something reverential. Yet her lips were softer than they'd ever been. Her skin beneath the pajama top was smoother than he'd ever imagined. Her legs around his waist were tighter, begging him, owning him before he'd even entered her.

He felt more powerful than he ever had in his life as he carried her to his bed.

"Nothing could be sweeter than your taste." He let her fall to the bed and came down on top of her. She was so delicate beneath him and so strong.

He'd heard her siren's call for the last twelve years. And now he would make her his.

Her eyes were bright in the dim light of the lamp by the door, but he wanted more light. He wanted to see every inch of her. The last time, they'd done things in the dark. But he never wanted to be in the dark with her again. So he reached past her to flip on the bedside lamp, bathing her in soft golden light.

"I want to touch you everywhere. I need to taste every part of you."

She blinked. And then she whispered, her voice husky, sexy, "What are you waiting for?"

A piece of him wanted to go absolutely wild. But another, bigger part wanted to slow everything down and savor each moment.

"It's going to be so much better than before." He reached between them and flicked open the buttons of her polar bear pajama top. Instead of going for the gold, he trailed his fingers across her cheek, nibbled the tender flesh of her lobe, licked the shell of her ear.

Cammie shivered, reminding him of how much she liked that, how delicate and sensitive her ears were. With one last lick and a warm breath, he whispered, "There's so much more of you I want to see."

He kissed her neck down to the slope of her shoulder. He licked the hollow of her throat, and lying between her legs, he felt her thighs tighten around him in need.

They hadn't talked much the last time, but now he wanted nothing more than to hear her voice. "Tell me what you want, and I'll do it."

Her words were a hoarse murmur. "Touch me."

He trailed his fingers to the tip of her breast, circled the tight bead until she gasped. "Taste me."

Then she pushed him, her hand on the back of his head, guiding him down to where she wanted him. And that was something totally new as well. Before, she hadn't told him what she wanted, either with words or actions—but then, he hadn't asked.

"Anything you want." He looked up at her as he moved down her body. "Everything you want."

He closed his lips around the pearl of her breast, sucking her into his mouth, worrying her with his tongue until she writhed beneath him.

She gasped. "Dane, please."

As he spread her pajama top wide, he moved to the

other peak, taking it deep, reveling in her breathy whisper of his name. Twelve years ago, there'd been no names, and it had been freaking sexy. But this was so much hotter. And he was so much harder.

"Every inch of you," he whispered.

He tasted, licked, caressed all that beautiful, smooth, delicate skin, from her breasts all the way to her belly button, where a gentle lick made her laugh.

Her laugh could make a man lose everything.

Then he reached the tie of her pajama bottoms. And he looked at her.

He hadn't asked permission last time. And he didn't need it now—at least, not the words—because her scent told him how ready she was. But he wanted her to ask. He needed to know they were in this together.

"Tell me what you want." Shifting slightly to the side, he laid his hand just above her sex.

"I want you to pleasure me. I want it so badly," she said on a shaky breath. Then, on a whimper of need, she added, "If you don't do it, I'll have to do it myself."

Amazing visions floated through his mind, of her dreaming of him, of all those nights when she'd been just down the hall from him. Of her needing him, imagining that it was his touch on her body. Of her crying out his name.

He should have known, should have felt the power of her thoughts. Maybe he had. Maybe that's why he dreamed of her every night. Yes, every single damned night since she'd come to work for him. Even if he'd told himself it couldn't possibly be that often.

He slid off the bed, kneeling between her spread thighs as Cammie propped herself on her elbows to look at him.

She hadn't watched all those years ago. She'd loved it, lost herself in it, but she hadn't watched. And there was something so hot about her gaze on him now, something so erotic.

He slowly drew the polar bear pajamas down her legs, throwing them aside until only her panties remained. The damp patch between her legs beckoned him, and instead of tearing them off, he leaned over her, breathed warm air on the fabric, covered her with his mouth. She ground against him, and he took her that way, right through her panties, reveling in her taste, her scent, her moisture, her heat.

As sweet she'd been then, she was sweeter now. As wet as she'd been then, she was wetter now. As hot as she'd been, she was on fire now.

He couldn't wait another moment. Ripping the panties off her, he took her with his lips and his tongue the way he'd dreamed of so many times.

★ ★ ★

Cammie cried out his name the moment his mouth found her and his tongue delved deep.

He'd been so good before—no one had ever been

better. His touch had burned itself into her brain. His taste had lived inside her, his scent filling her head whenever she closed her eyes and thought of that night.

But his mouth on her now was like nothing she'd ever felt before. Maybe it was all the years she'd dreamed of it. Wanted it. Needed it. He clamped his big warm hands on her derriere and lifted her so he could taste more and more of her.

And she watched, relishing the sight of his dark head between her thighs, his closed eyes as he drank her in, his powerful shoulders spreading her thighs wide. Entering her with two blunt fingers, he flipped her world upside down. Just the right touch. So perfect. So—*oh my God*—

His mouth buried against her, he opened those blue, blue eyes.

And she exploded, crying out his name, chanting, "Dane, Dane, Dane."

She'd made sounds for him before, moans, groans, sighs, but now, with his mouth on her, his fingers inside her, his tongue playing her, her cries slammed up into the ceiling, raining down on her again.

And she came for him endlessly.

Chapter Twenty-Two

It was like believing she'd been awake all along, only to realize she'd sleepwalked through her entire life.

He ran his mouth over her thighs, kissed her hot skin, worked his way up her body until he held her in his arms, kissed her. It was like a communion, his taste and her taste mingled, creating a whole new flavor she'd never before known.

"I thought I remembered how good it was," she whispered, looking up into his beautiful blues. "But I never remembered it like *that*."

He chuckled, stroking her hair back from her temple and cupping her cheek. "I've imagined it all a thousand times." He dropped a kiss on the corner of her mouth. "And it's never been this good."

Her heart rolled in her chest, upside down and right side up again. He was still there, still holding her, still gazing at her with what she told herself could only be love. Even if he hadn't said the word. He would—one day, he would.

She trailed her hand down his chest. He'd been

shirtless when she knocked on his door, and she followed the arrow of dark hair down to the waistband of his sweats. "You have on way too many clothes. And I'm nowhere near done with you yet."

He gave her the Harrington lady-killer smile. This time, it was all for her. She wouldn't think about how it had been for anyone else, ever.

He stood, grinning. "I can remedy that ASAP." He stripped, the soft sweats sliding down his legs until he stepped out of them.

She could only breathe out a simple exclamation. "Oh my."

Of course she remembered how stunning he was. They swam in the Caribbean all the time, as well as his Pebble Beach pool. And there'd been the hot tub on his San Francisco terrace. But now the room's lamplight painted his sculpted muscles with bronze, and his tight boxer briefs cupped him intimately. The way she wanted to cup him.

His male beauty stole the breath from her lungs, until she grew dizzy from lack of air. And from her need for him.

He circled a finger at her. "You're still wearing polar bears."

She laughed, and pushing herself up, she shimmied out of the pajama top. Then she sat on the edge of the mattress and tipped her head back to look at him. "Let me do the rest. I want to unwrap you like you're the most precious gift I've ever received."

Desire flickered in his eyes. No, need. Need was wholly different from desire. It was a flame that burned inside him, sparking an answering flame deep within her.

Reaching for him, she slipped her fingers inside the elastic of his briefs. Slowly, ever so slowly, she rolled the fabric down. First, it was just his crown. Her mouth watered. He was so hard. So ready. He could take her now. She wanted that.

But more than taking him inside her, she needed *this*.

Inch by inch, she revealed all his hard, male splendor begging for her touch, her lips, her tongue.

Could it be possible he was even bigger than she remembered? Maybe it was knowing each other so much better now. Inside and out. The emotion growing right along with the physical, making everything bigger, brighter, better.

The briefs fell to the floor, and he stepped out of them. She could have tasted him then, but she wrapped her hand around him, felt the weight of him, the thickness, the length.

His guttural rasp rolled down to her. "Please. Don't tease me."

She looked up into his burning gaze. "I am so done teasing."

The last twelve years had been one long, agonizing, exquisite tease.

And now it was over.

She bent her head and wrapped her lips around his crown, sucking for a long moment, loving the gasp and groan that exploded from him.

He swore, and she loved that too.

For long, incredible moments, she licked him, tasted a drop of his essence, swallowed it, and wanted more.

Then she swallowed all of him, taking him deep.

Shoving his fingers through her hair, he swore and growled. "Please," he begged.

For what? For her to finish him? For her to throw herself back on the bed and beg him to take her?

Memories of the last time were suddenly so clear to her. All she'd known after he'd taken her to the peak with his mouth had been the need to have him inside her. She hadn't done *this* to him.

But now, she savored the taste of him, the feel of him between her lips, the tremble in his limbs, the tautness of his muscles. Gripping him in one hand, she squeezed his thigh with the other, her nails making small dents in his flesh.

If it was even possible, he grew bigger, harder, filling her mouth.

Until he pleaded, "Let me come inside you. I need that. I want that. I have to have it. Please. Cammie." Then he swore again.

She let him slide from her lips, sucking hard one more time, and looked up at him.

Then Dane said the thing that could have made the moment fall completely apart. "If I know my butler, he's left a necessary little packet somewhere around here for us."

But she wouldn't let the *necessities* ruin anything, and she stood then, went up on her tiptoes to wrap her arms around his neck. "I'm on the pill." She didn't explain it helped her cramps. "I don't need the little packet if you don't."

He looked at her with eyes such a vivid blue she thought he could see all the way to her marrow. To her heart.

"I haven't been on a date since you went on family leave," he said. "I couldn't. Not while you were dealing with everything. All I could think about was you. That's why I called you on video chat all the time. So there's been no one else for so long. I want to feel all of you. And I want you to feel all of me."

Her heart burst wide open. She hadn't wanted to think he'd been out there dating nameless, faceless women while she'd sat by her uncle's bedside. And she'd savored every one of those nightly video chats.

"Then don't make me wait another second," she whispered against his lips.

He twisted then and fell back on the bed with her on top, his skin caressing her from breast to thigh.

"I feel like I've done this a thousand times," she told him. "Every night in my dreams."

He tangled his fingers in her hair. "In my dreams, it was just me inside you and nothing between us." Then he pulled her down for his kiss, that unique combined taste—him, her—filling her up.

She wanted to taste it for the rest of her life.

He let her go, whispering, "Take me. All of me. Please."

Looking into the ocean-blue depths of his eyes, into the flames burning there, she felt as if the words meant so much more than just the physical. They offered up his heart and his soul too.

And she took him.

* * *

She came down on him, taking him deep. And he felt as though she was the home he'd always longed for.

He groaned as she threw her head back, letting out a long, low moan of need and pleasure.

Then she leaned forward, bracing her hands on the bed, her lips only inches from his, her hair falling over him, her breath sweetly bathing him. "I want slow. Real slow. Until I need it fast."

"Take me any way you want me."

He wondered if he'd always been the one to take, if he'd never given. Except that one night with her. How could he have been so blind? But maybe that was why this joining was so precious. Because it had taken so long to get here. Because he'd dreamed away the last twelve years.

And now she was real. *This* was real.

The short glide she performed on him was enough to drive him completely out of his mind. He wanted his hands on her hips, wanted to slam into her, to roll her beneath him and thrust so deep they both saw stars.

Yet, even more, he needed whatever way she chose.

As she rolled her hips on him, she moaned, her eyes drifting closed as she lost herself in the pleasure. The slow ride was exactly what her body craved. She tensed around him, released, again and again. And threatened to blow off the top of his skull.

"That is so good," she said in a voice he'd only ever heard once, that night, in the throes of her passion.

He wanted to hear that voice forever.

Eyes closed, she whimpered, chanted, "Oh, oh, oh."

His gut knew what would make this even better. Reaching between them, he put his finger on the tight button between her legs. And he stroked her.

The chanting stopped, taken over by groans of exquisite pleasure and of her desire for him. Only him. He knew it, felt it in every clamp of her body around him.

Her legs began to quiver, and her arms, supporting

her on the bed, trembled. Her eyes scrunched closed, and her breath fell in sharp gasps from her lips.

He remembered those sounds. He'd heard them every night for twelve years. And he remembered how excruciatingly good that night had felt. Yet now, with all his senses heightened, he felt every vibration of her body, her tension rising, dragging him with her. His own blastoff was so close, it took every ounce of willpower to hold off, to wait for her. This was altogether different from before, so much more—the slipslide of her against him, on him, the way she gripped him so tightly, the way she lost herself in ecstasy.

She bowed her head, puffed out her breath, fast, harsh. Then she cried out as her body clamped down on him. He felt her orgasm as if it were his own. With barely a rational thought, he rolled her to her back, pulled her legs up around his waist, and pounded into her. Her whole body vibrated, her beautiful rose-gold hair flying across her face, her mouth open, gasping out her satisfaction in two words. "Don't stop." Then three more. "Please don't stop."

He couldn't have stopped even if the world were ending around them. He took them both to a place they'd only glimpsed the last time. And prayed they would stay there forever.

★ ★ ★

Her words came out part laughter, part tears. "That

was…" She couldn't complete the thought.

He finished it for her. "Exquisite."

She nodded. "Yes. That's it. Exquisite. Stunning."

"Life-altering. Mind-blowing."

"Out of this world."

"Freaking unbelievable."

They laughed together. She rolled her head to meet his gaze as she lay curled against him. "Are you trying to outdo me with words?"

He shook his head, grinned. "I could never outdo you, sweet lady. You drive me crazy."

She rubbed her cheek against his shoulder. "Is that a good drive-me-crazy or a bad drive-me-crazy?"

He rolled on top of her. "It's the most amazing crazy I've ever felt in my life." He kissed her quick, even though she wanted him to linger. "And I only want it to get crazier."

Then he rolled off and strolled into the bathroom, his butt muscles rippling.

He was so beautiful. So perfect.

She crawled to the bottom of the bed, searched for her panties, and was stepping into them when he returned. "Come on, Lord Lazybones. I'm starving."

He grinned like a naughty kid. "Me too, Lady Lazybones."

She loved the banter. She loved being lady to his lord. They dressed, then ran down the stairs hand in hand, giggling like children.

The kitchen was state of the art, yet it still had a touch of the old, with the range built into the ancient hearth and the refrigerator designed to look like an old-fashioned icebox. Sitting on stools at the granite counter opposite the sink, they finished the rest of the roast beef, Dane feeding Rex the tidbits Fernsby would yell about.

Narrowing his eyes, Dane said, "I'm still hungry."

She found a Sainsbury's packaged fish pie in the freezer and heated it up in the microwave. Seated once again at the counter, she smiled. "I like eating junk food sometimes. It's so deliciously salty."

He grinned. "I agree, but you still taste better." And he pulled her off the stool, angling her to stand between his legs.

Kissing her, he slid his hands beneath her pajama top, cupping her breasts, tweaking the tips until she groaned. Then he slipped into her waistband and palmed her bottom. Not to be outdone, she glided inside his sweats, pulling on him to stand up long enough for her to slide them down to his ankles.

"Get on the counter," she demanded.

He happily agreed while she sat on the stool between his legs. She made love to him with her mouth until he begged her to stop. Then he hauled her up on the counter and spread her thighs, thrusting between her legs and touching her in every perfect spot until she was the one who screamed.

And of course, they couldn't let it end there.

★ ★ ★

Dane couldn't count how many times they made love in the night. He held her close, waking up hard and ready against her backside. Lifting her leg over his thigh, his fingers deep inside her, he played her for long moments until she cried out, shattering. Then he entered her, taking her hard and sweet. And the taking was mutual.

Waking to bright morning sun breaking through the slit in the curtains, he wanted nothing more than to stay there with her forever.

Except that she wasn't in the bed.

It couldn't have been a dream. Not like he'd been dreaming all these years.

He went in search of her and found her in the kitchen, where she'd already made coffee and toast.

Over the delicious aroma of rich coffee, he could smell her, that uniquely sweet and spicy scent that could only be Cammie.

And he wanted more of her, right there on the kitchen countertop where he'd had her last night.

★ ★ ★

Over slightly burnt toast, Dane said, "That was amazing."

Cammie almost faltered. "It was awesome," she

agreed.

But why did everything have to look different in the morning light?

They drank coffee and ate their toast slathered with marmalade. She popped two more pieces into the toaster, one for each of them.

And he didn't say it.

"Fernsby won't return for a while. We should go back to bed. Or maybe take a shower." He winked.

She stared at him for a long moment. And somehow managed to laugh. "We can't let T. Rex miss his morning walk."

He grinned. "Then after the walk."

After last night, she'd expected him to say it. She wanted him to say it. And somehow it was like a knife stabbing straight through her heart when he *didn't* say it.

Dane would never lie. And that was the problem. He wasn't going to say anything he didn't truly feel. He would be honest. He wanted her. He desired her. Maybe he even needed her. And yes, deep down, she thought he loved her.

But he couldn't say it.

And didn't that mean they were right back where they'd been before she'd knocked on his door last night? Right back where they'd been all along? With her wanting more than he could ever give?

★ ★ ★

Okay. He could handle this. He wanted to go back to bed and make love to her all over again. Make her scream all over again.

But she wanted to take the dog for a walk.

All right. He could deal with that. He wouldn't pressure her. Especially after last night. He couldn't push her and ask if what they'd done last night meant as much to her as it did to him. Last night, she'd said he was the missing piece to her puzzle. He'd taken that to mean so much.

But maybe it hadn't meant as much as he wanted.

That was okay. He'd give her time. He wouldn't push. He wouldn't make her run away. And tonight he'd take her to bed again and show her over and over how much she meant to him.

But that would be tonight. For now, he said, "You know, we really need to hire an assistant for you. With you being in charge of the new project, we're going to need more help. I'll start looking for someone."

He couldn't read her expression. It was suddenly flat, not a single indication of what she was thinking.

Then she smirked. "Oh, no. I'm choosing my own replacement."

She put both hands on the counter and levered off the stool. "I'll take a shower and get dressed. Then I'll take Rex for a walk before we get to work."

Just like that, in the space of a moment where he hesitated about what to say, she was gone. He watched the empty doorway through which she'd disappeared.

Mentioning the assistant had been his way of giving her time. And letting her know she was his equal. It hadn't been a way to avoid talking about his feelings.

But she was running away. Even though he could swear he hadn't pushed her. But maybe he'd pushed over dinner, telling her the next move had to be hers. Setting up an expectation. And she had made her move. Except that this morning, she regretted it.

That day after the Maverick meeting when he'd thought she'd been about to quit on him was the closest to a heart attack he'd ever come.

Don't push too hard, don't ask too soon, just play it low-key.

All he could do now was wait and see. Even if the wait might kill him.

Chapter Twenty-Three

Cammie couldn't flat out ask Dane, *Do you love me?* She just couldn't. It would break her to ask. She'd laid her heart on the line last night when she'd told him he was the missing piece to her puzzle. What else could that mean except that her heart was only complete with him in it? Yet, even as perfect as last night had been, as out of this world, he hadn't said he loved her.

Was Dane even capable of love after his upbringing? His parents had pretty much abandoned him and all his siblings when they were young. Something like that left irreparable damage. If that were so, they didn't have a chance.

It hurt her head to think about it.

Sitting at her computer, she busily searched for an assistant for them both while she managed the special needs resort. The office suite, formerly the library, was a darkly paneled room, with bookcases floor to ceiling, a massive fireplace, and only two smallish windows looking out on the garden. Which made the entire room dark.

She could barely concentrate.

Especially with Dane sitting at his desk busily throwing a rubber ball for Rex. The dog went crazy, running into walls, rolling across the carpet, sliding on the hardwood that wasn't covered by the rug. At any other time, she would have laughed at T. Rex's antics. And Dane's.

But it wasn't any other time. It was the morning after he'd made glorious love to her.

And she could think of nothing else but why he hadn't said he loved her.

The slam of the front door made them both jump.

"Good God," Dane said, sitting up straight. "That can't possibly be Fernsby."

Of course it wasn't. Fernsby would never slam a door. Yet who else could it be?

A moment later, the man himself stood in the office doorway. Grinning. The man who never smiled was actually *grinning*.

"I'm one of the contestants on the show." His fist moved as if he wanted to punch the air and only barely held himself back. "I beat that scourge of the earth, Digbert." He laughed, a raspy sound, as if his throat muscles didn't know how to laugh. "He actually made *croissants*." Glee trickled through his voice. "How did he get past the first round? Even one of your sister's vegan monstrosities would have been better."

Cammie had never—absolutely never—seen this

side of Fernsby. It was uncanny that sheer happiness had freed him. Or had victory over his nemesis brought it out?

She wasn't about to miss this opportunity. Not for anything.

She jumped out of her chair and hugged him.

Then, miracle of miracles, Fernsby, the staid, stern butler, waltzed her around the library.

Who even knew the man could dance?

* * *

Dane had expected Fernsby to start in on him the moment he walked through the door, pulling him aside to ask what the heck had happened with Cammie. Because they obviously weren't all lovey-dovey the way Fernsby had predicted. They were still miles apart at two separate desks.

If Fernsby even noticed, he didn't say a thing. He was too happy.

Fernsby and *happy* had never before gone together in his lexicon. But Fernsby danced Cammie around the library, his face lit up with irrepressible joy.

Dane must be dreaming. Or it was a nightmare. He couldn't tell which.

Suddenly releasing Cammie, Fernsby seized Dane, waltzing him around the room just as he'd waltzed Cammie.

It was like something out of *My Fair Lady*. The horror remake.

Yet Dane couldn't help laughing—loud, uproarious sounds welling up his throat.

Fernsby grabbed Cammie again, whirling them both hand in hand as if they were dancing around a maypole. Until Fernsby abruptly let go, and the only way Dane saved himself from falling was by latching on to Cammie and dancing across the floor with her.

All he wanted to do was hold her close, kiss her luscious lips, and drag her upstairs to his bed.

The maniacally happy Fernsby—or maybe just maniacal—danced his way out of the room. Cammie pulled away from Dane.

And that was that.

* * *

Fernsby stopped outside the door, overhearing Camille say, "I'm so happy for him. But we still need to find that assistant."

He'd given them the most romantic setting, the perfect food, the best champagne, all of it whispering romance into the air. And now… nada.

Fernsby muttered, "A butler's job is never done."

What had he said to the Mavericks? Ah yes, that he was the only butler who could handle a boss too big for his britches.

Dane obviously still needed a kick in the pants.

★ ★ ★

Maybe he should have carried her upstairs the moment Fernsby frolicked out of the library. Or kissed her senseless. Maybe waiting her out was a mistake.

But his cell rang. Cammie pushed him toward the phone lying on the desk. "You'd better get that."

He grumbled, wondering if it was just an excuse to pull out of his arms.

But then he looked at the screen. "It's Daniel Spencer. It must be three o'clock in the morning back home. What the hell?"

Her eyes widened. "It's got to be important."

He put the phone on speaker and demanded, "Why are you calling me at three in the morning? You should be sleeping."

"Because I knew you were in England," Daniel said, as if that revealed everything. "And this can't wait. I've been going over the numbers all night."

"Which ones?"

"I've found the perfect property right on Lake Tahoe." He laughed, sounding as if he were buffing his fingernails on his shirt. "We all agreed that Tahoe is healing—the beautiful waters, the clean air—and that we want a place relatively on its own away from the big casinos."

"Tell us everything," Cammie said, Daniel's excitement vibrating all the way across the air waves and grabbing her. Or maybe that had been the dance around the library.

"It's on the waterfront with an amazing stretch of beach and its own dock. It backs into the forest, with hiking trails, and there's a ski resort and snow park close enough to send kids on bus trips for the day."

Cammie pelted him with questions. This was her show. "What's on it now?"

"An old resort, defunct for ten years. There's sewer, power, all the infrastructure."

Cammie gasped, hand over her mouth. "Are there any hazardous waste issues? Asbestos?"

"Nothing disclosed. Though we'll still do a survey. It's on the market only because a real estate development company was renovating, and they've run out of money. We'll probably need to tear down the existing structures and start over, but that's no big deal. That's what the development company should have done instead of working with what was already there. You run into all sorts of trouble with that. But we need to jump on this now. It won't last long."

Dane leaned over the phone, fists on the desk. "We'll get right on the plane and head back to you ASAP."

"Good. Like I said, this won't last long."

"Thank you, Daniel," Cammie added, smiling at the phone as if Daniel could see her. "I knew you'd find the perfect spot."

"It's what I love to do. I can't wait." Then he was gone, probably wanting to get to bed after pulling close to an all-nighter.

Dane wanted to waltz around the room all over again.

"Let's get packed." He looked at his watch. "We can be on our way in ninety minutes."

Then he'd have a ten-hour flight to work on her.

* * *

She stared at Dane. So smart, so competent, so assured. But this was her project. If Dane went along, everyone would defer to him, just as Daniel had called him instead of her even though Dane had already informed the Mavericks that she was in charge.

If he was there, she'd look to him for approval the entire time.

She had to take charge. Without Dane as backup. Otherwise, she'd always be Dane's little assistant.

Even more than proving to everyone else that she was good enough, she needed to prove it to herself.

That made her straighten her spine. She *was* good enough.

As Dane headed for the door, she said, "Since I'm one hundred percent in charge of this project, I have to take charge of it completely. Which means I have to do this myself."

He stopped dead and looked at her. "What does

that mean?" His voice sounded bewildered, his brow scrunched in puzzlement, his head tipped slightly, as if he were Rex asking why Dane had stopped throwing the ball.

"Can you understand?" She paused a long moment. "I have to do this without you."

★ ★ ★

He was doing it again. Holding her back. He hadn't given her a promotion years ago. And now, he was rushing to do the very thing she needed to do herself.

Yet he couldn't help asking, "You don't even want me to fly home with you?" He sounded like a little boy begging her not to leave him behind. The way he'd so often begged his parents when he was young.

But this was different. He had to tell himself that.

"If you do, we'll talk about it the whole way, and my plan will turn into your plan." She put her hand to her chest. "This needs to be all me."

"Of course it does," he said softly, wanting so badly to touch her and knowing he couldn't. "You're right." Then he picked up his phone. "I'll make the arrangements. You go pack."

She looked at him one long, last moment and whispered, "Thank you."

As she walked out of the office, he shoved away the thought that if he let her go now, it would be for good.

But sometimes the only choice you had was to set a

person free to do what they needed to do. And pray it led them back to you.

He had to set her free, like so many of the animals he'd nurtured when he was a kid. And pray she'd return. Even if none of the creatures or the people he'd loved before ever had.

★ ★ ★

Cammie had finished packing. She hadn't brought much, since most of what she needed was already here. She snapped the carry-on closed and hefted it to the floor. Rex lay on the bed, looking up at her with the saddest pair of eyes she'd ever seen. Sort of like Dane had downstairs. The dog whimpered as she pulled up the bag's handle.

She scratched him behind the ears. "I won't be gone long. I promise."

The dog licked her hand as if saying he understood.

"Are you going somewhere?"

She jumped at the sound of that deep, stern voice. Bracing herself, she faced Fernsby in the doorway and said, "Daniel just called. I'm heading back to California. He's found the perfect property in Lake Tahoe, and I need to see it. Since I'm managing the project, it's my job and my decision."

It was funny, or odd, how Fernsby just seemed to know things without being told. He knew all about the new resort and her promotion.

He raised his hands to applaud her. "You'll do a smashing job, Camille. I'm very proud of you." His expression turned even more grave, if Fernsby could actually be more grave than usual. Except when he was waltzing. "I must talk to you before you go. In private," he added ominously.

Her heart dropped all the way to her toes. A shiver ran through her bones, and she trembled like a teenager at boarding school being brought before the headmistress. Fernsby had never asked to speak with her privately before.

She wondered if she'd come out of this alive.

And she tried to forestall the dressing-down. "But the plane is waiting."

Daniel had called back to say he'd chartered a plane for her and would meet her when she arrived in California. She couldn't take Dane's plane, of course. How would he, Fernsby, and Rex get home?

But Fernsby said unequivocally, "The plane will just have to wait."

What choice did she have? When Fernsby made a demand, you had to obey.

"Is it about the baking show? You want to make sure you can have the time off? Dane's totally behind you on this." She prayed that was what Fernsby wanted to talk about.

He'd been so out of character this morning. Something was going on.

But Fernsby merely strode across the room and squished his tall frame into an armchair. Then he pointed to the other chair on the opposite side of the table, where she liked to read.

She had no option but to sit.

And Fernsby began. "Once upon a time…" He paused for effect.

Cammie stared, wide-eyed.

"There was a woman." He gazed at her with unblinking gray eyes. "I made a mess of it."

Oh yes, this was totally out of character. His sudden soul-baring made her twitch. "I'm so sorry." She didn't know what else to say.

He looked at her, his silvery eyes silencing her. He would say what he had to say no matter what she did. "I have never spent a day when I didn't regret losing her." He held his hand up, almost as if he were examining his fingernails. The hand where a gold band might have rested. "If I could change that, I would in a heartbeat." That couldn't be a smile twitching on his lips. No, not Fernsby, despite his display in the library. "I know you don't believe I actually have a heart."

She had to refute that. "Of course you have a heart. You absolutely adore Rex. And I think you love Dane too."

If Fernsby was capable of an eye roll, which she didn't believe, the expression in his eyes could have been just that. "I don't like dogs. I don't even like people." He waited a beat of the heart he claimed he didn't have. "But I will admit to having a soft spot for that." He pointed at the bed where Rex lay, giving him the evil eye. "And I have a soft spot for Mr. Harrington."

Good Lord. Fernsby admitting to a soft spot? Unheard of. She knew it existed, just as she knew his heart existed, but to have him say it aloud?

"As I was saying." He looked at her, his gaze adding the words *before I was so rudely interrupted*. "If I could go back in time and change things…" He didn't finish the sentence. "But I can't. I had so many reasons it wouldn't work. She had so many reasons it wouldn't work. By the time you get to my age, you realize all those reasons are poppycock."

Cammie wondered how old he really was.

"The truth is that we were just afraid to fail at love. And now I see you doing the same thing to yourself." He gave her another stern look. "Please don't make my mistakes. We both know the truth about where you belong." His pause closed around her heart. "And who you belong with."

She didn't know what to say. Was there really anything *to* say? Fernsby had actually been in love. Once upon a time. It was almost unfathomable. Even more unfathomable was that he'd told her about it. She felt like Alice in Wonderland. Was Fernsby the Cheshire Cat? Or the Mad Hatter?

"Fernsby," she said, trying to keep her voice as calm as possible and not sure she accomplished it, "I'm afraid you might be misreading things."

He raised one long finger and wagged it at her. "You and I both know the truth. I realize you wish to deny it. Just like I wanted to deny the truth all those years ago. But while you're gone, I want you to think about everything I've said." His hard gray gaze made her shudder.

She wanted to tell him that she knew exactly what she wanted. She just wasn't sure Dane wanted the same thing, even after they'd made love. Because that wasn't the same as *being* in love. And what if Dane could never admit it? She couldn't discuss any of that with Fernsby. She certainly couldn't admit they'd made love last night. That was beyond the pale, even after Fernsby's uncharacteristic confession.

Fernsby stood then to tower over her. He intoned like a judge on the bench, "I have faith in you. You will know what to do when you come back."

Then he rolled her suitcase out of the bedroom.

What if he was right? What if she was just afraid to fail at love?

★ ★ ★

A car waited in the driveway, ready to take her to the airport. Fernsby had already laid her case in the trunk.

There was nothing to do but walk away. And yet,

she couldn't. She and Dane had left so much unsaid.

Cammie turned to find him right there, so close she could breathe him in. He gazed at her with his heart in his eyes. At least, she wanted to believe that.

He cupped her face in his big hands. "I know you can do this," he whispered. "I believe in you with every fiber of my being."

Then he kissed her—the sweetest, most beautiful, most heartfelt kiss she'd ever known. It wasn't dueling tongues and passionate lips. In its simplicity, it was so much more. It was the splendor of what they'd done last night and the tenderness of his arms around her as her uncle lay dying. It was the thoughtfulness with which he bought her flowers when her heart was crushed and the sensitivity when he eased her pain by bringing her the cutest puppy ever. It was the purity of friendship.

When he stepped back only an inch or two, she said, "Thank you for understanding that I need to do this on my own."

He brushed his lips across her forehead. "Of course you do. I should have seen that without you telling me."

Then she climbed into the car and let it carry her away from him.

God, how she loved that man. Turning in the seat, she looked back at him, still standing in the drive long after Fernsby had gone inside.

She'd wasted the morning being angry with him for not saying the words she wanted to hear. They could have made love again.

But she knew he loved her. He understood what she needed, and he accepted it. If he didn't love her, he could never have let her go. Dane liked to be in control. He was always smack in the middle of everything. He was a decision-maker.

It must be killing him to let her make this tremendous decision without him.

It was another of the many reasons she knew he loved her, knew it straight through to her heart and deep into her soul.

As the car turned the corner on the long, long drive, Dane disappeared behind a hedgerow, and the manor house vanished from view.

She needed to complete this deal. She didn't have to prove herself to Dane. She had to prove it to herself. He'd mentioned once that he'd held her back, but she was the one who'd held herself back.

Not anymore. This deal was hers.

Then she'd return and persuade Dane to admit he loved her, that he couldn't live without her.

Exactly the way she felt about him.

Chapter Twenty-Four

With that tender kiss, he let her go. He'd played it cool, hadn't pushed. He understood why she had to do it. But he couldn't help the fear. What if she didn't come back? Or what if she did, and they had to start over again from the beginning? What if she didn't quit, but wanted the rules reinstated? Or even added new ones to the list?

Dane had barely closed the front door behind him when Fernsby attacked.

Though with Fernsby, the word *attack* was relative. He was his usual severe self—gone was the impish man who'd waltzed around the library—and a light burned in his silver-gray eyes that turned them to ice.

"Sir," he said with a hard edge like a slap, "it's obvious you have FUBARed the entire operation."

If Dane hadn't been so miserable, he would have laughed at Fernsby's use of the WW2 acronym. But it was true. Dane had effed up beyond all recognition. Though he wasn't sure exactly what he should have done.

Fernsby was on a roll. "I did my part." He waved his hands in the air. "No details, sir, but you clearly did something wrong. Because the two of you are *not* together." He enunciated each word sharply. "And I'm not talking about the fact that she's off to do this amazing new job, which we both know she was meant to do. And at which she will excel." If possible, Fernsby grew even taller, until he was almost Dane's height. "I saw the two of you before I entered the library. It was obvious."

It was obvious even to Dane. "I told her I wanted us to be together." The flagstone floor beneath his feet suddenly felt incredibly hard. And cold.

Fernsby eyed him critically. "Did you get down on one knee and tell her she is the perfect woman for you?" When Dane shook his head, he went on, "Did you tell her she is the most important person in your life?"

He said very quietly, "No."

Fernsby spoke without raising his voice. His frustration was all in his clenched fists. "Did you tell her you love her?" The words were said in capitals and underlined five times. "Or did you just tell her you wanted to have sex with her?" More capitalized words, with extra-extra underlines.

Dane fought back. "I certainly did *not* tell her all I wanted from her was sex."

Fernsby's wrinkled brow and glowering gaze said,

What the hell did you say, you imbecile? But he only asked, "Do you love her, sir?"

There was only one answer. "Yes, I do."

"Do you love her with every cell in your body?"

The answer was simple. Just repeat. "Yes, I do."

Fernsby exhaled like a fire-breathing dragon. "Then why can't you tell her, man?" Not *sir*, not *Mr. Harrington*. Not *Lord Bradford*. Not even *Lord Braindead*.

Dane had no choice but to admit the truth. "Because I don't want to push her so hard she runs away."

Fernsby's head jerked slightly, like an automaton who suddenly understood its programming. "Haven't you figured out that not telling her how you feel is the exact thing that *will* drive her away?" His lips flattened into a grimace as he added, "Sir."

"But in my experience—" Dane stopped, not only because of Fernsby's flesh-flaying glare.

"Camille is nothing like your parents," Fernsby prompted.

You always want too much from people, Dane.

In his experience, people you loved always left. Especially if you loved them too much.

Fernsby said in the mildest tone he'd used yet, "Your parents were rather self-centered, in my opinion."

He knew that. He'd said often enough that they were bad examples. He'd blamed his siblings' lack of relationships on them. But even so, somewhere deep inside, he'd always thought that if he'd done something differently, his parents might have been different too.

Dane cocked his head. "Cammie knows how to love."

Fernsby stretched his lips in a facsimile of a smile. "She showed us that time and again with her devotion to her uncle."

"Where Cammie's concerned, there can never be too much love." Dane said it almost with wonder. As if the thought had never occurred to him before, when he'd actually known it almost from the day he'd met her.

The day he'd fallen in love with her.

Cammie would come back. Absolutely. But she'd only stay if he gave her his heart. If he had the courage to let his love envelop her.

He pounded his fist into his palm. "Damn it, I totally screwed up."

He loved her with all his heart. But for all he'd told himself he was protecting her, the truth was, he was safeguarding his own heart. "The other day, you told me she was my heart's desire. And she is. And yet—" He tore his gaze away from the flagstones and looked at Fernsby. "When it came right down to it, I didn't open my heart all the way for my own selfish reasons."

Fernsby looked on him now with something that might have been kindness. Which was so un-Fernsby-like it threw him off.

"Camille will always tread lightly upon your heart. She will never stomp it."

"I know that." He shot out a determined exhale. "She and I need to be together. She's my other half." He remembered her words to him. "She's the missing piece of my puzzle."

Fernsby raised his eyes to the ceiling. "Thank the Lord you finally see that, sir."

Dane didn't have time to think about it. More important things were at hand. He hadn't bared his soul to her. But she had given hers to him completely. That metaphor revealed her love for him. He hadn't said it back. Instead, he'd tried to get out of it by showing her with his body.

"You're right," he told Fernsby. "I haven't been honest. I didn't tell her everything I felt about my parents."

Sitting at the dining table last night, Cammie had told him of her fears, how hurt she'd been by the men in her life, how hard it was to put herself out there again. But he hadn't reciprocated by revealing how hard it had been to grow up with parents who didn't care. Or how hard it was now to lay his heart in another person's hands. Even hers.

Yet that was what Cammie deserved to hear.

Standing taller, he vowed, "I'll tell her everything. I'll fly out there right now."

Fernsby opened his mouth.

Dane held up a hand. "But... I know I can't. She asked me to let her do this on her own. I have to abide by that. But when she's done, I'll be right there like a shot."

Raising both arms, Fernsby seemed to strain forward, almost as if he wanted to waltz around the front hall the way he had in the library. But his hands dropped. And he said with a deep intonation, "A wise decision, sir."

Dane could swear his eyes twinkled. Almost as if he were a fairy godfather.

★ ★ ★

Each minute that dragged by was torture. Dane had never been good at waiting. And every time the grandfather clock in the hall chimed out another hour, he wanted to shout—or punch something.

But as badly as he wanted to fly to her, he couldn't. For her sake. She needed this. He had to give it to her.

She'd proven to him how well deserved this promotion was, proven over and over again the full scale of her capabilities. She'd had the courage to tell him what she wanted, not just in his bedroom, but that day after the Maverick meeting when she'd asked him to promote her.

Still, he couldn't help constantly refreshing his phone, waiting for a text to magically appear.

Fernsby brought in a tray of something that probably tasted delectable. Dane didn't want even a bite as he stared at the screen.

Until Fernsby reached over the desk and tore the phone from his hands. "Sir, you must let her do this. This is what she's always needed. And she can do it."

After a harsh exhale that burned his throat, Dane said, "I know. But the wait is killing me."

As he raised a brow, the corner of Fernsby's mouth twitched. If Dane didn't know better, he'd say a smile was trying to claw its way out. Although the man had actually danced.

"You can't rain on Camille's parade, sir," Fernsby said, quoting the old song. "But there's no reason we can't fly home now and wait for her call there. That way, it won't take you so long to get to her."

Dane jumped up from his desk to throw his arms around Fernsby. "My dear man, you're a lifesaver."

Fernsby stepped back, brushing away the wrinkles Dane had left in his bespoke suit. "I've taken the liberty of informing your pilot," he said, nose in the air.

Dane would have hugged him again if Fernsby hadn't already been walking away.

"I knew there was a reason I kept you around all these years," Dane called after him.

Without turning, Fernsby raised his hand. Was that the man's middle finger? Then he looked again, and no, there were all his fingers, waving. Dane must have imagined it.

★ ★ ★

The jet was flying over the Rockies when Cammie called. And if Dane had ever doubted he had a heart, he knew it now, because it was just about ready to burst out of his chest.

Her voice was like a caress over every single nerve in his body. "It's a done deal," she said. Joy and triumph infused her voice. And maybe a bit of wonder too. She flew off into a soliloquy, her words almost merging together. "This place is perfect. It's got practically a mile of private beach. There's room for a baseball diamond. A volleyball court on the beach. Basketball, tennis, pickleball, just about anything you could think of, Dane. I walked the perimeter back by the trees and counted at least a dozen trailheads. There's even a trail up to a gorgeous waterfall. You're going to love it. I've already got contractors and inspectors en route, and as soon as we're done, I can come back to England."

She told him the price she'd negotiated, and Dane whistled. "You are brilliant."

He heard her smile all the way over the mountains. "I detailed for the developers all the work we'd have to put into tearing down existing structures, getting new construction permits instead of renovation permits, yadda, yadda. And suggested that perhaps we should look for something else that already had the structures we needed and necessitated only the barest minimum of modification." Then she laughed. "They had no idea how desperate I was to grab it before it was gone."

So excited for her, he blurted, "Damn it, you're freaking amazing, and I love you."

After a three-second silence, she laughed it off. "You always say that when I make the perfect deal."

All right. She didn't want to hear it now. But she would soon. Very soon. "Congratulations. Only you could have made this deal. You didn't need my assistance at all."

She whispered, "Thank you."

Then, before he could blurt out everything he felt, because it simply couldn't be done over the phone, he told her, "We're on our way back, but I'll have the pilot divert us to Tahoe." He looked at his watch. "I should be there in a couple of hours."

"You're going to love it," she told him.

"I already do." She was talking about the property, but he meant so much more.

He'd fallen for her on a golf course. And he'd never recovered.

It had just taken him a long, long time to admit he never wanted to recover.

* * *

Dane had followed the sun home to her, arriving at the Tahoe airport by midafternoon. Fernsby took T. Rex to the hotel along with the bags, while Dane drove out to the site.

It was just as Cammie had said. Perfect. The property sloped down to the beach on the lake and far back up into the mountains. The sun was bright, the May day warm, the peaks still snow-covered. Tahoe had been blessed with a good snow year, and there was still skiing on the highest slopes.

The buildings were old, a seventies-style that didn't fit the beauty of the land. Cammie was right, as was Daniel, that demolishing the existing structures and building a new resort that fit the landscape and the needs of its guests was the only way to go. The cracked and weedy parking lot was full of work trucks with a variety of logos, from contractors to demolition experts to inspectors. When he rounded one of the building's crumbling cornerstones, he saw her.

Cammie wore a tailored suit that hugged her curves and made his mouth water. Not because it was sexy or revealing, but because it was her.

He'd never salivated over her. He hadn't let himself, because they'd had their rules. But now they'd broken every single one. His body knew it, his brain knew it, and so did his heart. His every cell wanted her. Not just in lust, but in need.

He needed her in his bed, in his life, in his heart. Forever.

Holding a clipboard, she was surrounded by a gaggle of men and women who hung on her every word. He overheard a smattering of phrases, like *hazardous materials* and *bringing things up to code* and *confirming sewer lines are sound* and *power lines are connected*.

His beautiful girl Friday directed, questioned, instructed. She was the capable, confident woman she'd always been. But she was a girl Friday no more. In fact, she'd never been his girl Friday. She'd always been in charge—of him, of his life, of his work, just as she was in charge of the men and women standing before her now. She was his idea genius and his right hand.

His partner.

And she charmed the group as easily as she'd charmed him from the moment he'd first seen her.

Why had they waited twelve years? But he knew the answer. This was how it was meant to be. They needed to be workaholic colleagues and best friends and equals. They needed to know each other inside and out.

They needed to love each other *before* they fell in love.

As he watched her now, totally in charge, respect gleaming in the faces of the professionals surrounding her, he realized this was what they'd been working toward. A partnership of equals.

With a smile and a wave of her hand, the group broke up, off to do the tasks she'd assigned them. He couldn't wait another moment. Even as a contractor turned back to her with a question, Dane commanded her attention.

Before the man could open his mouth, Dane said, "Excuse us. We'll be back in a moment." Grabbing her hand, he pulled her into a copse of trees near the lake.

She looked up at him with her beautiful green eyes, perfectly at home among the wildflowers surrounding them. "What are you doing?" she whispered. "I'm in the middle of a meeting."

"You have them completely corralled. They all have their tasks. You've set everything in motion and handled it all." Still holding her hand, he said, "And now it's my turn." He went down on one knee in the moist, sandy soil.

She gasped. "You're getting your suit filthy."

"I don't care." Because a five-thousand-dollar suit was replaceable.

But Cammie, the love of his life, could never be replaced.

* * *

Cammie put both hands to her mouth. She wanted to laugh. She wanted to cry. This was everything she'd ever wanted. But she whispered, "Get up."

He held her gaze a long moment, his true-blue eyes compelling. "Not until I bare my soul."

"But, Dane—"

"Shh," he whispered. Her heart wanted to burst.

Then he told her everything. "For so long, I was focused on taking care of the family. Clay and Troy and Gabby were so young when our parents died."

She'd seen how hard he worked to make sure their needs were met. When she came to work for Dane, Troy had just won his first gold medal and was poised to win so many more. After attending night school, Ava had graduated from college. Clay was a sophomore at university. And Gabby was heading for cooking school.

Dane had navigated all of that with his siblings, always cheering in their corner.

She said softly, "I know how hard you worked. You and Ava did an amazing job raising them."

He'd given up so much to do it—his dreams of being a veterinarian, dropping out of college to handle the financial debacle his parents left behind, then working at a resort just to keep food on the table and pay for his siblings' college educations. He'd worked so his siblings could achieve all their dreams while he had to give up his own.

"I admired you from day one," she admitted. "Especially when I learned everything you did for them."

He put up a hand. "I'd do it all again. They're my family. But I could never give them the love of good parents, much as I wanted to."

She wanted to drop to her knees and hug him close. "You gave them all the love they needed to help them grow into the most incredible adults."

Something sparkled in his eyes. It might even have been tears. But she knew better than to point it out.

"The thing I couldn't give them was the example of a loving family. Of parents who cared for each other, supported each other, parents who wanted to spend time with their children. Parents who inspired them. Like Susan and Bob Spencer."

She held out her hand. And he took it. "Don't you know you always inspired them?"

"But not in all the ways I wanted to. Look at them. Not one of them has had a meaningful relationship."

"They have loving relationships with you and with each other." She pulled him to his feet. He was just too far away from her down there on the ground.

Dane shook his head, his hair falling over his forehead. "But I could never show them how to love. Because I was afraid." He put his finger to her lips as though he thought she'd deny it for him. "I drifted from woman to woman, never knowing what I truly wanted or needed."

She squeezed his fingers. "You have so much love in you, Dane. Look at everything you've done for them. And everything you've done for me."

His eyes melted to baby blue, sadness creeping into them. "I never gave you the piece of my heart you deserved."

"Did you ever think that maybe I wouldn't let you?

That it was a two-way street? We had our rules because we both needed them. But you showed me how you loved me all along in everything you did for me and Uncle Lochlan. You moved me into your homes so I'd have more money to take care of him. You were always there, listening to me, comforting me. And you made it possible for me to make the last years of Uncle Lochlan's life the best they could be."

He laughed, a sharp sound in the quiet. "For God's sake, I didn't even give you the promotion you deserved. I never let you manage a project. And the worst is that I didn't even realize you truly wanted to."

All she could say was, "Dane, please."

He shook his head as he barked out his anger with himself. "You deserved so much more than I gave you. You were the one who showed me how to put heart into all my projects. That wasn't me. It was all you."

"You always gave me everything you could." She wanted to throw herself at him, hold him. But he had to let all his feelings out before she could.

He shot out a harsh breath. "I didn't give you my love. And Cammie, I've loved you since the moment I met you. I loved you that first night. If you hadn't come into my office the next day, I would have searched heaven and earth to find you. I should have told you that the moment you sat down. I don't know why I didn't. Maybe I couldn't recognize what I felt back then. Maybe I knew all along I'd screw it up."

He tightened his fist; she was afraid his nails would break the skin of his palm.

"If I had been a better man, I would have offered you not only the job, but also myself." He tipped his head back and closed his eyes as if the spring sun burned his irises. Then he looked at her again. "I have fallen more in love with you every day since. And every day, I told myself we had our rules, the perfect working relationship. That you were my best friend. That I shouldn't ask for more. Because I didn't believe I deserved more. There's always been a part of me that believed that my parents ran away from *me*." He laid his hand over his heart. "That somehow, I didn't know exactly how to go about loving, and I pushed them away because I smothered them. I never wanted to smother you."

She laid her hand over his and whispered, "You've always had a huge heart. And you could never have loved your parents too much. Real love can't smother. They were the ones who let you down."

He nodded. "I figured that out. Yesterday. After you left the manor." He smiled. "And with a little pep talk from Fernsby."

Cammie laughed. "He gave me a pep talk too."

Then he said the thing she'd craved to hear for twelve long years. "I love you, Cammie. And I don't care about our damned rules." He held her hand in his, right over his heart. "I know we can't possibly screw this up. Because I love you too much. I want you too much. And I will do everything in my power never to disappoint you. To always hold you close. To think of you first, to love you, to be the man you deserve."

She wanted to throw herself at him. "And I love you because you've always had heart. You didn't need me to show you that. You've always deserved love. I've always known how focused you are on taking care of the family and what a terrible example of love your parents gave you. But you learned how to love in spite of them."

He smiled, his heart shining in his eyes. "Now you know everything there is to know about me."

"I've always been afraid of losing what I had," she admitted. "I needed the rules because I was afraid to risk. I was afraid of not being good enough. I've been afraid of asking for too much, just the way you have."

He trailed his hands up her arms, then cupped her face. "I would give up the entire business for you. I'd give up everything in the world for you, everything I do and everything I am, if I could be the perfect man for you."

"You *are* the perfect man for me. You don't need to give up a thing, because I've loved you from the first moment I saw you too." She leaned against him, letting his warmth soak into her body, and tipped her head back. "Let's make a new rule that takes precedence over all the other rules. Let's make a rule that we'll never need any more rules. That we won't be afraid to say what we need or ask for what we want."

"And that we'll love each other for the rest of our days," he said, pulling her close enough to see streaks of blue flame in his irises. "That all we need is each other."

"And our family."

"And to watch it grow." Then he kissed her, his taste so sweet, so loving, so beautiful. The taste of love.

Dane looked down at her. "The moment I saw you on the putting green all those years ago, I knew there would never be another woman for me. I'm sorry it took me so long to admit it. But Fernsby was right. I was afraid. I was a coward."

She smiled. Fernsby. Of course. "A man of so few words," she said. "But what he says is everything we need to hear."

"Except to have you say you love me."

"I love you," she whispered.

He wrapped her tightly in his arms, his words drifting through her hair. "I have always loved you. I love you now. And I will love you endlessly."

Chapter Twenty-Five

Fernsby looked down at his phone the second after it chirped. He didn't have to open the text to read it. The three brief words shouted from the screen: *You were right!*

Fernsby did not punch the air. Another man might have, but he was much more subdued, in keeping with his persona as the best butler any billionaire could ever have.

Despite his frenzy of dancing in the library.

Holding Lord Rexford in his arms, he whispered to the dog, "Fernsby is always right."

He surveyed the room, making sure he'd missed nothing. He'd turned down the bed, neatly folding the duvet at the bottom. On the way back to Lake Tahoe's most distinguished hotel, he'd stopped to buy some necessary supplies.

Fernsby always thought ahead. He hadn't had time to prepare a meal fit for lovers, but room service had delivered quite an excellent meal. He stepped back to assess his work. Yes, everything was in order.

Only then did he type back a reply: *Your room is ready, sir.* He included the room number and passcode. While other plebeians in the hotel might receive key cards, the luxury suites on the top floor each had a lock which could only be accessed with the designated code.

He'd canceled Camille's room and had her suitcase transferred. She would never need a separate room again.

Fernsby backed out with one last appraisal. It was perfect. Then, looking both ways along the hall and finding no one in sight, Fernsby allowed himself a smile. Bending his head to Lord Rexford in his arms, he murmured, "Did I not tell you that true love always wins?" He grinned down at the little dachshund. "A butler's job is to knock a few heads together until they realize what's best for them."

Then he fished a treat out of his pocket for the dog, who had been so good today while Fernsby worked his magic.

* * *

Standing at the bedroom door, Cammie gaped. "Did you have all this set up?"

Dane could say only one word. "Fernsby."

The suite had Fernsby's fingerprints all over it. The scrumptious meal for two on a dining trolley, a candle and bud vase in the center. The rose petals sprinkled on the sheets. The candles sweetly perfuming the room from almost every flat surface, on the sideboard and the tables surrounding the cushy sofa, the bedside tables and the bureaus, even in the bathroom.

"You told him *everything*?" Her eyes sparkled, as polished as a piece of jade.

Dane grinned. "Fernsby told *me*. He said he knew all along we were meant to be together."

She glided across the plush carpet to loop her arms around his neck. "Fernsby. He's a man of many talents."

"He's a magician."

"He's an all-knowing seer."

Dane couldn't wait another moment to lower his head to hers and take her lips. The kiss was so sweet and yet so hot. It turned him upside down. The way she had that night. The way she had in his dreams.

He whispered, "That delectable meal is a Caesar salad topped with salmon. And it's cold."

Those beautiful eyes of hers twinkled at him like stars. "Which means we don't need to dine until later."

He kissed the tip of her nose and backed her toward the bedroom. "My thoughts exactly."

When the backs of her knees hit the bed, he began undoing the buttons of her elegant business suit.

"What are you doing?" she asked with the sexiest lilt in her voice.

"I'm undressing you."

When the last suit button popped, she reached for

his jacket, deftly sliding it off his shoulders. "Two can play this game, Mr. Harrington." She started on the buttons of his shirt.

He busied himself undoing the gold cufflinks Ava had purchased for him after he'd made his first million. Before Cammie had helped him find his heart.

The cufflinks made no sound on the carpet as she thrust his shirt down his arms and threw it aside.

Staring at his cotton-clad chest, she murmured, "I decree that you shall never wear a T-shirt under your dress shirt ever again."

He raised one eyebrow, Fernsby-like. "Why not, pray tell?"

She ran her fingers over the soft cotton undershirt. "Because I don't want any more impediments than necessary when I undress you."

He picked her up then, swinging her around the room until she giggled. Then he set her back on her feet and dragged the T-shirt over his head. "I don't intend to let you be dressed at all." He went at the buttons of her silk blouse with gusto.

"You want me to work in my robe?"

"In your robe with nothing underneath." His heart leaped with all the needs and desires racing through his body. "Or your workout clothes. Don't you know that's why I never worked out with you? Those tight leggings of yours damn near drove me insane."

She laughed, a low, husky tone that made him

twitch. "And here I was dying to see you get all sweaty and sexy while you lifted weights."

"I can see a lot of workouts in our future." He kissed the tip of her nose. "Here's another idea for office attire. One of those sexy sundresses you always wear on the island. Those little dresses haunted my dreams."

She ran her finger down his chest to the waistband of his slacks. "Did you know you have this sexy line of hair that goes right down here? I saw it every time you raced into the ocean for a swim." She trailed her fingers over the outside of his slacks.

At her touch, he surged to full strength.

"Oh, that deserves payback," he growled, pushing aside the lapels of her blouse to stroke her breasts through the tantalizing lacy bra.

She moaned as he unsnapped the front clasp. Then he did what he craved, bending to take a tight pearl into his mouth.

His name fell from her lips on a groan. "Dane." Then she pushed him to a standing position once more, her skin glistening where he'd licked her.

"Do you know how many times I've cried out your name in the night?" she whispered.

And here he'd thought she had her emotions under lock and key. "I never heard you."

"I was very quiet. But I never stopped thinking about that night. I never stopped wanting it again."

He framed her beautiful face with his hands, her skin smooth against his palms. "I thought about you every night. I wish now we hadn't waited so long."

She swirled his chest hair beneath her finger. "We needed to know each other inside and out." And Lochlan had needed to be her priority.

"We needed everything that happened in the last twelve years to teach us there's no one else in the world for us but each other." He whispered, "I love you."

Then, as if every minute of all those years had just caught up with him, he kissed her with all the passion inside him, all the lost nights, all the fantasies that filled his dreams, all the moments he'd looked at her across the office and wanted her, needed her.

Even with his lips locked to hers, he reached behind her and unzipped her sexy pencil skirt, letting it fall to the carpet. And she worked his belt buckle, unzipping and pushing his slacks over his hips. Her bra fluttered to the bed as he slid the straps down her arms.

Then he toed out of his shoes and socks, never letting her lips slip from beneath his as he plundered her mouth. As she plundered his. Finally, even the last scraps of fabric that kept them apart—his boxer shorts, her silk panties—fell to the floor.

And he dove on her.

★ ★ ★

She'd waited so long to feel Dane's weight on her. He'd made love to her at the manor, and that had been beautiful and perfect. But he hadn't said he loved her. And she hadn't been able to confess she loved him.

Now, there was nothing between them, nothing held back. He kissed her with the passion of her dreams. He kissed her with the memory of that night so long ago, when it had been so good she'd needed rules to make sure it didn't happen again. He kissed her with the love they shared.

Pulling back slightly, he dazzled her with the laser blue of his eyes. "I need to taste every bit of you, like I've never tasted you before."

To beg was a delight. "Please."

He helped her back onto the rose petals Fernsby had scattered across the sheets, the sweet scent rising up to mesmerize her. Or maybe that was the feel of Dane's silky dark waves beneath her fingers as he kissed his way down her body. His tongue on her throat made her tremble, his mouth on the tight bead of her breast dragged a moan from her lips, his fingers trailing down her abdomen drew a shiver of need from deep inside. Then he fell into the vee of her legs, looking up, his gaze so hot it scorched her flesh.

"Put your legs over my shoulders," he urged her.

She opened for him, locking her ankles behind him. He touched her then, one finger sliding down her center until she quivered with desire. And she whispered, "You naughty, naughty man."

He looked at her steadily. "I'm the man you want me to be. You gave me heart. You gave me back my soul, though I was afraid I'd lost it years ago. You made me who I am."

She reached down to hold his face in her hands, loving the sexy look of him between her legs and the emotion in his eyes. "You've always been the man I want you to be. The man I admire. The man I love."

He looked at her with so much love in his eyes, love she'd never expected to see, love she could never again live without. "All I want right now is to make you feel good."

"Just make me feel, Dane. That's all I want. Just to feel what you do to me."

Then he took her with his mouth.

It had been so good that first night, so unforgettable, then even more glorious when she'd come to him in the manor house.

But it had never been like this. His lips, his tongue, his fingers did crazy things to her, things she'd never have imagined. Her body climbed, higher, higher, until she felt as if she could touch the sky, as if she could feel heaven, as if her body were no longer tethered to the earth, but tethered to him. She climbed to a beautiful somewhere only Dane could take her to.

He closed his hands on her bottom, holding her tight against him, and the pleasure was more than she could bear. She cried out, clamping her fingers in his hair, twisting the silky locks, unmindful of the pain she might cause him. But he never stopped. He didn't let her go, didn't let her come down, didn't even let her breathe. Until the climax slammed into her like a rogue wave, tumbling her head over heels, the sensation so powerful she thought she might have lost consciousness.

Then Dane climbed her body, holding her as she trembled with aftershocks. He lay between her legs, hot, hard, ready.

She trapped his face between her hands and whispered, "I love you. I want all of you. Now." She raised her legs to his waist, and he lifted slightly so she could wrap her hand around him, guiding him inside.

He entered her then, giving her all that he was. "This is what I've always wanted." He held her gaze. "You. Me. Together just like this. Forever."

He moved gently inside her, taking the gift she offered him and giving her the gift of himself. Pulling him down, she kissed him, her lips on his as he filled her up with everything she'd missed for twelve long years.

He was strong, powerful, yet he took her with a gentleness that only love could bring. Clamping her legs around him, she begged, "Take me. Please. I need you to make me all yours."

Going up on his elbows, his hands framing her face,

he gave her more than she could ever have dreamed of.

As he whispered, "I love you," they went over the cliff edge together. Always together and never apart again.

★ ★ ★

He'd never known another woman like her. He'd loved her from the moment he first saw her. And he would never let her go again.

As she lay soft and sweet in his arms, he murmured into her hair, "You know, I was always rooting for you in your relationships. I never wanted you to be sad and alone. You're my best friend, and I always wanted your happiness." He kissed her forehead. "But I always secretly hoped those relationships would fail."

She leaned up to meet his lips. "Me too. I wanted you to be happy, but I never wanted you to fall for any of those women."

His gaze traced every feature of her face, from her forehead, to her lush lashes, to her sweet lips. "You know the reason why I could never truly get into a relationship?"

She smiled. "Because you loved me the whole time, just the way I always loved you."

Truer words had never been spoken.

"Absolutely, Lady Brilliant." He kissed the tip of her nose.

"Ooh. Lady Brilliant. I love it." She raised an eyebrow. "Does that mean your real title is Lord Brilliant?"

"If the shoe fits." Then he rolled her beneath him and showed her just how brilliant they were together.

And, like the stars, the night was endless.

Epilogue

Two months later

The Maverick and Harrington clans filled Dane's home theater. He dimmed the lights for a crystal-clear screen, his gaze roaming the assembly. Next to Fernsby, Susan sat with Bob in the front row. He thought they might be holding hands.

His heart did a two-step as Cammie slipped her hand into his and laced their fingers, the two-step turning into a waltz. He didn't want to get ridiculously romantic about it, but his heart waltzed like Belle and the Beast in Cammie's favorite movie.

Not that he would ever admit that to anyone. Maybe not even Cammie. Although he had watched the movie twice with her.

The opening credits came up on the season finale of *Britain's Greatest Bakers*.

Everyone in that room had sworn, even pinkie sworn, not to watch the episode. It was actually why he'd agreed to back-to-back showings of both the animated and live-action versions of *Beauty and the Beast*. It had been the only way to placate Cammie.

He'd been on saccharin overload ever since. But it had kept him from watching the last episode of *Britain's Greatest Bakers*.

They'd chosen Pebble Beach for the viewing. It was Fernsby's home territory and Fernsby's show. And it was the first time Dane had hosted the weekly barbecue. Correction—it was the first time he and Cammie had hosted.

Fernsby sat in the place of honor, front and center. Even Noah and Jorge didn't squirm in their seats the way two seven-year-olds normally would when faced with a baking show.

In the second row, Paige and Evan each held a baby. Miracle of miracles, both Keegan and Savannah slept soundly.

Dane had led Francine Ballard to a seat on Fernsby's other side. The two appeared to get along famously.

He was happy to see Troy and Clay had made it, too, as well as his sisters. Dane felt surrounded by family, and the thought made him slip his arm around Cammie, holding her close.

As the show began, Bob and Susan put their heads together, whispering, and it struck him how utterly adorable they were. That a couple who'd been together as long as they had could still whisper and giggle together like new lovers amazed him.

His heart filled up completely, Dane took the opportunity to plant a kiss on Cammie's hair. She smiled up at him, so sweetly that he felt his insides get all jumbled up just knowing she was his and he was hers.

The opening credits ended, the show began, and all the whispering stopped.

Fernsby actually looked pretty damn good up there on the big screen. It wasn't quite movie-theater size, but it was still ginormous. Dressed in a chef's apron and a chef's hat cocked jauntily on his head, he looked twenty years younger. He actually seemed to smile.

Cammie tugged on Dane's hand, pointing at the screen, and mouthed, *Is that a mirage?*

Flummoxed, Dane wasn't sure he even recognized the smiling man. Fernsby had to be acting. Obviously, they couldn't have a staid, taciturn butler-type on the show. No one would vote for him.

He hadn't even smiled like that the day he'd returned from filming.

Yeah, it was totally an act. It had to be. But then Dane remembered that waltz in the library. Who knew?

But there was Fernsby, smiling, up on the big screen. Even though it was vegan day. Yes, Fernsby had to make a vegan dessert. It was crazy. Dane was suddenly terrified the man hadn't won after all. Because he certainly hadn't gone to Gabby, the vegan and gluten-free expert, to ask for advice.

As the show unfolded, Dane held Cammie's hand the entire time, both of them crossing their fingers. Because, really, what would happen if Fernsby wasn't the winner? The thought had never occurred to Dane. And the man himself had locked his lips on the secret.

Except for the voices and sounds up on the screen, the theater was entirely silent. He couldn't even hear anyone breathe.

Then it happened. The judges tasted and reviewed, talked and gabbed, going on forever, making Dane want to jump up and shake his fist at how long it was taking. Couldn't they just fast-forward?

Until the moment the head guy—Dane hadn't even listened to his name, which was very unlike him—stopped in front of Fernsby. Then he held out his hand. Fernsby shook it. It was as if the entire show on screen and the entire theater went into meltdown, jumping, shouting, Susan pulling Fernsby out of his seat and actually hugging the man, who remained undeniably stiff.

And Cammie whispered in Dane's ear, her sweet scent washing over him, reminding him of all the sweet nights in his big bed and all the definitely hot moments when he made her scream wildly, endlessly.

"The handshake means he won!" She practically bounced out of her seat.

You'd never be able to tell by Fernsby. Even as Susan gave him that resounding hug. But then Fernsby whispered something in her ear, and Susan Spencer laughed. It was crazy. It was Fernsby. Always full of surprises.

Francine Ballard patted him on the hip—all she could reach from her seat. And Fernsby turned, taking her hand in his and bowing low to brush a kiss across her knuckles.

Cammie whispered, "Will wonders never cease?" Then she looked at Dane. "Did he tell you about his lost love?"

Dane was reeling from all the shocks, but this one might have landed him on the floor if he hadn't been holding her hand. "A lost love? *Fernsby*?"

She nodded, leaning in to kiss the side of his mouth. "You're gaping, Lord Blowfish."

"He told *you*?" His voice rose on the last word.

Cammie sighed. "Let's just say he felt compelled to. But it's his story." She pecked him on the nose. "You'll have to ask him about it."

He would never ask Fernsby about it. He turned, gazing at his butler, who was taking all the backslapping and hugs and congratulations without breaking his composure.

"We can't just wait here," Cammie said. Then she rushed down to the front and threw her arms around Fernsby in a bear hug, or at least as bearish a hug as someone smaller and shorter could give.

Was that a slight bending of the man's spine?

No. Dane must be imagining it.

The hugs and congratulations continued, Cammie edging farther out of the way to give Fernsby room.

Then it was Dane's turn. He strode down the aisle to the front, as if he wasn't flabbergasted. As if he hadn't had the rug torn out from under him. And all the other clichés he could think of.

"Fernsby, congratulations."

Just when Dane thought all he'd have to do was stick out his hand and shake Fernsby's for all the man was worth, he suddenly found himself enveloping his butler in a manly hug.

It was probably the craziest thing he'd ever done. Besides taking twelve years to tell Cammie he loved her.

Oddly, maybe wondrously, Fernsby actually hugged him in return.

Dane stepped back, his hands still on Fernsby's shoulders. "I knew you could do it."

Fernsby, with the sternest, straightest face the man had ever exhibited, said, "I had faith you could do it too, sir."

Then, with yet another miracle of miracles—could there be more than one miracle of miracles?—Fernsby looked at Cammie. And smiled.

★ ★ ★

Good Lord. Cammie glanced at the ceiling to make sure it hadn't fallen in. Fernsby had smiled. An undeniable, endless smile. The hug her two favorite men shared hadn't shocked her as much, even though she'd never seen Fernsby hug anyone, ever. But this was Fernsby's day.

And that hug had the flavor of father-son bonding. Whatever the two had said to each other, it had made Fernsby look at her.

And smile.

Cammie wouldn't dream of smothering her answering smile. She had everything she'd ever wanted. Dane professing his love for her and trusting her in every decision she made for the new resort. Dane taking her hand as they hiked the trails of Pebble Beach or walked along the beach with the waves pounding the shoreline. Dane beneath her on his soft mattress, whispering all the naughty things he wanted to do to her, then actually doing all those naughty things.

Even now, her cheeks flushed with the glorious memories.

Her cheeks grew even warmer when she looked at Evan and Paige with their beautiful babies, now three months old, a reminder of that barbecue when she'd realized she wanted Dane and love and family. All the pregnant ladies, Lyssa, Ari, and Rosie, were also a sweet reminder. And they were very pregnant now—huge, in fact, all far into the third trimester. As if the women were triplets, they each held their hands on their bellies, their faces glowing.

Someday, she thought, automatically searching for Dane. She found his gaze on her, and he smiled. Then he glanced from her to the pregnant ladies and back. She understood his meaning. He wanted what these wonderful Mavericks had as badly as she did.

As if there weren't several heads and bodies between them, he mouthed, *I love you.*

She mouthed the words back at him.

Back in January, watching the Harringtons take on the Mavericks on that soccer field, she could never have dreamed of this. She couldn't even hope for it.

But Dane would always be hers. Just as she'd always been his, right from the beginning, before she even knew his name. They belonged to each other. From this moment on. Forevermore.

Then she simply couldn't stop her feet from carrying her to him or her arms from winding around his neck, pulling him down for a kiss. Not a showy, blatant kiss, just the soft, gentle touch of lips on lips that sealed their love.

When she surfaced, Fernsby was once again smiling.

* * *

Now that was a *lot* of very pregnant ladies. Lyssa Spencer looked as if she could have her baby right here.

So did Rosie. And Ari couldn't be far behind.

Ava resisted the urge to shudder. The gooey looks their respective partners gave each of them were a tad frightening.

The entire group assembled out on the patio. The July sun beamed down on them from a cloudless sky. Flowers bloomed in the beds surrounding the pool deck, and from beyond came the distant sound of golf clubs whacking golf balls and the incessant shush of the waves hitting the beach. The little dachshund barked wildly at Charlie Ballard's Zanti Misfits hiding in the rock garden.

Following his onscreen triumph, Fernsby had laid out a spread that had every mouth watering. Today's centerpiece was his winning vegan, gluten-free Victoria sponge.

Ava was sure it had never been done before. But Fernsby, a man with depths more profound than she could have imagined, had done it.

And now he did the honors before any of them could even tackle the rest of the gourmet banquet. "You must not be full for this tasting," he announced. "This isn't the end of our meal, it's the beginning." How proud he was of his lighter-than-air sponge.

The mini dachshund ran up to sit at Fernsby's feet, as if he might receive a slice, or even a crumb. But Fernsby offered the first piece to Gabby, his sternest critic. Even the televised handshake would be nothing compared to Gabby's assessment.

A hush fell over the Mavericks and Harringtons, as if they were one big family rooting for one of their own. Somehow, since January's soccer game, Ava, her siblings, even Fernsby and T. Rex, had become Mavericks as well. They'd been accepted. Susan Spencer, standing beside her, linked fingers with Ava, as anxious for Gabby's opinion as anyone who'd known Fernsby for the last fifteen years.

The Maverick matriarch was a tall woman. Ava topped her by only half an inch.

She felt something in their clasped hands—energy flowing between them. The synergy Dane talked about. Ava knew in her heart that this group of Mavericks, which included all the Harringtons now, would do great things together.

But now they needed Gabby's judgment.

First, she sniffed. Then she tested the cake's texture with a finger. Finally, she sliced into the Victoria sponge with a dessert fork, just the tip of the piece Fernsby had cut for her, and raised it to her mouth.

Ava could almost feel Fernsby vibrating.

Other than her chewing, there was no expression on Gabby's face. Ava wanted to laugh as her sister played Fernsby to the hilt.

With another bite, she allowed a thoughtful frown to gather between her brows.

Fernsby's fists clenched, as if he might have to

throttle her if she didn't offer her opinion soon.

Though she hadn't finished her piece of vegan, gluten-free Victoria sponge, Gabby looked at Fernsby.

Ava defied the entire assemblage to read her sister's expression. Gabby gave nothing away. Until finally, she said, loudly enough for everyone to hear, "I know we've had our differences over the years, Fernsby." She paused dramatically, everyone wanting to scream at her to hurry up. "But I must grovel at your feet and ask you to create a Fernsby special for my cafés. It would be my greatest honor."

Emotion flickered in Fernsby's normally detached expression. Ava was sure, if there had been no one else to witness it, he would have picked Gabby up in his arms and whirled her around the pool deck. Instead, holding himself rigid, he intoned, "My dearest Gabrielle, I will make a Victoria sponge for you." Then something glittered in his gray eyes. "But I also have something even bigger in mind."

The entire Maverick group, including the two boys, Noah and Jorge—perhaps even the babies—held their collective breath.

Until Gabby couldn't hold it a moment longer. "What? What will you make?" She took a big gulp of air.

"A butter tart." Fernsby paused a long beat, as if waiting for Gabby to deflate. Only to blow her up again with his next words. "A butter-free butter tart."

Gabby gasped, her hands flying to her mouth, covering the shriek that wanted to burst out.

Then Fernsby smiled. Again. Shocking Ava to her core. Again.

"It will be the most delicious tart any of you have ever tasted," he declared with ultimate confidence.

And Gabby threw herself into Fernsby's waiting arms.

"Oh my God. What's happened to Fernsby?" Ava said without even thinking. "And what's happened to my sister?"

Susan squeezed her fingers and whispered, "Synergy."

It was so true. After all the years since they'd lost their parents, maybe even long before that, she and her family had finally found a home.

Maybe it was the Maverick synergy that had shown Dane the way to Cammie. She looked at them now, hand in hand, beaming like newlyweds. What had happened to her brother was almost too hard to believe. Not that Ava hadn't known Dane was in love with Cammie almost from day one, especially after he went ballistic when Troy simply asked her out. But she'd truly believed her brother would never figure it out. It had taken so long that Ava had come to believe he was exactly like her, that he knew how bad relationships could be, and he wanted none of it.

Yet here he was, looking at Cammie as if he was

starstruck.

And Cammie gazed up at him so adoringly that, had Ava been a different woman, she might have been moved to tears. Just the other week, she'd told Cammie she didn't need to pay back any of her uncle's care fees. And yet, Cammie had made a bank transfer and said she'd go on doing so until the debt was paid. She even insisted on paying Dane too.

That was Cammie. A woman of her word, a woman who never forgot what someone else had done for her. A woman Dane deserved.

And yet, despite all evidence to the contrary surrounding her here at this Maverick barbecue, Ava knew relationships didn't always work out. Especially not for her.

She felt eyes on her then and searched the crowded patio, only to find those eyes belonged to Fernsby. Deliberately, he turned his gaze on Dane and Cammie. And back to her once more.

Then he winked.

Oh my God, Fernsby isn't thinking about matchmaking for me, is he?

It was enough to strike terror into her heart.

★ ★ ★

ABOUT THE AUTHORS

Having sold more than 10 million books, Bella Andre's novels have been #1 bestsellers around the world and have appeared on the *New York Times* and *USA Today* bestseller lists 93 times. She has been the #1 Ranked Author on a top 10 list that included Nora Roberts, JK Rowling, James Patterson and Steven King.

Known for "sensual, empowered stories enveloped in heady romance" (Publishers Weekly), her books have been Cosmopolitan Magazine "Red Hot Reads" twice and have been translated into ten languages. She is a graduate of Stanford University and has won the Award of Excellence in romantic fiction. The Washington Post called her "One of the top writers in America" and she has been featured by Entertainment Weekly, NPR, USA Today, Forbes, The Wall Street Journal, and TIME Magazine.

Bella also writes the *New York Times* bestselling "Four Weddings and a Fiasco" series as Lucy Kevin. Her sweet contemporary romances also include the USA Today bestselling "Walker Island" and "Married in Malibu" series.

If not behind her computer, you can find her reading her favorite authors, hiking, swimming or laughing. Married with two children, Bella splits her time between the Northern California wine country, a log cabin in the Adirondack mountains of upstate New York, and a flat in London overlooking the Thames.

NY Times and *USA Today* bestselling author Jennifer Skully is a lover of contemporary romance, bringing you poignant tales peopled with characters that will make you laugh and make you cry. Look for *The Maverick Billionaires* written with Bella Andre, starting with *Breathless in Love*, along with Jennifer's new later-in-life holiday romance series, *Once Again*, where readers can travel to fabulous faraway locales. Up first is a trip to Provence in *Dreaming of Provence*. Writing as Jasmine Haynes, Jennifer authors classy, sensual romance tales about real issues such as growing older, facing divorce, starting over. Her books have passion and heart and humor and happy endings, even if they aren't always traditional. She also writes gritty, paranormal mysteries in the Max Starr series. Having penned stories since the moment she learned to write, Jennifer now lives in the Redwoods of Northern California with her husband and their adorable nuisance of a cat who totally runs the household.

Newsletter signup:
http://bit.ly/SkullyNews

Jennifer's Website:
www.jenniferskully.com

Blog:
www.jasminehaynes.blogspot.com

Facebook:
facebook.com/jasminehaynesauthor

Twitter:
twitter.com/jasminehaynes1

Printed in Great Britain
by Amazon

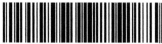